D0117689

Also by Elizabeth Somer

Age-Proof Your Body
Nutrition for a Healthy Pregnancy
Nutrition for Women
The Nutrition Desk Reference
The Essential Guide to Vitamins and Minerals

FOOD & MOOD

FOOD & MOOD

The Complete Guide to
Eating Well and Feeling Your Best

SECOND EDITION

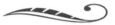

ELIZABETH SOMER, M.A., R.D.

AN OWL BOOK

HENRY HOLT AND COMPANY · NEW YORK

The nutritional and health information presented in this book is based on an in-depth review of the current scientific literature. It is intended only as an informative resource guide to help you make informed decisions; it is not meant to replace the advice of a physician or to serve as a guide to self-treatment. Always seek competent medical help for any health condition or if there is any question about the appropriateness of a procedure or health recommendation.

Henry Holt and Company, LLC
Publishers since 1866
115 West 18th Street
New York, New York 10011

Henry Holt® is a registered
trademark of Henry Holt and Company, LLC.

Library of Congress Cataloging-in-Publication Data
Somer, Elizabeth.
Food & mood: the complete guide to eating well and feeling your best /
Elizabeth Somer.—2nd ed.
p.   cm.
"An Owl book."
Includes bibliographical references and index.
ISBN 0-8050-6200-9 (pbk.)
1. Nutrition   2. Mood (Psychology)   3. Nutritionally induced diseases.   I. Title.
RA784.S647   1999   99-29065
613.2—dc21   CIP

Henry Holt books are available for special
promotions and premiums. For details contact:
Director, Special Markets.

Second Edition 1999

Designed by Paula Russell Szafranski

Printed in the United States of America

9   10   8

For Patrick,
my lifelong partner, who sticks by me
no matter what my moods

Contents

Acknowledgments

Food & Mood is the product of team effort. I am deeply grateful to all the people who offered help, advice, feedback, and suggestions with this project. In addition, without the wealth of excellent research being conducted around the country and throughout the world, and the willingness of those researchers to explain their findings to me, I never would have grasped the complexity and interconnectedness of how food affects how we feel, think, sleep, and behave.

First, I'd like to thank those who helped on a daily basis, including Jeanette Williams, whose culinary expertise was invaluable in developing the recipes; my assistant, LeAnn Kaufman, who always said yes to every request; Janet Haley, who painstakingly reviewed every word of the manuscript and always kept her sense of humor; Miriam at Salem Public Library, who has located hundreds of hard-to-find research articles; Victoria Dolby, who relentlessly retrieved the other few thousand studies from the Biomedical Library; David Hale Smith, my agent, for his moral support, invaluable feedback, and support; Shelly at DHS Literary, who typed anything I asked; Amelia Sheldon, who graciously and enthusiastically worked on every word, every line, and every detail; and Jessica Klein, for her work on the resource list.

A special thanks to the thousands of researchers and clinicians whose work formed the foundation of this book, especially those who took time out of their busy schedules to answer my endless questions. These include: Dr. George Armelagos at Emory University; Francis Berg; Dr. Jeffrey Blumberg at the U.S.D.A. Human Nutrition Research Center at Tufts University; Elizabeth Burrows, M.S., R.D., at the Cancer Prevention Research Center; Dr. C. Wayne Callaway at George Washington University; Dr. Larry Christensen at the University of South Alabama; Nancy Clark, M.S., R.D.; Dr. Fergus Clydesdale at the University of Massachusetts; Caroline Smith DeWaal, at the Center for Science in the Public Interest; Dr. Adam Drewnowski at the University of Washington; Dr. S. Boyd Eaton at Emory University; Dr. Irvin Emanuel at the University of Washington; Dr. Mary Enig at Enig Associates; Dr. Mark Friedman at the Monell Chemical Senses Center; Dr. Paul Gold at the University of Virginia; Dr. Michael Green at the Institute of Food Research in the United Kingdom; David Harvey at the U.S. Department of Agriculture; JoAnn Hattner, R.D., M.P.H., at Stanford University; Dr. Joseph R. Hibbeln at the National Institute on Alcohol Abuse and Alcoholism at the National Institutes of Health; Dr. Gretchen Hill at Michigan State University; Dr. Jan Johnson-Shane at Illinois State University; Dr. Darshan Kelley at the Western Human Nutrition Research Center; Deborah Keston, M.P.H.; Dr. Sarah Leibowitz at Rockefeller University; Dr. Richard Mattes at Purdue University; Dr. Mark Messina, Ph.D., at Loma Linda University; Dr. Simin Nikbin Meydani at Tufts University; Carol Munter; Dr. Gary Myers at the University of Rochester; Dr. James Penland at U.S.D.A.'s Human Nutrition Research Center; Dr. Ed Pierce at the University of Richmond; Dr. William Pryor at Louisiana State University; Dr. Judith Rodin at the University of Pennsylvania; Dr. Barbara Rolls at Pennsylvania State University; Dr. Norman Rosenthal at the National Institute of Mental Health; Dr. Robert Russell at Tufts University; Dr. Adria Sherman at Rutgers University; Dr. Barbara Smith at Johns Hopkins University; Dr. C. W. Smith at the University of Arkansas for Medical Sciences; Evelyn Tribole, M.S., R.D.; Dr. Thomas Wadden at the University of Pennsylvania; Dr. Walter Willett at Harvard School of Public Health; Dr. Zoe Warwich at the University of Maryland; and Dr. Gary Zammit at St. Luke's Hospital.

Foreword

You are your own best mood and mental-health barometer. You know yourself better than anyone else, and you know when something is not quite right with your energy, your moods, your thinking, or your health in general. You know when stress is taking its toll, you're not sleeping right, you can't shake a gloomy mood, or you're more irritable than usual. You know when your eating habits are out of control, your food cravings are at their peak, or your energy level isn't what it used to be. As a physician and surgeon, I suspect that some of you reading this are like many of the patients I see every day: You often ignore these subtle red flags. You feel under the weather, but don't feel bad enough to seek medical attention. But why settle for less when your life, health, and energy could be so much more? Why just get by when you could be living life to its fullest?

Taking charge of your health begins by being proactive and educating yourself. As Medical Correspondent for ABC's *Good Morning America* and *20/20*, I am well aware of what a daunting task it can be to sift through the conflicting advice about health care, diet, foods, vitamins, and herbs, trying to glean what's fact and what's fiction.

That's why *Food & Mood* is such a valuable resource. Finally there is a fact-based, comprehensive, easy-to-read book you can trust. Elizabeth Somer has summarized the vast and still-growing scientific literature from more than two thousand recent studies on how our diets affect our moods, mental health, sleep patterns, energy levels, and even our ability to manage our weights. From basic advice to eat breakfast, cut back on coffee, and exercise more to the latest research on natural serotonin boosters, memory-enhancing supplements, and energizing herbs, she separates the facts from the hype and provides the essential "take-home" messages about what really works, what doesn't, and why.

Food & Mood distills complex scientific information into practical tips and suggestions that are easy to incorporate into even the busiest lifestyles. Most importantly, Ms. Somer explains how to adopt habits gradually to make real, substantial, and lasting changes in our health, our energy levels, and our lives. Even in serious cases of clinical depression or other mental-health problems where medical attention is warranted, following the dietary advice in *Food & Mood* is an excellent supplement to good medical care.

Nancy Snyderman, M.D.

Introduction

While researching the first edition of *Food & Mood* in 1994, I was amazed at the wealth of evidence linking what we eat with how we feel. Yet many of us have grown accustomed to feeling "under the weather" or "not up to par"; some of us are grumpy, tired, or muddled; and still others are unable to control their food cravings and are frustrated by weight gain. Many people unknowingly choose foods that aggravate depression, insomnia, fatigue, food cravings, stress, and memory loss, and prevent general good mental and emotional health. Others have developed food habits that are setting them up for uncontrollable cravings and weight gain. Yet making even small changes in what and when we eat can have profound effects on how we feel right now, tomorrow, and in the future. In many cases there's no reason to put up with feeling bad, mindlessly overeating, or thinking poorly.

The link between food and mood is cyclical. If poor eating habits are the initial problem, then depression, mood swings, poor concentration, or fatigue can develop as a result of dietary deficiencies and excesses, which in turn result in more poor food choices. On the other hand, most people don't make the effort to eat well when they're depressed, tired, or stressed, and poor nutrition aggravates these emotional conditions. Before you know it, you feel bad, don't know why, and have no idea what to do about it.

Consequently many people put up with feeling bad, ignore the warning signs, and live with the discomfort of getting by rather than feeling great. Granted, we know that what we eat affects our health: Fail to drink calcium-rich milk and we're likely to develop osteoporosis; eat too much red meat and other foods high in saturated fats and we're likely candidates for heart disease. The consequences of these choices, however, take decades to develop. Many people don't realize how immediate is the food-mood connection. What you eat (or don't eat) for breakfast will affect how clearly you think, whether or not you battle a food craving, and what your energy level will be a few hours later. What you chose to eat two hours ago is having an effect on your mood right now. You are much more likely to feel great, think clearly, sleep well tonight, and have the energy you need to live life to its fullest if you are fueling your body with the foods it needs. Why put up with feeling or thinking anything less than great when a natural solution is as easy as making a few simple changes in your food choices?

Of course your diet also is having long-range effects on your mood, thinking, and energy level. Protect your brain cells from damage by eating antioxidant-rich fruits and vegetables and taking the right supplements and you're likely to sidestep age-related memory loss in years to come. Stockpile your body and brain's nutrient stores and you'll handle stress better when it hits unexpectedly. Boost your intake of iron-rich foods and you might prevent fatigue in the future.

Even when what you eat is not directly related to how you feel, think, and act, improving your nutritional status *always* will help you feel better, give you more energy, and help fend off colds, infections, and other illnesses related to emotional problems. In short, if you want to feel your best, you have to eat the best.

What's Changed in the Last Few Years?

In the six years since *Food & Mood* was first published, the research on the relationship between mood and food has increased exponentially. In the early 1990s a handful of known appetite-control chemicals were orchestrating our appetites; that list increased substantially by the turn of the century. The simplified approach to curbing appetite by regulating one chemical, such as serotonin, has been abandoned as we become increasingly aware of how chemicals and hormones from both the brain and the body work intricately together. Diet often can do what no medication can: gently and simultaneously rebalance your appetite-control chemicals.

Dietary approaches to manage naturally your brain chemistry and appetite also have changed with the times. Even five years ago carbohydrate-rich cookies or a bagel were considered the only way to raise serotonin levels. New research shows that a special type of fat also curbs cravings, boosts mood and brain power, and even reduces suicide rates. Significant gains have been made in understanding how our diets affect mental function, suggesting that the decline in memory and thinking once thought to be a natural consequence of aging is really a natural consequence of poor diet and other health habits. A new supplement even shows promise in turning back the hands of time when it comes to memory.

We also have a better understanding of why our appetites run amok, leading to overeating, uncontrollable cravings, and weight problems. Most importantly there are a wealth of effective solutions for curbing an out-of-control appetite. For example, recent studies from the University of Pennsylvania report it's the weight of food, not the calorie content, that tells us we're full. A pound of food, either chocolate or broccoli, will do the trick; however, the high fat and sugar in the chocolate supplies more than 2,000 calories, while an equal weight of broccoli supplies only 127 calories. Working with this new information is as simple as consuming foods that weigh a lot but are low in calories, such as soups, stews, and smoothies.

The New Edition

This edition of *Food & Mood* has been completely revised to include the latest research. New information on what herbs and supplements are effective is included in each chapter. You'll also find all-new snack and breakfast ideas, ways to trim fat without sacrificing taste, smart foods and calming foods, an updated Feeling Good Diet, a week's worth of new menus, fifty new recipes, two new chapters on managing appetite, and much more. Every chapter has been updated to include the latest research on:

- Why you crave carbohydrates, chocolate, ice cream, and salty foods, and how you can satisfy these cravings without sacrificing your waistline or your health (chapters 2 and 3).
- How to naturally fight fatigue (chapter 4).
- How to curb the symptoms of premenstrual syndrome (PMS), and why carbohydrates are not always the best choice for treating seasonal affective disorder (SAD) (chapter 5).
- The natural solution to depression, including new sections on exercise and the omega-3 fatty acids (chapter 6).
- How to manage stress, including new facts on how diet can reduce the effects of the stress hormones, why fish might help reduce

hostility and anger, and how stress affects mineral levels in your body (chapter 7).

- Why dieting makes you dumb, why fish really is brain food, and why a new supplement dramatically boosts brain power (chapter 8).
- How food allergies affect sleep, how coffee and alcohol influence insomnia, a new serotonin-boosting supplement and how it affects sleep, why a glass of warm milk might not put you to sleep, and all-new late-night munchies (chapter 9).
- How to manage out-of-control appetites, including how flavor and aroma influence your food choices, why women crave chocolate and men crave steak, self-tests, tips, and suggestions for putting know-how into practice (chapters 10 and 11).
- Why you should take supplements no matter how well you eat, how to choose the best supplement program for you, answers to the most-asked questions on supplements, and the fifteen nutrients you can't do without (chapter 14).

How to Break the Cycle

The basic premise of this book is that you not only are what you eat, but you also eat what you are. Your food choices have profound effects on your energy level, mood, sleep habits, ability to cope with stress, and more. On the other hand, how you feel is intricately linked to what you choose to eat from one meal to the next. Poor eating habits establish patterns in the brain chemicals that regulate appetite and mood, which set you up for mood swings, food cravings, poor sleep habits, and other emotional problems that are not inherent in your personality.

The commonsense eating habits outlined in this book are a compilation of tried-and-true recommendations and hot-off-the-press findings based on scientific evidence. Rather than putting up with chronic fatigue, erratic moods, sleepless nights, or out-of-control cravings and generally allowing your life to slip through your fingers because you couldn't muster the energy to live it to the fullest, I hope that reading this book and following the Feeling Good Diet will help you take back your life, your moods, and your energy level by making the first step toward feeling your best for the rest of your life!

Salem, Oregon
March 1999

FOOD & MOOD

I.

THE FOOD-MOOD LINK

CHAPTER ONE

How Food Affects Your Mood

What a miracle you are!

- With little or no effort, you can remember simple and complicated facts and events, so that by the time you have reached adulthood, you are a rich canvas of experiences, memories, and relationships.
- You can feel a wide array of emotions, from ecstasy and grief to boredom and apathy.
- You can solve problems, untangle puzzles, develop plans, and form opinions.
- You have a unique sense of humor and a one-of-a-kind personality, as well as personal dreams and hopes for the future.
- You are unique in the foods you love, the foods you hate, the foods you crave, and the foods you eat daily. Even how you decide what food satisfies a craving and how you go about soothing that need is peculiar just to you.

At the very foundation of each of these traits, talents, and preferences is an orchestra of cells and chemicals that allow your basic nature to develop and interact with the world. Who you are depends on how well that orchestra, called your nervous system, plays its music.

Getting to Know Your Neurons

The smallest functioning unit of the nervous system is the nerve cell, or *neuron*. This cell "talks" to other nerve cells and tissues by relaying electrical messages within the brain and back and forth through the nervous system to the rest of the body. To instinctively pull your hand away from a hot burner on the stove, blink an eye, feel hunger, decide what to eat, prepare a meal, hear a noise and recognize its origin, memorize a song, smell cinnamon and know it's coming from the bakery down the street, or perform any of the millions of thoughts, feelings, and actions you do every day requires that thousands of your 100 billion nerve cells and an equivalent number of support cells (called *glia*) communicate efficiently.

The neuron is not your typical cell. Most cells in the body are relatively spherical, but the nerve cell is shaped more like a tree. On one end are its branches, called *dendrites*, which allow the nerve cell to receive incoming messages from other neurons. These messages are relayed down the "trunk" of the nerve cell (called the *axon*), much like voice messages are carried on telephone wires. The axon can vary in length, from a fraction of a millimeter to three feet long (see Illustration 1.1). The messages eventually reach the "roots," or *axon terminals*, of the nerve cell, which bump against dendrites on other nerve cells. Nerve cells don't touch. Instead they are separated by tiny spaces that flow between the axon terminal of the sending nerve cell and the dendrites of the receiving nerve cell. This tiny space is called the *synapse*.

In order to relay the message from one nerve cell to the next, the sending nerve cell must find a way to "jump" the gap, or synapse, to get to the other side. Without some way to transmit messages across this gap, messages would stop at the end of the sending nerve cell, and all processes dependent on the nervous system, from moods to movements, would come to a halt.

To ensure this does not happen, nerve chemicals called *neurotransmitters* are stored in tiny sacs at the end of the axon terminals. The electrical message (such as a thought or a feeling message) traveling down the axon arrives at the terminal and causes some of these sacs to release their neurotransmitters. These nerve chemicals flow across the synapse, tickle the receiving nerve cell, and keep the message moving from one nerve to another, much like handing the baton to the next runner in a relay race. Once the neurotransmitter has relayed its message, it is broken down or reabsorbed back into the receiving nerve cell's storage space to be used again. In this way, neurons communicate with each other and send "state-of-the-union" messages from the body to the brain, and back again. The brain processes this information by

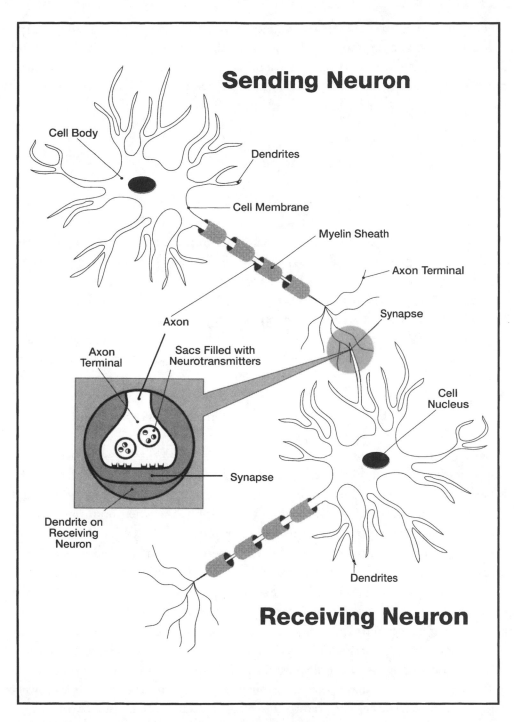

Illustration 1.1   How Our Nerves Communicate

sending messages back and forth among its billions of nerve cells and then releasing orders for action to the muscles and organs of the body—all within a split second and with no conscious effort on your part. Every dip or rise in mood, every hunger pang, every thought, every response—in short, who you are—is orchestrated by these nerve cells and their neurotransmitters.

A Symphony of Chemicals

Until recently, scientists had identified only a few chemicals and hormones that regulated body and brain processes, including insulin, adrenalin, noradrenaline, and glucagon. But in the past twenty-five years the chemical story has become considerably more complex with hundreds of newly identified compounds that regulate everything from your mood and what you want to eat to whether or not you experience headaches or develop heart disease.

The participants in this chemical symphony include neuropeptides such as neuropeptide Y (NPY) and galanin; amines; prostaglandins such as the prostacyclines and thromboxanes; the leukotrienes; and numerous hormones, from cholecystokinin (CCK), estrogen, and testosterone to cortisol, prolactin, and adrenocorticotropic hormone (ACTH). It is likely these and many other chemicals we've discovered recently are just the beginning and that many more compounds will be identified in the future.

At least seventy neurotransmitters have been identified that regulate nerve function, including memory, appetite, mental function, mood, movement, and the wake-sleep cycle. Table 1.1, "Some of the Chemicals That Influence When and What You Eat," on pages 9–11 provides a partial list of these neurotransmitters and other hormonelike compounds along with their effects on appetite. Disruption of even one neurotransmitter dramatically alters nerve cell function and instigates a cascade effect on other neurotransmitters, which can have profound effects on one or more of our physical, emotional, and mental processes. In essence, if an electrical message comes down the axon but there are insufficient amounts of the correct neurotransmitter at the terminal, then the message is not communicated to the next neuron, and the information flow stops. For example, too little of the neurotransmitter acetylcholine results in memory loss, while too little of the neurotransmitter norepinephrine causes depression. Too much of other neurotransmitters can overcommunicate a message. For example, excessive amounts of norepinephrine causes the mental disorder called mania.

Table 1.1 Some of the Chemicals That Influence When and What You Eat

CHEMICAL	WHERE?	INFLUENCE?
Cholecystokinin	GI tract	Reduces food intake
Bombesin	GI tract	Reduces food intake
Gastrin-releasing peptide (GRP)	GI tract	Reduces food intake
Somatostatin	GI tract	Reduces food intake
Litorin	GI tract	Reduces food intake
Motilin	GI tract	Increases food intake
Neuromedin B	GI tract	Reduces food intake
Thyrotropin-releasing hormone (TRH) & derivatives	GI tract	Reduce food intake
Calcitonin gene-related peptide	GI tract	Inhibits appetite
Oxytocin	Brain	Reduces salt cravings Reduces appetite
Insulin	Pancreas	Increases food intake
Glucagon	Pancreas	Reduces food intake
Glucocorticoid hormones	Adrenal glands	Increase food intake
Cortisol	Adrenal glands	Increases fat intake
Aldosterone	Adrenal glands	Increases food intake
Progesterone + Estrogen	Ovaries	Increase food intake

CHEMICAL	WHERE?	INFLUENCE?
Testosterone	Testes, ovaries, adrenal glands	Increases food intake
Leptin	Fat tissue	Reduces food intake
Fatty acids	Fat tissue/liver	Increase food intake
Satietins	GI tract	Reduce food intake
Opioids (endorphins)	Brain	Increase fat intake (might be triggered by taste on tongue)
Growth hormone-releasing hormone	Brain	Increases food intake
Serotonin	Brain	Low—increases carbohydrate intake; High—decreases carbohydrate intake
Norepinephrine	Brain	Increases intake of sweets
Neuropeptide Y (NPY)	Brain	Increases carbohydrate intake
Galanin	Brain	Increases fat intake
Corticotropin-releasing hormone (CRH)	Brain	Inhibits appetite
Neurotensin	Brain	Inhibits appetite
Vasopressin	Brain	Decreases food intake
Dopamine	Brain	Inhibits appetite
Pancreatic polypeptide	Pancreas	Increases food intake

CHEMICAL	WHERE?	INFLUENCE?
Neuropeptide YY	Brain	Increases food intake
Orexins (A and B)	Brain	Increase food intake
Peptide YY	Brain	Increases food intake
Melanin-concentrating hormone	Brain	Increases food intake

To further complicate the symphony, these neurotransmitters are housed in central regions of the brain—such as the hypothalamus—that also regulate reproduction and communicate closely with other brain centers—such as the amygdala—that control emotions. Our food preferences, desires, cravings, and loves are literally hardwired into our basic instincts for survival, safety, and love!

What You Eat Affects How You Feel

What you eat directly and indirectly affects all these nerve chemicals, which in turn influence your moods, energy level, food cravings, stress levels, and sleep habits. For example:

1. Many neurotransmitters are composed of either amino acids—the building blocks of protein obtained from the diet—or a fatlike substance called choline, also obtained from food. When you consume too little of one or more of these dietary building blocks, your body limits production of the neurotransmitter dependent on their availability, and you experience changes in mood, appetite, and thinking. For example, the nerve chemical histamine is built from the amino acid histidine. Histamine is important in regulating alertness; brain energy metabolism; the release of hormones; appetite; and coordination.
2. Vitamins or minerals, such as the B vitamins, vitamin C, vitamin E, iron, selenium, and magnesium, are assembly-line workers in the manufacture of neurotransmitters; some aid neurotransmitter activity, as in the case of iron, and some protect neurotransmitters

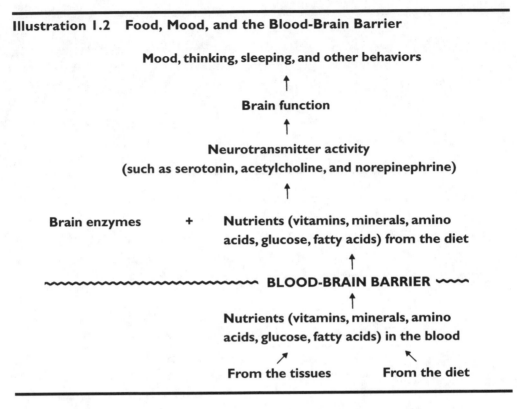

Illustration 1.2   Food, Mood, and the Blood-Brain Barrier

Mood, thinking, sleeping, and other behaviors

↑

Brain function

↑

Neurotransmitter activity
(such as serotonin, acetylcholine, and norepinephrine)

↑

Brain enzymes   +   Nutrients (vitamins, minerals, amino
acids, glucose, fatty acids) from the diet

↑

~~~~~~~~~~~~~~~~~~~~~~ BLOOD-BRAIN BARRIER ~~~

↑

Nutrients (vitamins, minerals, amino
acids, glucose, fatty acids) in the blood

↗   ↖

From the tissues   From the diet

from damage, as in the case of vitamin E. If your diet does not supply ample amounts of these "helpers," neurotransmitters are not made or stored in sufficient amounts, and you feel grumpy or can't think straight. Correct these deficiencies, and mood and thinking improve.

3. Some neurotransmitters become more or less active depending on dietary intake. Either overconsuming or dramatically restricting a particular food, such as fats or carbohydrates, can trigger imbalances in neurotransmitters that can contribute to depression, irritability, food cravings, mood swings, and thinking problems (see Illustration 1.2, above).

4. Nutrients such as protein, zinc, vitamin B_6, iodine, folic acid, and vitamin B_{12} are essential for the normal development of the nervous system. Insufficient intake of these nutrients from conception through the early years of life results in potentially irreversible dam-

age to the nervous system, thus permanently altering personality, mental function, and behavior.

5. Some food additives, such as monosodium glutamate (MSG), and chemicals, such as tyramine (found in aged cheeses), can influence brain activity and result in mood changes, or can interfere with the manufacture or release of neurotransmitters. Other additives can block neurotransmitters so the receiving neuron is unable to understand the message. Still other additives alter the structure of a neurotransmitter, increase your cells' output of neurotransmitters, or affect the enzymes that normally regulate how much neurotransmitter remains in the gap between nerve cells. Any of these changes can have profound, yet sometimes subtle, effects on your mood and thinking.

The Diet-Made Chemicals: Serotonin, Dopamine, Norepinephrine, and Acetylcholine

The manufacture of most neurotransmitters is controlled by the brain. But some are directly influenced by what you eat, especially the amino acids (the building blocks for protein). For example, there are five neurotransmitters whose origins can be directly linked to the food we eat. Tryptophan, an amino acid found in meat and milk, is the building block for serotonin, and dopamine and norepinephrine are influenced by the amount of tyrosine in the diet. Histadine intake helps regulate production of histamine, and threonine is the building block for a nerve chemical called glycine. Some fatlike compounds also turn on production of nerve chemicals. For example, eating choline-rich foods boosts acetylcholine production. The levels and activity of these neurotransmitters are sensitive to food intake, and changes in dietary patterns can have profound effects.

Serotonin: General Mood Regulator

The neurotransmitter serotonin performs a variety of functions. High serotonin levels boost your mood, curb your food cravings, increase your pain tolerance, and help you sleep like a baby. Low levels of serotonin result in insomnia, depression, food cravings, increased sensitivity to pain, aggressive behavior, and poor body tempera-ture regulation.

No other neurotransmitter is as strongly linked to your diet as is serotonin. This neurotransmitter is manufactured in the brain from an amino acid called trypto-phan, with the help of a variety of nutrients including vitamins B_6 and B_{12}, and folic acid. As blood and brain levels of tryptophan rise and fall and as vitamin intake fluctuates between optimal and deficient, so follow serotonin levels. Serotonin levels rise twofold when people take tryptophan supplements, which reduce the time it takes for an insomniac to get to sleep; boost mood in people battling depression; calm people prone to violence; increase tolerance to pain; and help curb carbohy-drate cravings. People who take medications—such as fenfluramine, for weight loss—that boost serotonin activity also report improvements in mood and a drop in calorie intake. This serotonin-stimulating drug also increases alertness and sociabil-ity and decreases feelings of tiredness and irritability. (A cousin to tryptophan avail-able in supplements is 5-hydroxytryptophan [or 5-hydroxy-L-tryptophan (5-HTP)], which improves mood in some people, but whether it is safe or effective for other symptoms of serotonin deficit is unknown.)

From Food to Mood and Back to Food:

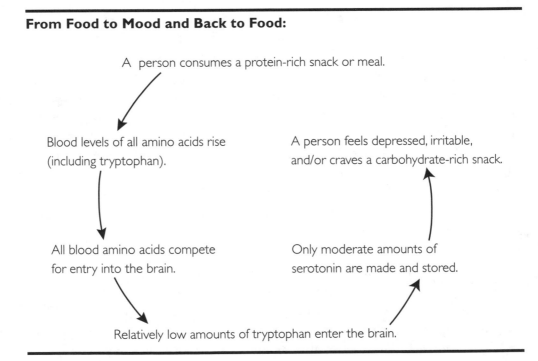

A person consumes a protein-rich snack or meal.

Blood levels of all amino acids rise (including tryptophan).

A person feels depressed, irritable, and/or craves a carbohydrate-rich snack.

All blood amino acids compete for entry into the brain.

Only moderate amounts of serotonin are made and stored.

Relatively low amounts of tryptophan enter the brain.

Ironically, eating a protein-rich meal *lowers* brain tryptophan and serotonin levels, and eating a carbohydrate-rich snack has the opposite effects. Tryptophan is a large amino acid that shares an entry gate into the brain with several other large amino acids, such as tyrosine. When you eat a protein-rich meal, you flood the blood with both tryptophan and its "competing" amino acids, and they fight for entry into the brain. Tryptophan gets crowded out, and only a small amount gets through the blood-brain barrier (the series of membranes, enzymes, and blood vessels that separate the brain from the body and, as a whole, act as the gatekeeper protecting the brain from harmful substances, such as some drugs, radioactive compounds, and disease-causing viruses). (See Illustration 1.2, on page 12.) As a result, serotonin levels do not rise appreciably after a meal or snack that contains protein, even if that food is high in tryptophan.

From Food to Mood:

A person consumes a carbohydrate-rich snack or meal.

The pancreas releases insulin.

Mood improves and carbohydrate cravings subside.

Blood levels of all amino acids, except tryptophan, drop as these amino acids enter muscle cells.

Serotonin is stored in high amounts in the nerve cell.

Tryptophan (with the help of vitamin B_6, vitamin B_{12}, and folic acid) is converted to serotonin.

Tryptophan levels remain high in the blood.

Tryptophan enters readily into the brain.

In contrast, a carbohydrate-rich meal triggers the release of insulin from the pancreas. This hormone causes most amino acids floating in the blood to be absorbed into the body's (not the brain's) cells—all, that is, except tryptophan, which remains in the bloodstream at relatively high levels. With the competition removed, tryptophan can freely enter the brain, causing serotonin levels to rise. The high serotonin levels increase feelings of calmness or drowsiness, improve sleep patterns, increase pain tolerance, and reduce cravings for carbohydrate-rich foods. (See "Diet and Serotonin Levels," on page 17.)

Dopamine and Norepinephrine: Mood and Energy Elevators

Dopamine and norepinephrine (also called noradrenaline) are manufactured from the amino acid tyrosine with the help of several other nutrients, including folic acid, magnesium, and vitamin B_{12}. When your dopamine and norepinephrine levels drop, you're more likely to feel depressed, irritable, and be moody; consuming more tyrosine boosts levels of these neurotransmitters and improves mood, alertness, ability to cope with stress, and mental functioning.

Like tryptophan, tyrosine is found in protein-rich foods. Unlike tryptophan, tyrosine levels in the blood and brain rise when a person consumes pure tyrosine or, to a lesser extent, eats a protein-rich meal. The same processes that lower tryptophan levels—that is, high levels of competing amino acids and no insulin—are the very processes that favor tyrosine. Consequently, tyrosine and tryptophan are at odds with one another: For tryptophan/serotonin levels to rise, tyrosine levels must be low; conversely, when tyrosine and its corresponding neurotransmitters are high, tryptophan levels are moderate to low.

This seesaw relationship between tyrosine and tryptophan results in a similar effect on appetite. Eat a carbohydrate-rich breakfast, such as pancakes or waffles, and serotonin levels rise, which will shut off the desire to eat more carbohydrates. At the next meal you'll be more likely to select a low-carbohydrate, high-protein selection, such as a tuna sandwich with milk, which raises dopamine/norepinephrine levels. And so we swing back and forth from carbohydrates to proteins throughout the day, in part because of fluctuations in these neurotransmitters. To examine your own mood swings and energy levels, try Quiz 1.1, "What You Eat and How You Feel," on page 19.

Diet and Serotonin Levels

Different food components have different effects on serotonin.

Sugar (sweets): Triggers quick release of insulin that lowers blood levels of most large amino acids except tryptophan, which remains in the blood and can enter the brain. As a result, serotonin levels rise, but blood-sugar levels also rise and fall dramatically.

Refined starch (white bread, white rice): Triggers release of insulin that lowers blood levels of most large amino acids except tryptophan, which remains in the blood and can enter the brain. As a result, serotonin levels rise, but blood-sugar levels also rise and fall, sometimes to levels too low.

Whole-grain starch (whole wheat, brown rice, oatmeal): Triggers a slow, sustained release of insulin that lowers blood levels of most large amino acids except tryptophan, which remains in the blood and can enter the brain. As a result, serotonin levels rise gradually, and blood-sugar levels remain stable, without the rise and fall experienced with sugar or refined grains.

Vitamin B_6: Aids in the manufacture of serotonin. A deficiency of this B vitamin reduces serotonin production and affects mood and food cravings.

Estrogen: Might inhibit vitamin B_6 status and decrease brain serotonin levels by its effects on neuropeptide Y (NPY).

Tryptophan: Raises blood levels, then brain levels of tryptophan, which increases serotonin production.

Protein: Raises blood levels of all large amino acids. As a result, only small amounts of tryptophan enter the brain, serotonin levels do not rise, and cravings for carbohydrates might increase. A person also might feel energetic and more clearheaded as a result of lowered serotonin levels.

Fat: Omega-3 fatty acids in fish oil raise serotonin levels, although how they do this is unclear.

Raising blood levels of tryptophan always increases the manufacture of serotonin in the brain, but raising blood levels of tyrosine increases dopamine and norepinephrine levels only if:

1. The nerve cells are using these neurotransmitters and need more; or
2. Nerve cell numbers are reduced, as in aging.

In the second case, fewer cells are working harder (that is, sending more messages and needing more neurotransmitters) in an attempt to compensate for the dwindling

From Food to Mood:

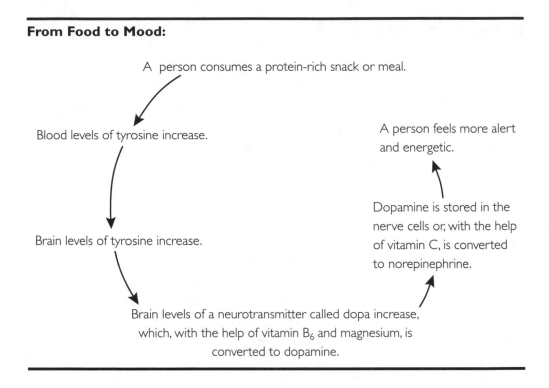

A person consumes a protein-rich snack or meal.

Blood levels of tyrosine increase.

A person feels more alert and energetic.

Brain levels of tyrosine increase.

Dopamine is stored in the nerve cells or, with the help of vitamin C, is converted to norepinephrine.

Brain levels of a neurotransmitter called dopa increase, which, with the help of vitamin B_6 and magnesium, is converted to dopamine.

numbers of cells. Tyrosine supplements boost dopamine levels in Parkinson's disease patients with degeneration of the nerves that produce dopamine.

A building block for tyrosine, the amino acid phenylalanine, is found in the brain in small amounts. Although its structure resembles that of amphetamines, it is unknown whether phenylalanine can affect behavior or curb appetite. However, a few studies show that this amino acid might help curb depression and improve symptoms of attention deficit disorder in adults.

Acetylcholine: The Memory Manager

When it comes to choline, the food-and-mood link is straightforward. Unlike amino acids, which must compete for entry into the brain, the fatlike substance choline has no competitors. The more you consume, the more it makes its way into the brain, where it is converted to a neurotransmitter called acetylcholine. This nerve chemical is important in memory and general mental functioning; dwindling acetylcholine levels, which are common with aging, result in memory loss and reduced thinking ability. Choline also might be effective in the treatment of tardive

Quiz 1.1   What You Eat and How You Feel

Rate your mood before and after you eat to monitor how your diet might affect even temporary mood and energy levels. Rate each mood between 0 (does not apply) and 5 (strongly applies) before you eat lunch. Then rate yourself again within one hour after eating.

MOOD	BEFORE LUNCH	AFTER LUNCH
Agreeable		
Alert		
Calm		
Clearheaded		
Clumsy		
Content		
Coordinated		
Discontented		
Drowsy		
Energetic		
Excited		
Feisty		
Friendly		
Full		
Happy		
Hostile		
Hungry		
Interested		
Lethargic		
Muddled		
Quick-witted		
Relaxed		
Sad		
Sluggish		
Tense		
Tired		
Tranquil		
Troubled		
Withdrawn		

What did you eat for lunch? _____

From Food to Mood:

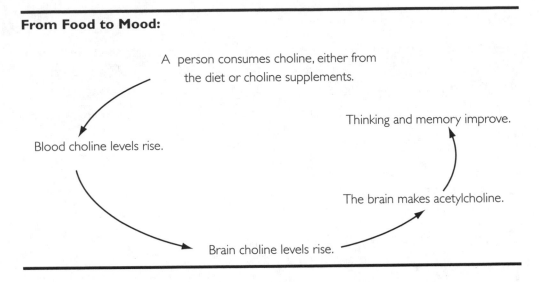

A person consumes choline, either from the diet or choline supplements.

Blood choline levels rise.

Brain choline levels rise.

The brain makes acetylcholine.

Thinking and memory improve.

dyskinesia (a nerve disorder characterized by uncontrollable movements), mania, and possibly Alzheimer's disease. You can boost brain levels of choline by consuming choline-rich foods such as wheat germ and eggs, taking lecithin or choline supplements, and/or taking nicotinamide (a form of the B vitamin niacin), which enhances brain concentrations of choline.

The Survival Chemicals:
Neuropeptide Y (NPY), Galanin,
and the Endorphins

As we have seen, single nutrients in the diet can make or break your mood. An army of nerve chemicals produced by the appetite-control center in your brain, called the hypothalamus, have the same sort of influence. The nerve cells that regulate sexuality and the group of nerve cells that control eating are in constant communication. When these cells receive messages that fuel stores are threatened (as a consequence of strict dieting or even after an overnight fast), they release an array of appetite-stimulating neurotransmitters, including neuropeptide Y (NPY), galanin, and the endorphins, to perk up our desires to eat. According to Sarah Leibowitz, Ph.D., professor of psychology at Rockefeller University, it is no coincidence that this region of the brain also is the control tower for reproduction. The ability to reproduce, and thus keep our species alive, requires that we maintain well-stocked energy and fat stores.

The Role of Neuropeptide Y (NPY)

NPY—in combination with blood-sugar levels, serotonin, noradrenaline, and another nerve chemical, called gamma-aminobutyric acid (GABA)—turns on your desire for carbohydrate-rich foods. In essence, as NPY levels go up, so do your cravings for sweets. The link is clear. Inject NPY into the hypothalamuses of animals, and they start munching grains and sweets and ignoring fatty foods; the higher their NPY levels, the more they enjoy their carbs, while their carbohydrate cravings dwindle as NPY levels decrease. A quick-weight-loss diet is likely to send NPY levels soaring, so don't be surprised after starting such an eating plan if you are soon battling uncontrollable food cravings.

NPY jump-starts the eating cycle in the morning. Sugar stores (glycogen) in the muscles and liver are drained during the night as we sleep; waning blood-sugar levels send a message to the brain to release NPY. This neurotransmitter subtly convinces us to eat waffles, pancakes, toast, jelly, doughnuts, and other carbohydrate-rich foods for breakfast.

Stress also triggers NPY production. In this case, a stress hormone, corticosterone from the adrenal gland, triggers NPY production and activity. Elevated

From Mood to Food:

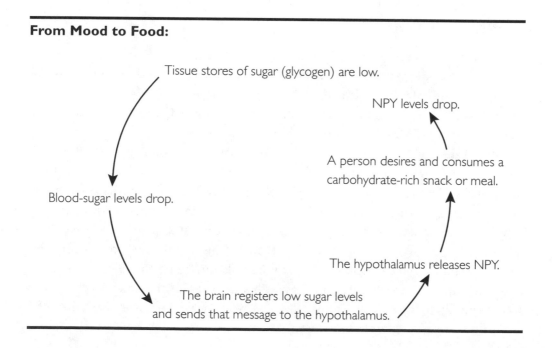

Tissue stores of sugar (glycogen) are low.

NPY levels drop.

Blood-sugar levels drop.

A person desires and consumes a carbohydrate-rich snack or meal.

The hypothalamus releases NPY.

The brain registers low sugar levels and sends that message to the hypothalamus.

From Mood to Food:

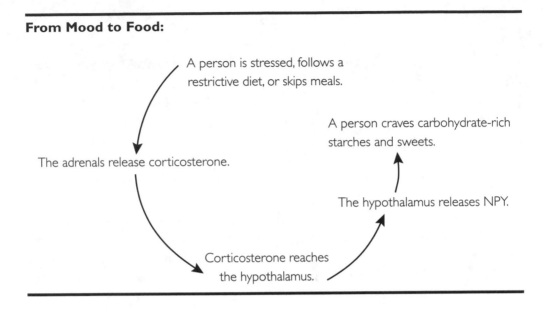

NPY levels also are found in obese people, suggesting that this nerve chemical might contribute to excessive food intake and weight problems.

Galanin at a Glance

A different set of nerve chemicals from the hypothalamus often influences whether and when you want fatty foods. These neurotransmitters include galanin and the endorphins. As galanin levels rise, so does your desire to eat foods that contain fat, such as salad dressing, chocolate, meat, or potato chips. Quite simply, the more galanin your hypothalamus produces, the more fat you eat.

What causes galanin to be released? The breakdown of body fat, which occurs during dieting or when several hours have passed between meals, releases fat fragments (called free fatty acids) into the blood that travel to the hypothalamus in the brain and trigger the release of galanin. Elevated galanin levels, in turn, trigger cravings for fat-containing foods, from ice cream to a hamburger. Reproductive hormones such as estrogen, the stress hormones including cortisol, elevated insulin levels, and possibly the endorphins also turn on galanin, while the neurotransmitter dopamine might turn off galanin release. This can explain the cravings that often accompany premenstrual syndrome (PMS) in women, which occur when estrogen levels fluctuate throughout the menstrual cycle.

From Mood to Food:

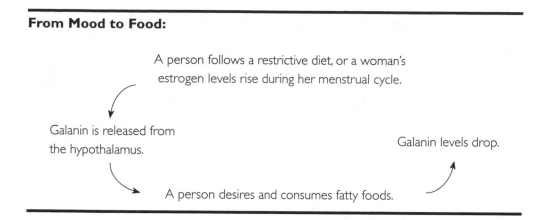

A person follows a restrictive diet, or a woman's estrogen levels rise during her menstrual cycle.

Galanin is released from the hypothalamus.

Galanin levels drop.

A person desires and consumes fatty foods.

Galanin works in concert with other neurotransmitters, such as the endorphins and serotonin, and might have a slight stimulating effect on your carbohydrate intake. In addition to increasing our cravings for fat, galanin affects how much of that dietary fat is stored as body fat—again.

As you might imagine, NPY and galanin levels fluctuate during the day. While NPY levels are high in the morning, galanin levels begin to rise by early afternoon and peak in the evening. The NPY-induced desire for carbohydrates provides quick-energy fuel in the morning, and the galanin-induced desire for fattier foods later in the day is possibly the body's attempt to store longer-term energy in anticipation of the overnight fast (see Illustration 1.3). Managing these neurotransmitters to curb cravings, boost mood, and manage your weight will be discussed in the chapters 2, 3, 5, 6, 10, and 11.

The Endorphins: The Natural High

The endorphins are your body's natural morphinelike chemicals that help boost your tolerance to pain, calm you during stress, and produce feelings of euphoria and satisfaction. They are released during intense exercise and are the underlying cause of "runner's high"—that feeling of joy and peacefulness that many athletes experience during and following exercise. Laughter, soothing music, meditation, and other pleasurable experiences also raise endorphin levels.

Endorphins make eating tasty, sweet, or creamy foods fun. When animals are injected with a medication that increases endorphin levels, they eat more; medications that block endorphins curb the desire for tasty foods. Similarly, endorphins in our bodies have no effect on our regular eating habits (they won't encourage you

Illustration 1.3   The Ups and Downs of NPY and Galanin

Under ideal conditions, when NPY and galanin are functioning in balance, these two neuro-transmitters rise and fall in a seesaw fashion during the day. NPY levels are highest in the morning and drop off in the afternoon as galanin levels are rising. Stress, strict dieting, and other conditions can offset this balance, which can trigger changes in eating habits and mood.

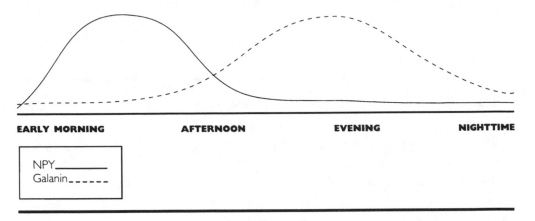

EARLY MORNING   **AFTERNOON**   **EVENING**   **NIGHTTIME**

NPY_____
Galanin_____

to eat more wheat germ or broccoli!); they only increase our desire for cakes, cookies, ice cream, and creamy candy. Satisfying those endorphin cravings is self-perpetuating because these foods further raise endorphin levels in the brain, which explains why you want to eat an entire box of chocolates once you start! The very taste of something sweet on the tongue immediately releases endorphins in the brain, making the sweet treat instantly enjoyable.

Elevated endorphins also contribute to a pregnant woman's longings for certain foods (in conjunction with the female hormone progesterone); a woman's uncontrollable cravings the two weeks before her period; a sweet tooth during times of stress; cravings for alcohol in an alcoholic; and overeating in obese people, binge eaters, and bulimics. The pleasurable feelings associated with eating tasty foods are further enhanced by other neurotransmitters, such as gamma aminobutyric acid (GABA).

From Mood to Food and Back to Mood:

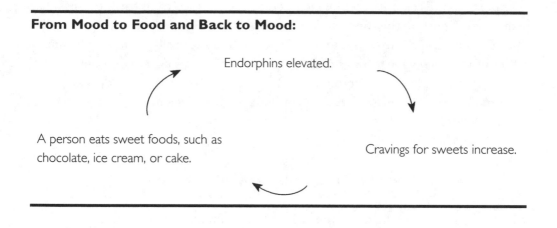

Endorphins elevated.

A person eats sweet foods, such as chocolate, ice cream, or cake.

Cravings for sweets increase.

Beyond the Brain

The symphony of nerve chemicals that dictate your food preferences and mood are not housed exclusively in the brain. Some play their music from distant regions in the body, such as the digestive tract, pancreas, adrenal glands, and fat tissue. Cholecystokinin (CCK) is a hormone found in both the brain and the small intestine that aids in digestion and contributes to feelings of satiation. The female hormone estrogen enhances CCK's effectiveness. The more CCK that is released, the slower you digest food, the faster you feel full, and the less food you eat. Studies show that animals lose their interest in sugar when CCK is injected into their brains. In studies on people, we see that low levels of CCK are found in those with eating disorders, such as bulimia, which might partially explain why they don't feel full even when they've eaten huge amounts of food. In contrast, AIDS patients with high CCK levels and low endorphin levels are likely to lose their appetites, which contributes to the wasting syndrome associated with this disease. The amino acid phenylalanine increases CCK levels, which has led to its inclusion in some weight-loss supplements but still has not made them effective for weight loss.

Somatostatin and glucagon also are released from the digestive tract in the presence of food, and they signal the brain to stop eating. Somatostatin slows digestion, which distends the stomach and gives us the feeling of fullness. Starvation results in excessive somatostatin in anorexics, which might explain why they feel full after eating tiny amounts of food. Obese people, on the other hand, secrete small amounts of somatostatin during a meal, so they are more likely to overeat. Glucagon tells us when we've had enough protein.

Enterostatin is another hormonelike compound released from the intestines that reduces fat consumption and, at least in animals, helps reduce body weight by "burning" fat tissue. Although its role in digestion is not fully understood, enterostatin might encourage feelings of fullness, so a person eats a little, but not a lot. It is likely that enterostatin, serotonin, galanin, and the endorphins work in concert to raise and lower cravings for fatty foods, from salad dressing and mayonnaise to meat and chocolate.

The Highs and Lows of Blood Sugar

Blood sugar is at the helm of your appetite and mood control. An army of hormones, including glucagon from the pancreas, epinephrine and the glucocorticoids from the adrenal glands, and thyroxin from the thyroid gland, raise blood-sugar levels when they fall below normal concentrations. Insulin balances the effects of these hormones by lowering blood-sugar levels when they rise too high.

When we digest the food we eat, our bodies break down sugars and starches into their simple units of glucose or fructose. These simple sugars enter our bloodstreams and trigger the release of insulin from the pancreas. Insulin—with the help of other nutrients such as chromium, magnesium, and manganese—ushers blood sugar into the cells of our bodies, thus supplying energy to the tissues and maintaining normal blood-sugar levels.

However, not all carbohydrates are created equal. Insulin secretion mirrors blood-sugar levels. Unprocessed, complex carbohydrates (starches such as the carbohydrates found in whole-grain breads and cooked dried beans) are made up of hundreds of glucose units linked together like high-energy pearls on a string. They are broken down slowly in the digestive tract and gradually enter the bloodstream, producing a mild and progressive elevation in blood-sugar and insulin levels. Processed starches, such as white bread or white rice, and concentrated sugars, such as table sugar or sweets, are more rapidly converted into simple sugars that enter the blood and trigger a larger release of insulin from the pancreas. When you eat a sweet snack, insulin funnels the excess sugar out of the blood and into the cells, decreasing blood-sugar levels, sometimes below normal levels, while elevated insulin levels linger for hours. The sugar-induced rapid rise in insulin might arouse your hunger signals as well, according to Judith Rodin, Ph.D., professor of psychology and psychiatry at Yale University. Her research shows that people are hungriest and like

The Effects of Dietary Habits on Blood Glucose

Skip a meal: Blood glucose levels drop slowly and, in the case of breakfast, might only partially rise to normal levels if food intake is delayed too long.

Skip two meals: Limited glycogen stores are mobilized to maintain blood-sugar levels; stores are exhausted within twenty-four to forty-eight hours of fasting. The release of fat fragments results in increased levels of galanin, which triggers cravings for fatty foods.

Eat only sugar or sweets (desserts, candy): Blood sugar quickly (within ten to fifteen minutes) rises to above-normal levels, followed within twenty-five to forty minutes by a dramatic drop in blood sugar to subnormal levels.

Eat only refined starches (white bread, refined cereal): Blood-sugar levels rise less quickly than sugar, but still can rise too high, resulting in too much insulin released from the pancreas and a drop in blood sugar to subnormal levels, but not as dramatic as is experienced with sugar.

Eat whole-grain starches (whole wheat bread, whole-grain cereal): Blood-sugar levels rise slowly and steadily for up to four hours. Insulin is released in small, steady amounts from the pancreas, resulting in even blood-sugar levels and no dramatic drop in blood sugar as is seen with sugar or refined grains.

Eat a mixture of protein and carbohydrates (turkey on whole wheat bread): Blood-sugar levels stabilize for up to three to four hours.

Drink alcohol: Blood-glucose levels might be slightly reduced for a short time—less than one hour.

Drink caffeine (coffee, tea, cola, soft drink): Blood-sugar levels rise in the first hour, followed by a drop in glucose to subnormal levels.

sweet tastes more when their insulin levels are high. You can see from this cycle why it seems that the more sweets you eat, the more sweets you crave.

But the cycle does not stop there, since blood insulin levels also correspond to body fat stores. The more often and the longer blood insulin levels remain high, the more likely a person is to accumulate excess body fat and battle a weight problem. Since body fat is linked to galanin activity, and insulin is linked to serotonin, CCK, and CRH, it is likely these tissues, hormones, and brain neurotransmitters (and possibly hormones from the adrenal glands, such as the stress hormones, including cortisol) work as a team, with imbalances resulting in powerful urges to eat too much and gain weight (see "The Effects of Dietary Habits on Blood Glucose," above).

What Makes Us Stop Eating?

With such an orchestra of chemicals telling us to eat, you might be thinking that it's amazing we ever leave the dinner table at all! Fortunately, the brain has a feedback system that tells the body when it's had enough to eat. NPY levels drop and serotonin levels rise after we eat a waffle, putting a halt to our carbohydrate cravings. Galanin levels are kept in check by eating some, but not too much, fat. Other neurotransmitters, such as corticotropin-releasing hormone (CRH), curb hunger, especially during times of stress and long-term dieting. Inject CRH into the brains of animals and they cut back on their food intakes; drugs that block CRH return those animals to their normal eating habits. This chemical also reduces our desire to try new foods and is probably one reason why some people lose their appetites when they are stressed or are fasting.

The body also has checks-and-balances on brain activity when it has had enough to eat. CCK is released from the intestines after a meal and sends messages of satiation to the brain. It also interacts with CRH. Elevated insulin levels in the blood after a meal also switch off NPY levels and turn on CRH in the brain, which curbs appetite. In addition, leptin is released from fat tissue and tells the brain to shut off NPY and increase CRH. Estrogen released from the ovaries can turn off appetite by stimulating the release of CRH and suppressing the release of NPY as well. Of course we can tamper with these checks-and-balances by the medications we use (the birth control pill suppresses CCK; cortisone increases insulin levels), how much we exercise (physical activity helps normalize endorphin levels), how much stress we experience (stress elevates cortisol levels, which increases our preference for fatty foods), and what we eat. This will be discussed in more detail later in this book, especially in chapter 7.

The new wave of weight-loss medications is attempting to regulate this symphony of appetite-control chemicals. Drugs that raise CCK levels have come and gone as we have seen that the body develops a tolerance to orally administered CCK. Fenfluramine and another serotonin-boosting drug called dex-fenfluramine entered the market with mixed reviews and serious side effects, such as high blood pressure. Other serotonin-regulators and medications that decrease NPY levels are now being tested, and leptin is being considered as a potential drug for treating obesity. How useful these drugs will be in the long run is questionable when you consider the complexity of our appetite-control symphony of chemicals. As you have seen, no one neurotransmitter works alone, but rather each works in concert with numerous other neurotransmitters, hormones, and chemicals in the delicate and complicated task of regulating our eating. Tampering with only one or two of the players in that concert is likely to have an unforeseen cascade effect on other chemicals instead of directly influencing our food choices alone. As you read this book you will learn that gently and naturally nudging brain chemistry into balance can be accomplished, at least in part, by making a few changes in what and when you eat.

When Eating Becomes Unhealthy

Eating is a pleasure for most people, but for those people preoccupied with food and thinness, it is a nightmare. Anorexia nervosa (self-starvation), bulimia nervosa (excessive food intake, followed by vomiting or purging), binge eating (excessive eating episodes with no vomiting), and even obesity share many common causes, traits, and symptoms. No one knows exactly why some people develop eating disorders and others try dieting but return to normal eating. Eating habits rest on a continuum from healthy to deadly, with common habits like dieting sometimes spiraling into an eating disorder as the fear of being fat becomes an obsession that is fueled by diet-induced imbalances in the body's appetite-control chemicals. Even if emotional issues such as a desire to lose weight initiate an eating-related disorder, physical and chemical factors help perpetuate it. Studies have shown that hormones and nerve chemicals from growth hormone, prolactin, cortisol, and estrogen to NPY, the endorphins, serotonin, vasopressin, and CCK are turned topsy-turvy in people prone to obesity and in those suffering from eating disorders.

Upsets in CCK, Serotonin, NPY, and Endorphins

Erratic eating habits, such as dieting, starvation, or bingeing, send many of these appetite-control chemicals into a tailspin, thus perpetuating and escalating the problem. For example, CCK (see paragraph above) is released in small amounts in bulimics; consequently, their brains don't receive the signal to stop eating, or their systems become so desensitized to CCK that they eat faster and larger quantities of food before they feel satisfied. In contrast, semistarvation in anorexics oversensitizes their CCK system, so they feel full after eating even a few bites of food. Other neurotransmitters and hormones that are turned upside down in people who battle eating disorders or obesity include leptin, cortisol, bombesin (an appetite-suppressing chemical produced in the digestive tract), ACTH, CRH, and oxytocin (a neurotransmitter that aids memory and that might turn on and off our salt cravings).

Most bulimics report that a binge is triggered by cravings for specific foods, in particular sweets, and this is fueled by upsets in NPY and serotonin. In addition, NPY levels are elevated in anorexics who binge, and are very high in bulimics, which might override normal signals of satiety and contribute to their compulsion to overeat sweet and starchy foods. On the other hand, low levels of serotonin in bulimics encourage them to binge on sweets. Working with these fluctuations in neurotransmitters could help curb the symptoms of some eating disorders. Bulimics who have high blood tryptophan levels are more likely to stop the binge-and-purge cycle and suffer less depression than are bulimics who have low tryptophan levels. Knowing this, we can suggest that bulimics might sidestep a binge if they ate small amounts of carbohydrate-rich foods throughout the day to maintain a steady rise in serotonin.

Dr. Leibowitz suspects that imbalances in endorphins are common in bulimia, anorexia, and obesity, and might contribute to these eating disorders. For example, bulimic women who have low endorphin levels are more likely than people with higher endorphin levels to be depressed and to binge on sweet and creamy foods, such as ice cream, chocolate, and pie, possibly in an attempt to raise endorphin levels and elevate mood. Drugs that block endorphin levels in obese people, binge eaters, and bulimics also work to reduce food intake and binge eating, possibly by preventing wide fluctuations in endorphin levels that can lead to overeating. In contrast, anorexics can be addicted to the endorphin rush of starvation, which can sabotage treatment and result in an overwhelming desire to avoid food. The good news is that endorphin levels eventually return to normal in both bulimics and anorexics when they resume normal eating habits.

What's Wrong with Me?

Whatever begins the dieting spiral, it is likely that imbalances in this chemical stew are major reasons why eating disorders progress into the serious conditions that they do. A person might start out with a normal balance of nerve chemicals, but prolonged starvation or binge-and-purge cycles upset these appetite-control chemicals, which will normalize only when regular eating habits are resumed in both anorexics and bulimics.

However, there are some people who are born with imbalances in one or more nerve chemicals that genetically programs them to gain weight. Some in this category adopt bizarre eating habits in a desperate attempt to avoid obesity and remain fashionably thin. Other people have imbalances in appetite-control chemicals, such as endorphins and serotonin, that influence their hunger and satiety signals and make them more likely to develop eating disorders. Some people have imbalances in neurotransmitters that lead to emotional problems, such as substance abuse or depression, psychological problems that in turn lead to an eating disorder.

Knowing that the uncontrolled eating or self-imposed starvation is fueled by these powerful internal chemicals and their interactions can help remove some of the blame and guilt that often have been tied to eating disorders. This knowledge also has helped steer research toward developing medications that reset the nerve chemical balance and restore normal eating behaviors in anorexic and bulimic patients. However, the treatment of eating disorders continues to be multifaceted, encompassing counseling, dietary changes, and behavior changes. If attitudes and eating habits are changed and, in the case of anorexics, if weight is normalized, appetite-control chemicals also return to normal. If a person can conquer the initial hurdles in the treatment for eating disorders, there is hope that full recovery can occur.

Nature Versus Nurture

Just as you are born with a particular shape to your nose, a unique color to your eyes, and are destined to reach a certain height (assuming you are not malnourished), you also are born with an inherent neurotransmitter profile. In the laboratory, different rats with different personalities also self-select different combinations of foods. Some rats love fat and, if allowed to eat all they want of whatever they want, choose up to 60 percent of their calories as fat. Most of these fat-craving rats also are obese, but not all of them. Other rats love carbohydrates and ignore the fat. Most of these are lean, unless their preferences are for sweets, in which case they are likely to be overweight. Similarly, not all people's food preferences and responses to foods are created alike.

You can't change your genes and what they might dictate you to eat, but you can coax your neurotransmitters, through a few simple dietary and lifestyle changes, to influence what foods will appeal to you. Even slight changes in your appetite- and mood-control chemicals can have dramatic effects on your mood, eating and sleeping habits, ability to think and remember, and personality. If your eating habits are fueling any mood problems you have, even minor changes in when and what you eat can help you change your habits and begin to feel and think your best.

How Are You Eating?
A Self-Assessment

You can't decide where you are going until you know where you have been. So before reading further, take a few minutes to complete the following dietary self-assessment. Keep in mind that the more honest and accurate you are, the more feedback you will have on your current eating habits. This, in turn, will help you decide what eating patterns you have that might need changing and which ones support a healthy, active mind, body, and mood. The results of this assessment will be used in conjunction with the Food & Mood Journal on page 282 to help you tailor the Feeling Good Diet (see chapter 12) to your personal food preferences, lifestyle, and nutritional needs.

Quiz 1.2   A Self-Assessment of Your Diet

Choose the answer that most closely describes your eating habits, even if it isn't a perfect fit. There are no right or wrong answers. This self-assessment provides feedback on your current eating habits so you can compare what you currently are eating to the guidelines for the Feeling Good Diet in chapter 12. This is the starting point for planning how and what you want to change.

DIETARY QUESTIONS

1. What is the best example of your most typical eating style?
   a. I eat five or six mini-meals and snacks evenly divided throughout the day.
   b. I eat three square meals a day.
   c. I nibble all day, perhaps eating eight or more times in a day.
   d. I eat sporadically. One day I skip breakfast and lunch, then eat a large dinner. The next day I might eat breakfast and several snacks, but skip dinner.

2. What is your average calorie intake?
   a. More than 2,500 calories a day.
   b. 1,600 to 2,500 calories a day.
   c. 1,000 to 1,600 calories a day.
   d. Because I diet frequently, my calorie intake varies from fewer than 1,000 calories to more than 2,500 calories a day.

3. Do your eating habits fluctuate?
   a. Rarely. I usually eat about the same types of foods at about the same times during the day.
   b. Somewhat, although I skip a meal or eat larger/smaller meals a couple of times during the week.
   c. Often. My eating habits vary almost daily.
   d. Always. I regularly skip meals; grab snacks on the run; forget to eat all day, then eat a large dinner; and/or switch from one eating style to another.

4. Do you eat breakfast?
   a. Yes, always.
   b. Usually (at least four days a week).
   c. Sometimes (fewer than four days a week).
   d. Seldom.

5. If you eat a morning meal, which of the following best represents your typical breakfast?

    a. Cereal or toast, milk, fruit.

    b. Eggs, bacon, toast with butter, coffee.

    c. Doughnut and coffee.

    d. Coffee or tea.

6. Do you eat lunch?

    a. Yes, always.

    b. Usually (at least four days a week).

    c. Sometimes (fewer than four days a week).

    d. Seldom.

7. If you eat a midday meal, which of the following best represents your typical lunch?

    a. A grain such as pasta or bread, meat, and a vegetable, or a large salad that contains some meat or cheese and a roll.

    b. A large meal, such as a hot roast beef sandwich with gravy and mashed potatoes.

    c. A fast-food lunch, such as a hamburger, French fries, and a beverage.

    d. Coffee, candy bar, or soda pop.

8. Do you eat an evening meal?

    a. Yes, always.

    b. Usually (at least four days a week).

    c. Sometimes (fewer than four days a week).

    d. Seldom.

9. If you eat an evening meal, which of the following best represents your typical dinner?

    a. I keep dinner light and usually have small portions of fish, salad, pasta, and/or fruit.

    b. Dinner is my biggest meal and can include generous portions of meat, vegetables, and bread or potato.

    c. A frozen entrée or a meal-replacement drink.

    d. I usually skip dinner or grab something from a fast-food restaurant.

10. What do you eat most frequently for a snack?

    a. Fruits and vegetables, whole-grain breads, or yogurt.

    b. Cookies, potato chips, or granola bars.

    c. Candy bar, doughnut, or French fries.

    d. Nothing. I seldom or never eat between meals.

11. What types of foods do you consume between dinner and bedtime?
   a. Fresh fruits and vegetables, whole grains, or low-fat milk products.
   b. Snack foods, such as popcorn, crackers, potato chips, or other convenience foods.
   c. Chocolate, cola soft drinks, hot cocoa, or coffee or tea.
   d. I do most of my overeating in the evening, including large bowls of ice cream with chocolate sauce, or second servings of leftovers from dinner.

12. How frequently do you have strong cravings for starchy or sugary foods?
   a. Seldom.
   b. Only during certain times of the month or year, such as the two weeks before my period, or in the winter.
   c. Frequently.
   d. Daily, and the urges often lead to overconsumption of the craved food.

13. How many servings of unsweetened fruits and plain vegetables (fresh fruit and vegetables or fruits canned in their own juice and plain frozen vegetables) do you eat in an average day?
   a. Eight or more.
   b. Five to seven.
   c. Three to four.
   d. Fewer than three.

14. Of those fresh fruits, how many are vitamin C–rich selections, such as oranges, grapefruit, or cantaloupe?
   a. Three or more.
   b. Two.
   c. One.
   d. Fewer than one each day.

15. Of those fresh or plain frozen vegetables, how many are dark green, such as romaine lettuce, spinach, or broccoli, or dark orange, such as sweet potatoes and carrots?
   a. Three or more.
   b. Two.
   c. One.
   d. Fewer than one each day.

16. How many servings of grains, such as bread, cereal, pasta, noodles, rice, or tortillas, do you typically eat each day (one serving = one slice of bread, one tortilla, or ½ cup cooked grains)?
   a. More than eight.
   b. Six to eight.
   c. Five to six.
   d. Fewer than five.

17. Of these grains, how often are the choices whole grain?
   a. All the time.
   b. One out of every two choices is whole grain.
   c. Occasionally I select whole grains.
   d. Seldom or never.

18. Of these grains, how often do you choose crackers, waffles, sugarcoated cereals, tortilla chips, buttered popcorn, or other grains with added fat and sugar?
   a. Seldom or never.
   b. Occasionally (two or three times a week).
   c. Frequently (once a day).
   d. Most of the time (more than once a day).

19. How many servings daily of extra-lean red meat, chicken, fish, and cooked dried beans and peas do you eat (one serving = 3 ounces of animal flesh or ¾ cup of beans)?
   a. Three to four.
   b. Two.
   c. One.
   d. None.

20. When you eat meat, how often do you trim the visible fat, remove the chicken skin before cooking, and cook without using oils and fats such as butter and margarine?
   a. Always.
   b. Usually.
   c. Sometimes.
   d. Seldom or never.

21. How many glasses of milk or 8-ounce servings of yogurt do you consume in a day?
   a. Three to four.
   b. Two.

c. One.

d. None.

22. What type of milk products, including milk, yogurt, and cheese, do you usually consume?
    a. Nonfat (nonfat milk, nonfat yogurt, fat-free cheeses).
    b. Very low-fat (1 percent low-fat milk; yogurt made from a mixture of nonfat and low-fat milk; and low-fat cheeses).
    c. Low-fat (2 percent low-fat milk; yogurt made from 2 percent milk; reduced-calorie or "light" cheeses).
    d. Whole milk (yogurt made from whole milk; regular cheeses).

23. How often do you snack on cookies, candy, fruited-yogurt, and other sweets (one snack serving = two small cookies, one small candy bar, one 8-ounce yogurt, etc.)?
    a. Once a day or less.
    b. Twice a day.
    c. Several times a day.
    d. Several times a day, and often in large amounts; I'll eat half a bag or more of cookies in the evening.

24. What do you usually eat for dessert?
    a. I seldom eat dessert and if I do, it's fresh fruit.
    b. Small servings of nonfat ice cream or sorbet, oatmeal cookies, or angel food cake.
    c. Moderate-sized servings of ice cream, pie, pastries, cake, or cheesecake.
    d. Large servings of pie or cake and ice cream, candy, or other sweets. Sometimes I eat right from the cake or pie without portioning off a serving.

25. How often do you add sugar to your foods, including coffee or tea, cereal, and/or fruit?
    a. Never.
    b. Sometimes.
    c. Frequently.
    d. All the time.

26. What is your typical weekly consumption of soda pop, including diet sodas?
    a. None to three 12-ounce cans each week.
    b. Four to six 12-ounce cans each week.
    c. Seven to ten 12-ounce cans each week.
    d. More than ten 12-ounce cans each week.

27. How many cups (5-ounce servings) of caffeinated coffee or tea do you drink on a typical day?

    a. I don't drink caffeinated coffee or tea.

    b. Two to three 5-ounce cups or fewer.

    c. Four 5-ounce cups.

    d. Five or more 5-ounce cups.

28. What is your average alcohol consumption for the week? (One drink is a 6-ounce glass of wine, 1 ounce of hard liquor, or a 12-ounce can of beer.)

    a. I average less than five drinks a week, or do not drink at all.

    b. I average a drink a day.

    c. I average ten drinks a week.

    d. I average two drinks or more a day.

29. How often do you bake, steam, broil, poach, or grill food rather than fry, sauté, or use sauces and gravies that contain fat?

    a. Always.

    b. Usually.

    c. At least 50 percent of the time.

    d. Seldom or never.

30. How often do you sauté in water, broth, herbs, or other no-fat liquids?

    a. Always.

    b. Usually.

    c. Often.

    d. Seldom or never.

31. How often do you use tomato-based or no-fat sauces on pasta rather than creamy sauces or sauces with fatty meats?

    a. Always.

    b. Usually.

    c. Often.

    d. Seldom or never.

32. How much salad dressing do you use?

    a. I use fat-free salad dressing or use 2 teaspoons or less of oil-based dressing on my salads.

b. I use low-fat dressing and limit the serving to 2 tablespoons.

c. I use regular salad dressing and limit the serving to 3 tablespoons.

d. I use generous servings of regular salad dressings (more than 3 tablespoons) and eat salads regularly.

33. How often do you eat in fast-food restaurants?

  a. Less than once a week.

  b. Once a week.

  c. Twice a week.

  d. More than twice a week.

34. How often do you use butter, margarine, oils, whipping cream, sour cream, whipped toppings, mayonnaise, and shortening?

  a. Seldom.

  b. Once a day.

  c. Several times a day.

  d. I couldn't cook or eat without these foods.

35. How often do you read labels and select foods that contain 3 grams of fat or less for every 100 calories?

  a. Always.

  b. Usually.

  c. Often.

  d. Seldom or never.

36. How many glasses of plain water do you drink daily?

  a. Six or more glasses.

  b. Four to five glasses.

  c. Two to three glasses.

  d. I seldom drink water.

37. How often do you limit intake of salty foods and avoid using salt in food preparation or at the table?

  a. Always.

  b. Usually.

  c. Often.

  d. Seldom or never.

38. What is your current weight?
  a. I'm within 10 percent of my desirable body weight.
  b. I'm approximately 15 pounds or more overweight.
  c. I'm approximately 15 pounds or more underweight.
  d. I'm more than 20 pounds overweight.

39. How often have you dieted to lose weight in the past?
  a. I've been on fewer than three weight-loss diets in my life.
  b. I've been on four to six weight-loss diets in my life.
  c. I've been on seven to ten weight-loss diets in my life.
  d. I've lost count. I'm always trying new diets to lose weight.

40. What type of supplement(s) do you take?
  a. A daily multiple vitamin and mineral supplement, extra calcium, vitamin C, and/or vitamin E.
  b. A moderate-dose vitamin supplement.
  c. I'm not sure what to take, so sometimes I supplement and sometimes I don't.
  d. I know my eating habits are not the very best, but I either don't take supplements or I fluctuate between not taking anything and taking large doses of single-nutrient supplements.

GENERAL HEALTH QUESTIONS

41. How often do you feel, look, act, and function at your best?
  a. Most of the time.
  b. At least 50 percent of the time.
  c. I get by most of the time, or am down more often than I'm up.
  d. I seldom feel really good.

42. How frequently do you engage in planned exercise?
  a. Five or more times a week for at least thirty minutes each time.
  b. Three or more times a week for at least thirty minutes each time.
  c. Fewer than three times a week.
  d. I don't exercise.

43. How frequently do you take time out for yourself—e.g., read a book, take a walk in the woods, visit with a friend, take a hot bath, work on hobbies?
  a. Daily.

b. At least a couple of times a week.

c. Once a month.

d. I don't remember the last time I had a moment's peace.

44. How often do you discuss your personal concerns with a close friend or family member?
 a. Daily or at least several times a week.
 b. Occasionally, when things get bad.
 c. Seldom.
 d. I have no one to talk things out with.

The following questions are not part of the preceding quiz. Your answers to these questions will help you assess your eating habits.

45. Do your eating habits change when you are sad, irritable, depressed, or lonely; happy, excited, stressed, or with friends; or when you are tired, lacking in sleep, or not feeling up to par?
Yes __ No __
If yes, when and how do your eating habits change?

46. What foods do you avoid?

47. Why do you avoid these foods?

48. Are you currently seeing a physician for any disease or problem? Yes __ No __
If yes, explain.

49. Do you have a personal or family history of depression, insomnia, stress-related health problems, weight problems, premenstrual syndrome (PMS), Seasonal Affective Disorder (SAD), or other emotional or mood disturbances? Yes __ No __
If yes, explain.

50. If yes, were the symptoms serious enough to require medical attention? Yes __ No __

51. Do your eating habits change during certain times of the month or during the winter?
Yes __ No __
If yes, when and how do your eating habits change?

52. Do you frequently develop colds, infections, or other signs of a weakened immune system? Yes __ No __

53. Do you take any medications, including aspirin, the birth control pill or estrogen, antibiotics, or heart disease or blood pressure medications? Yes __ No __
If yes, which ones?

54. Do you use tobacco or are you frequently around people who smoke? Yes __ No __

Scoring:
Review your answers and tally your score for questions 1 through 44, giving yourself
   2 points for every *a* answer
   1 point for every *b* answer
   0 points for every *c* answer
   −1 point for every *d* answer
Remember: This assessment is only feedback on your current eating and lifestyle behaviors. As you read this book, return to this assessment to compare how you have been eating with the dietary recommendations for each emotional or mental problem. Which eating habits need changing? Which ones can stay the same? After reading this book and following the Feeling Good Diet, complete this assessment again (give yourself at least six months) and see how far you have come!

If you scored:
70 to 88: Congratulations! Your dietary habits are excellent. Review those questions on which you scored fewer than two points and see if you can find room for improvement.
51 to 69: Very good. Your diet is in the ballpark. A few changes could do wonders for your emotional and physical well-being. Find four questions where you scored fewer than two points and decide how you will change your eating habits to improve your score and your mood.
37 to 50: Caution. Your dietary habits are average, which means you probably consume too much of the wrong foods and not enough of the right ones. Your diet is likely to be a contributing factor to your mood problems. Take action quickly. Identify five or more questions where you scored fewer than two points and make some changes today to boost your score and your moods.
Fewer than 37: Warning. What and how you are eating are major contributing factors to how you feel. The good news is you have lots of room for improvement! Start slowly by picking two or three habits where you scored fewer than two points. Make changes to boost your

score, and when those patterns have become habit, select another two or three questions with low scores to make additional changes. Keep improving your eating habits until you score 69 or higher.

For questions 45 through 54:

45. If you answered yes, read chapters 4, 6, 7, 8, and 9.

46 and **47.** Read chapters 10 and 11.

48, 49, 52, and **53.** Many emotional problems stem from physical ailments or even nutrient-drug interactions. Your physician and pharmacist can explain how a medication, illness, or treatment might affect your eating habits and mood.

49 and **50.** For information on PMS and SAD, read chapter 5.

51. If you answered yes, read chapter 7.

54. Smoking is a primary factor in insomnia and stress. If you answered yes, read chapters 7 and 9.

CHAPTER TWO

Do You Crave Carbohydrates?

- Do you find it impossible to eat just one cookie?
- Do you wonder why you crave ice cream, pizza, Chinese food, chips, and pastries instead of spinach, tofu, and wheat germ?
- Are your cravings for sweets much greater since you quit smoking?
- Are you unable to concentrate on work knowing there is a candy bar in your desk drawer?
- When faced with a box of chocolates, a glazed doughnut, or a blueberry torte, do you find yourself in a tug-of-war between the angel of good intentions and the devil of desire?

Almost all women (97 percent) and most men (68 percent) occasionally find it hard to "just say no" to a sweet treat or other carbohydrate-rich snacks. Eighty-five percent of men and women give in to those cravings at least half of the time. You might crave a milk shake or fantasize about ordering French fries after a camping trip, be willing to die for a bagel after being on a "protein-only" weight-loss diet, or give in to a craving for ice cream after a tiring day.

However, some people battle cravings daily and are virtually addicted to carbohydrate foods. Seemingly levelheaded people become anxious or irritable if they don't have their morning doughnut or afternoon soda pop, and nothing will stand in the way of satisfying a cookie craving. Once they start nibbling, the battle isn't over, since it's difficult for them to stop at just one cookie or one chip. They will tell you these cravings are different from hunger, which is easily satisfied by a variety of

Quiz 2.1   Are You a Carbohydrate Craver?

Answer yes or no to the following questions.

_____ **1.** It is difficult to resist sweets and desserts.

_____ **2.** I would rather snack on bread, a granola bar, cookies, cakes, or other starchy or sweet foods than on peanuts, sliced meats, yogurt, or crunchy vegetables.

_____ **3.** When I am tired, depressed, or irritable, I feel like eating something sweet.

_____ **4.** I have a hard time stopping once I start eating sweets, starches, or snack foods.

_____ **5.** I am not satisfied after eating a meal or snack that contains only meat and vegetables.

_____ **6.** A breakfast of eggs, bacon, and toast is likely to leave me feeling tired and hungry for something sweet by midmorning.

_____ **7.** I feel better (more relaxed, more calm, or uplifted) after eating something sweet.

_____ **8.** After being on a strict diet, I indulge in sweets or starchy foods.

_____ **9.** I feel lethargic and irritable when I don't have a midmorning or afternoon snack.

_____ **10.** I prefer a simple meal with a dessert to a gourmet meal with no dessert.

_____ **11.** I feel more energetic after eating a starchy or sweet snack.

_____ **12.** I have a craving for something sweet or starchy almost every day.

_____ **13.** My cravings for sweets or starchy foods are so strong, I often am unable to resist giving in to them.

_____ **14.** The urge to eat sweets or starchy foods is greatest after a meal that contains only meat and vegetables.

_____ **15.** I've tried lots of diets, but have not had long-lasting success with any of them.

Scoring:

Total the number of yes answers to the above self-assessment.

5 or less: There is a low probability that you are carbohydrate sensitive.

_6 to 9:_ You might be moderately carbohydrate sensitive, but you often can control your cravings. Following the Feeling Good Diet is all you need to get back on track, although you might benefit from some of the dietary recommendations in this chapter (see "Carbohydrate Cravings Control Guidelines," on page 54).

10 or greater: Carbohydrate cravings are likely to be a problem for you, so adapting the Feeling Good Diet based on the dietary recommendations in this chapter would be helpful.

foods. When it comes to a craving, only one food or one type of food will do the trick—and if we have such a craving, we're often willing to go out in a storm to ful-fill it. If you suffer from such a craving, this is not necessarily a sign of weak willpower or a split personality, so put aside the guilt. A far more complex and deep-seated reason lies at the very root of your being and causes those irresistible urges. Do you think you might be plagued by carbohydrate cravings? Take the quiz on page 45 to find out for sure.

Biological Callings

Women have known for millennia that there is more to cravings than just hunger. Pregnant women are often flooded with food cravings, especially during their first trimesters. A woman who ate only whole grains and a low-fat diet prior to preg-nancy now craves macaroni and cheese, sandwiches made with white bread, and TV dinners. Another pregnant woman can't get enough deviled-egg sandwiches, even though she disliked eggs prior to pregnancy. Menopausal women also report food cravings and aversions, although after menopause, food cravings begin to subside, with older persons less driven by cravings.

Anyone battling uncontrolled food cravings knows that the cravings usually begin midafternoon and continue until bedtime. Cravings also magnify when we diet, are under stress, skip meals, feel depressed, or are premenstrual. It doesn't take a scientist to put two and two together and come up with a connection between changes in body chemicals and food cravings.

Serotonin Secrets

A desire for sweets is hardwired into the brain. As discussed in chapter 1, a carbohydrate-rich meal or snack stimulates the release of the hormone insulin from the pancreas, which lowers blood levels of all amino acids except tryptophan. Nor-mally, tryptophan must compete with other amino acids for entry into the brain, but insulin eliminates the competition, allowing tryptophan levels to rise in the brain. Tryptophan is then converted into serotonin, the neurotransmitter that regu-lates sleep, reduces pain and appetite, and generally calms you down and improves your mood.

Some people crave carbohydrates not because they lack willpower but because they suffer from an imbalance in serotonin. For example, dieters, obese people, and people who crave carbohydrates often have lower serotonin levels than do lean people or people who prefer protein-rich snacks. In contrast, a study from the Medical University of South Carolina found that people entering a weight-loss program who ate more carbohydrates showed less anxiety and depression than did other dieters who restricted carbohydrate-rich foods.

From Mood to Food:

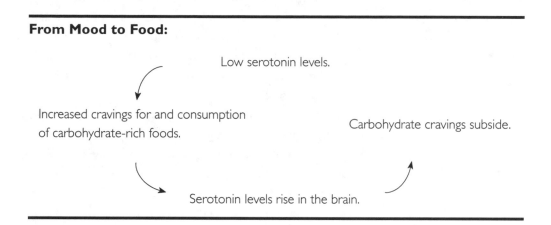

Low serotonin levels.

Increased cravings for and consumption of carbohydrate-rich foods.

Carbohydrate cravings subside.

Serotonin levels rise in the brain.

In essence, carbohydrate cravers turn to desserts, doughnuts, and other pastries, or even pasta and breads, to relieve dwindling energy levels, hunger, depression, and stress caused by their low serotonin levels. Their carbohydrate-rich snacks raise serotonin levels, curb the craving, and energize them. Cravers are therefore rewarded each time they indulge their cravings, because the food they eat increases their serotonin levels and makes them feel better. Just as Pavlov's dog learned to salivate in anticipation of food whenever a bell rang, carbohydrate-sensitive people become conditioned to crave desserts, breads, or other carbohydrate-loaded foods whenever they are tired, depressed, or anxious.

While the carbohydrate-rich meal or snack alters brain chemistry and provides temporary relief from mild depression or tension, a high-protein diet (even if it is rich in tryptophan), by supplying more of the competing amino acids, reduces tryptophan and serotonin levels in the brain. Consequently, carbohydrate-sensitive people who eat high-protein lunches, such as a turkey sandwich and a glass of milk, might experience fatigue or mood swings and "crave" a carbohydrate-rich mid-afternoon snack in an effort to raise brain serotonin levels and feel better. Low-carbohydrate weight-loss diets are doomed to fail for these people. Within days of cutting back on carbohydrates, the carbohydrate cravings amplify to the degree that leaves the dieter almost powerless against an all-out binge.

What's So Bad About a Little Sugar?

There is nothing inherently wrong in soothing your mood with a carbohydrate-rich snack. However, if that snack is usually a highly processed sweet or salty food, such as cookies or chips, and if you frequently munch on these foods, your cravings could set you up for weight gain. Eating a sugary diet reduces your chances of consuming enough of the 40+ nutrients you need for your body to function smoothly, and increases losses of chromium, a mineral essential for normal blood-sugar regulation and the prevention of weight gain. That's especially a problem for people who don't exercise daily and who can't afford to waste calories. Sugar also raises blood triglyceride levels, increasing the risk for developing heart disease.

Finally, sweets beget sweets. Animals eat more, have a greater increase in blood insulin levels, and gain weight when their diets are sweetened, which gives us a clue about one contributing factor in Americans' expanding waistlines. We eat 20 percent more sugar today than we did in 1986, or up to 152 pounds of refined sugar per person per year (up 25 pounds in thirteen years). As we know, most sugary foods also are high in calories. For example, a commercial cinnamon roll contains 12 teaspoons of sugar and 670 calories. Both sugar and starch supply 4 calories per gram, but starchy foods also contain mood-boosting nutrients, as well as water, which dilutes the calories. Sugar is just concentrated calories.

So What Can You Do?

To boost your mood without jeopardizing your waistline and your health, limit sugar to no more than 10 percent of your calories (that means about 10 teaspoons if you are on a 2,000-calorie diet). To reach this goal, limit soda pop to one or two servings a week (8 to 10 teaspoons of sugar in one can), candy to an occasional treat (another 5 to 8 teaspoons per candy bar), and cookies to a few small ones a week.

Further sidestep your sweet tooth by turning from highly sugared snacks to minimally processed, wholesome carbohydrates, such as whole grains and starchy vegetables. Snack on an English muffin topped with honey, or half a cinnamon-raisin bagel with jam, and you'll get the same serotonin boost that you'd get with jelly beans but without the blood-sugar drop. Also, be patient. You can't expect pasta to work like Prozac, at least not immediately. It will take two to three weeks of eating well before your body chemistry will adjust and you notice an improvement in your overall mood and a decrease in your cravings.

Endorphins, Sugar, and Instant Gratification

Serotonin is just one piece of the whole picture when it comes to managing your mood and carbohydrate cravings. People report an immediate calming sensation when they give in to food cravings, but it would take at least an hour for the diet-triggered release of serotonin to go into effect. There are obviously other chemical reactions at work when you have that cookie, chip, or chocolate bar at four P.M.

Food cravings also are fueled by an addiction to pleasure. Much like the high experienced after doing intense exercise, having a good laugh, or listening to good music, a euphoric or calming response is produced by certain foods that release morphinelike chemicals in the brain called endorphins. While the serotonin response from eating carbohydrates takes time to elicit, the mere touch of sugar on the tongue produces an immediate endorphin rush. Thus you feel good immediately after eating a doughnut, because of the boost in endorphins, which is followed by a lingering good mood induced by the slow-acting increase in serotonin.

Barbara Smith, Ph.D., professor of psychology at Johns Hopkins University in Baltimore, has researched the calming effects of sugar on newborns. "Healthy infants generally stop crying rather quickly when given small amounts of a [diluted sugar solution], and the calming effect persists over time, even when the sugar is removed," says Dr. Smith. As discussed in chapter 1, the endorphins probably enhance the pleasurable response to eating. In short, they make eating sweet foods fun and reassuring, which can put them at odds with your willpower.

Endorphins provide an example of the cyclical manner in which brain chemistry affects eating, which then affects brain chemistry. The endorphins are turned on when we consume sugary snacks, but they also turn on our cravings for sweet-and-creamy foods. Inject a rat with endorphins and he heartily devours fats, proteins, and sweets. Inject him with an endorphin-blocking drug called naloxone and his snack attack subsides. You can see that endorphins probably also play a role in regulating when and what you want to eat. Adopt a low-carbohydrate diet, and the resultant low blood-sugar levels trigger the release of endorphins, which increase our sweet cravings. Lose weight too fast, and fatty acids released from fat tissue also cause an endorphin rush that sends us to the refrigerator in search of a sweet or creamy snack.

The sugar-endorphin theory provides an interesting link between sweet cravings and several health conditions. For example, people with premenstrual syndrome

(PMS), bulimia, or Seasonal Affective Disorder (SAD) have more frequent cravings for sweets than is normal and report immediate relief from depression, tension, or fatigue after satisfying the craving. These people often say the cravings are accompanied by the thought "I need something to calm myself." The sugary snack provides a temporary quick fix, possibly because of its effect on endorphins, that worsens cravings in the long run since it strengthens the addiction to these morphinelike chemicals.

While simple carbohydrates such as sugar contribute to the problem, complex, minimally processed carbohydrates are part of the cure. Nutrient-packed whole-grain breads and cereals, crackers, brown rice, and starchy vegetables do not aggravate endorphin levels or blood sugar but they do satisfy serotonin needs. These nutritious foods help curb cravings and soothe moods. Later in this chapter you'll find guidelines on how to use this information to adjust your diet and curb your food cravings.

Sweet Addictions

The link between cravings and chemicals extends beyond food to other compulsive behaviors. People attempting to quit smoking report a range of symptoms, from fatigue and sleep disturbances to increased appetite and mood changes. Nicotine—the drug in tobacco—stimulates serotonin release. When people quit smoking, they turn to sweets to get the same serotonin effect. In essence, the sweet cravings of ex-smokers are an attempt to self-medicate and improve mood, diminishing the uncomfortable nicotine withdrawal symptoms they are experiencing. Bonnie Spring, Ph.D., professor of psychology at Chicago Medical School, found that ex-smokers in nicotine withdrawal are less likely to crave sweets and are more likely to stay off cigarettes if they consume high-carbohydrate diets—that is, lots of pasta, breads, cereals, and starchy vegetables, as outlined in the Feeling Good Diet (see chapter 12).

There also are links between alcohol abuse, food cravings, and mood. People who battle uncontrollable food cravings also are more likely to drink too much alcohol, struggle with weight problems, frequently diet, or frequently feel moody or irritable, all symptoms of serotonin imbalances. It's no surprise that alcoholics in the initial stages of recovery experience intense cravings for coffee, candy, sweets, and other carbohydrates. The sweets help counteract the depression, fatigue, and irritability associated with alcohol withdrawal by boosting their serotonin and possibly endorphin levels.

Carbohydrate cravings during tobacco and alcohol withdrawal probably are influenced by scrambled body chemicals, including blood sugar, serotonin, endorphins, and other hormones and nerve chemicals. When people undergoing withdrawal turn to sugary foods, they experience a temporary high, but within a few hours they feel tired, anxious, and irritable again (a condition called dysphoria) and return for another jolt of sugar and caffeine. The chemical roller coaster that results makes their recovery process that much more difficult and painful (see Illustration 2.1, below).

Illustration 2.1   Sugar and Caffeine: The Temporary Fix

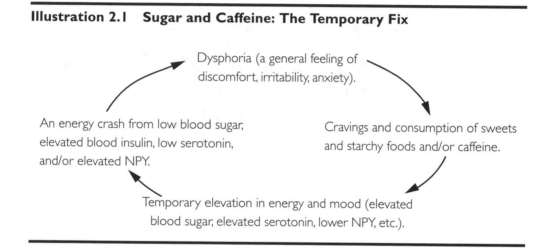

Dysphoria (a general feeling of discomfort, irritability, anxiety).

An energy crash from low blood sugar, elevated blood insulin, low serotonin, and/or elevated NPY.

Cravings and consumption of sweets and starchy foods and/or caffeine.

Temporary elevation in energy and mood (elevated blood sugar, elevated serotonin, lower NPY, etc.).

In contrast, an eating plan based on the Feeling Good Diet, which centers on small, frequent meals that contain some protein and some complex carbohydrates—such as whole-grain breads and cereals, crackers, pretzels, flavored rice cakes, and fruit and starchy vegetables—satisfies the cravings while helping the body rebalance the appetite-regulating chemicals. In short, people can use the right carbohydrates to fuel their recovery. See Table 2.1, "A Dozen Carbohydrate-Rich Snacks," on page 52, for ways to satisfy a craving without compromising health.

Table 2.1   A Dozen Carbohydrate-Rich Snacks

SNACK	CARBOHYDRATE (GM)
• 1 low-fat bran muffin topped with 2 tablespoons apple butter, served with 1 glass sparkling water flavored with lemon	52
• 1/4 cup hummus (made from boxed mix), 1/2 toasted whole wheat pocket bread, 10 baby carrots	33
• 1 slice whole wheat toast topped with 1/2 cup grated carrot mixed with 2 tablespoons raisins and 2 tablespoons fat-free mayonnaise	42
• 1/2 cup lemon sorbet topped with 1/3 cup cubed cantaloupe	51
• 1 whole wheat waffle topped with 2 teaspoons fat-free cream cheese, 2 teaspoons marmalade (preferably made with honey), and 1 tangerine, peeled, sectioned, and seeded	31
• 1/2 toasted cinnamon-raisin bagel, topped with 1 tablespoon fat-free cream cheese, 2 tablespoons crushed pineapple, and 1 teaspoon sunflower seeds	35
• 1 serving of Savory Cilantro Dip with Baked Tortilla Chips*	29
• 1/2 whole wheat bagel topped with 1 slice low-fat cheese, tomato, canned chili, and cilantro	23
• 2 cups Curried Squash Soup*	43
• 1 Thai Wrap*	30
• 1 slice Apple-Cranberry Upside-down Pie*	47
• 1 cup Curried Squash Soup* with 1 whole wheat roll	37

* See "Recipes for Feeling Your Best" at the back of this book.

Basic Instincts

The desire to eat sweets might spring from an even deeper internal well than a need for relief from anxiety or to feel good. The nerve cells in the brain that control eating are part of the body's elaborate plan for regulating energy balance and, fundamentally, for survival of the species. It is no coincidence, therefore, that the appetite-control center in the brain is next door to the reproductive center. Dr. Sarah Leibowitz, at Rockefeller University, believes the cycle of fat and sugar cravings coincides with reproductive needs.

Table 2.2 Our Favorite Foods

Men and women differ even in their food cravings. For one thing, women say they "crave" food, but men say they "prefer" foods. Semantics aside, men eat more barbecue potato chips, sausage pizza, chili, and beer, while women eat more yogurt, chocolate, taco salads, and cinnamon rolls. They both love pizza, cheeseburgers, French fries, and ice cream. It's not that the sexes own the rights to certain foods. Both women and men can crave a hot fudge sundae—it's just that more times than not it is craved by a woman. Although many women love a juicy steak now and then, their husbands and boyfriends don't consider dinner a meal unless it contains meat. In all cases, women crave foods more frequently than do men. Here's a partial list of the gender differences.

WOMEN'S FOOD PREFERENCES (IN ORDER)	MEN'S FOOD PREFERENCES (IN ORDER)
Chocolate	Beefsteak and roasts
Doughnuts, cookies, and cakes	Ice cream and frozen desserts
White bread, rolls, and crackers	Chicken or turkey
Ice cream and frozen desserts	Doughnuts, cookies, and cakes
Beefsteak and roasts	Spaghetti and pasta or white bread
Spaghetti and pasta	Fish
Cheese	Pizza
Chicken or turkey	Cheese or potatoes (not fried)
Pizza	Hamburgers, meat loaf, hot dogs
Potatoes	Eggs
Salty snacks	Chocolate candy
Hamburgers, cheeseburgers, and meat loaf	Salty snacks

"Nature is seeking reassurance that we have enough energy and body fat for survival of the species," says Dr. Leibowitz. For example, with their high estrogen levels, women consistently report more cravings than do men and are more likely to crave sweetened fats, such as doughnuts, cakes, and pies, especially during puberty and following ovulation (the cravings experienced with PMS). These calorie-packed foods are ideal for building up energy stores in preparation for pregnancy. Men, with their species-survival need for greater muscle mass, prefer protein fats, such as roast beef sandwiches, hamburgers, or meat loaf with gravy. (See Table 2.2, "Our Favorite Foods," above.)

Table 2.3   Carbohydrate Cravings Control Guidelines

The trick is to work with your cravings and appetite-regulating chemicals, not against them. The Feeling Good Diet (chapter 12) is the foundation for keeping your neurotransmitters, hormones, and peptides happy and balanced. Here are twenty-two suggestions for curbing—and perhaps even eliminating—a craving.

1. Keep hunger at bay by eating small meals and snacks evenly distributed throughout the day. This will keep NPY and serotonin levels in the normal range.

2. Eat breakfast and include at least one serving of whole grains and one serving of fruit. Skipping breakfast will only escalate NPY levels and increase cravings later in the morning.

3. Avoid fatty meals and snacks midday, since they give galanin an extra boost and set you up for more fat cravings at night. Snack on fresh fruits and vegetables, low-fat yogurt, pretzels, or a bagel with fat-free cream cheese rather than candy or cheese in the late afternoon. See chapter 3 for more on fat cravings.

4. Use alternative flavorings, such as vanilla, nutmeg, spearmint, cinnamon, and anise, to appease a sweet tooth.

5. Identify your trigger foods. What foods are you most prone to overeating? Plan ahead when you anticipate situations that will tempt you with these foods.

6. Seeing is craving. So avoid the temptation by steering clear of the dessert tray, buffet table, doughnut shop, or bread basket.

7. Think before you snack. Ask yourself what specific food would satisfy your craving. Then serve a moderate-sized portion of that food. This helps prevent grazing.

8. Plan your snacks. Allot a certain number of calories for a small, sweet snack and make it low-fat/nonfat frozen yogurt, fruit ices, vanilla wafers, or fig bars. Abstinence leads to binge eating, while allowing small servings of your favorite food helps curb the cravings.

9. If habit, not chemicals, is at the root of a craving, find more nutritious, low-calorie foods or develop a new habit that provides the same pleasurable or rewarding effect. Soak in a hot bath, go to the gym, or play ball with the dog during the vulnerable time(s) of the day.

10. Exercise. While couch potatoes are likely to make regular trips to the refrigerator and struggle with their weight, people who exercise regularly maintain a more constant weight and are less prone to bingeing and cravings. Exercise also is an alternative to sugary foods for getting the pleasurable endorphin rush and for reducing stress.

11. Drink plenty of water. Often a desire for sweets in the evening is actually a signal that the body needs fluids. Some people report that their cravings for ice cream subside within a few minutes after they drink one to two glasses of cold water. Try drinking water as you

clean up the kitchen and prepare dessert; you might feel less of an urge to indulge as a result.

12. Don't eat in response to stress and emotions. Ask yourself if you are really hungry or if you are eating to soothe a mood. If you are not physically hungry, then find a nonfood outlet for your emotions, such as calling a friend, listening to soothing music, or taking a walk.

13. Wait it out. Wait fifteen minutes before giving in to a craving. You might find that it goes away on its own.

14. Pay attention to portions. Soothe a craving with a little, not a lot. One oatmeal cookie is fine; the entire bag is a binge.

15. Watch out for coffee. The caffeine in coffee can upset blood-sugar levels, leaving you fatigued and longing for a quick-pick-me-up snack. Limit coffee to two cups a day.

16. Set minigoals. People have a limited capacity for self-control. Setting too many goals or expecting miracles overnight overwhelms willpower and nerve chemistry. Instead, set small, easy-to-achieve weekly goals, such as cutting back on potato chips from the whole bag to half a bag (throw the rest away or put it down the garbage disposal).

17. Keep tempting foods out of the house. If you can't resist it, don't buy it.

18. Keep a cravings journal. Write down the time of day and the circumstances, as well as your mood, that surround a craving. Look for patterns, triggers, and specific food cravings. Then develop a plan to appease the craving while nourishing your mood and health.

19. Keep nutritious foods on hand. Bring foods with you to work so you aren't faced with only the vending machine to soothe a craving.

20. Cut out all sweets for a week. You might find that the cravings you have for them dwindle or even vanish.

21. Watch your self-talk. Do you hear yourself saying, "I must have that cookie"; "A little won't hurt"; or "That's it, I've blown it, I might as well eat all I want"? These thoughts escalate cravings and urges to overeat. Replace them with positive thoughts such as, "I feel satisfied"; "I don't need that ice cream. What I really need is something to quench my thirst"; or "I ate more than I wanted to, but I'll stop now and get back on track."

22. Change your attitude. Stop labeling foods "good" or "bad." Stop denying yourself favorite foods. Stop obsessing over food or your weight. Dieting and restricting favorite foods only lead to more wanting and eventually overeating. Plan to include favorite foods in moderation. Focus on healthful eating, not dieting.

Dr. Leibowitz's research has uncovered a consistent daily cycle in two brain chemicals that whisper sweet cravings in our ears: NPY and galanin. Both people and animals have elevated NPY levels in the morning, which apparently jump-start

---

From Mood to Food:

An overnight fast leaves the body's glycogen stores low.

NPY levels drop

Blood-sugar levels drop.

Elevated NPY levels increase the desire for and consumption of carbohydrate-rich foods.

The hypothalamus in the brain is sensitive to these low blood-sugar levels and releases NPY.

---

the day's eating cycle by dictating a preference for carbohydrates (possibly with help from the endorphins). Laboratory animals eat more carbohydrates when NPY levels are high or when NPY is injected into their brains. Waffles, toast, pancakes, and cereal satisfy this NPY-induced craving and replenish carbohydrate stores drained after an overnight fast.

NPY levels also are high during times of stress or dieting. According to Dr. Leibowitz, these are the times a person is most likely to crave carbohydrates, which explains why people crave sweets after dieting, during PMS, and in depression. This would be a natural reaction to high NPY, as we have seen. NPY also is linked to serotonin, estrogen, and stress hormone levels, and the combined appetite-stimulating effect of all of these can be overpowering.

Stress magnifies food cravings. Interestingly, the stress hormones, such as norepinephrine (a cousin to adrenalin) and cortisol, both secreted from the adrenal glands during stress, raise NPY and galanin levels, which increase food cravings, overeating, and weight gain.

From Food to Mood:

Stress, dieting, or skipping meals.

Increased stress hormones, such as corticosterone and/or norepinephrine, from the adrenal glands.

Increased desire for and consumption of carbohydrate-rich foods.

Triggers the brain to release NPY.

Doing the Blood-Sugar Boogie

The most clearly defined connection between sugar and cravings involves blood sugar (glucose) and insulin, its regulating hormone. As discussed in chapter 1, during digestion sugars and starches are broken down into their simple units of glucose or fructose. These simple sugars enter the bloodstream and trigger the release of insulin, a hormone that regulates blood-sugar levels. A mixed meal of protein, complex carbohydrates, and fats—such as a roast beef sandwich on whole wheat bread—causes a moderate release of insulin and maintains a steady blood-sugar level. A meal of refined starches—such as a pasta dish made with egg noodles—produces a slightly more elevated rise in blood-sugar levels and a greater amount of insulin released from the pancreas. Sugary foods raise blood-sugar levels even higher and trigger a large release of insulin from the pancreas. As a result, blood-sugar levels drop, sometimes below normal levels, while elevated insulin levels linger for hours.

Judith Rodin, Ph.D., at the University of Pennsylvania in Philadelphia, believes the sugar-induced elevation in insulin might stimulate appetite and repeated sugar cravings. Her research shows that people are hungriest and like sweet tastes more when insulin levels are high. When people snack on sugary foods, their insulin levels rise, and they eat more food and calories at the next meal than do people who snack on other foods or drink water. Why, then, isn't everyone a carbohydrate craver? Because some people are "hyper-responders" and are more sensitive to insulin. Insulin levels in this group jump even at the sight or smell of food as their bodies gear up for a meal even before the food reaches their mouths.

Fortunately, a taste for sugar is often learned, which means it can be unlearned or replaced by a new habit. "You see a doughnut, you eat one, and your insulin levels jump to the occasion. Before long you expect a doughnut at the morning break, and your body learns that insulin levels go up when pastries are around, much like Pavlov's dog learned to salivate when a bell was rung," reports Dr. Rodin. The good news is that people with habits like this can curb the insulin response by following the Feeling Good Diet in chapter 12 and the guidelines outlined on pages 62–63 and 65.

The Fructose Fix

Fructose is a sweet alternative to sugar. Unlike refined sugar, fructose found in fruit does not trigger the insulin response and the food cravings. For example, in one study, people drank a beverage sweetened with either fructose, glucose, or aspartame (which goes by the brand name Equal or NutraSweet). Those people who drank the fructose-sweetened beverage ate fewer overall calories and less fat than did the other people.

Why? Fructose is absorbed more slowly than glucose or sucrose (which is 50 percent glucose and 50 percent fructose). It must travel to the liver to be converted to glucose before it can enter the blood. Thus fructose alone or with a meal stimulates insulin, but not as dramatically or as rapidly as glucose or table sugar. These three differences—slower absorption, the stopover in the liver, and a more gradual release of insulin—mean that you can help curb your cravings and avoid overeating at the next meal simply by switching from a sucrose-laden doughnut to a fructose-filled orange.

But don't get carried away. Concentrated fructose—which can be purchased in health food stores, found in honey, or is also called high-fructose corn syrup (HFCS) in processed foods and soda pop—is no substitute for more nutritious, naturally occurring fructose in fruits or complex carbohydrates in grains and vegetables, because:

- Whole grains, starchy vegetables, fruit, and other minimally processed, carbohydrate-rich foods come packaged with vitamins, minerals, fiber, water, and other essential nutrients, while highly refined sweets are high-calorie, nutritionally poor alternatives.

- Some people have trouble digesting fructose and develop diarrhea, gas, and abdominal pain when they eat small doses of concentrated fructose in honey or HFCS. The fructose in fruits is diluted with water, vitamins, and fiber and does not cause these health problems.
- When fructose is in excess of 20 percent of the total calories in our diets, it also might raise blood triglyceride, cholesterol, and LDL-cholesterol levels, thus increasing the risk for heart disease.
- Fructose won't raise brain serotonin levels, so don't expect to get a mood boost from this sugar.

The bottom line is that eating fruit and a little honey is one way to avoid the blood-sugar roller coaster produced by most processed sweets and desserts. Just be careful not to overload on HFCS-sweetened processed foods, pure fructose from the health food store, or excessive amounts of honey.

How Sweet It Is

The artificial sweetener story grows increasingly complicated as new sweeteners enter the marketplace. Saccharine (in Sweet'n Low) is on the "potentially hazardous to your health" list, having produced cancer in laboratory animals who were fed huge amounts of this sweetener. Sucralose (Splenda) and acesulfame-K (Sunett) appear safe, although it might be too soon to tell the long-term health effects, since these sweeteners have not been thoroughly tested. Aspartame (Equal or Nutra-Sweet) also appears relatively harmless to health in tests and general use. The down side is none of these sweeteners boosts mood, helps curb carbohydrate cravings, or manages weight.

If you are hoping sweeteners are a solution for weight loss, think again. A few studies show that using sweeteners might help in initial weight loss, but other studies report that aspartame-sweetened beverages increase appetite and food intake, possibly contributing to food cravings and weight problems. The reasons for this are unclear, but it could be that the body craves a certain amount of calories or sugar and is not tricked by artificially sweetened drinks and food.

It is thought by some that aspartame even might interfere with weight loss and weight maintenance. One study showed that people who ate chocolate sweetened with aspartame had higher rises in endorphin levels than did people who ate chocolate sweetened with sugar. Since elevation in these pleasurable nerve chemicals is associated with increased food intake, it could be that artificially sweetened foods and beverages stimulate appetite by upsetting the brain's chemistry. However, other studies have not found them to have an appetite-stimulating effect.

Until the controversy is resolved, it is wise to avoid aspartame if you have the disorder phenylketonuria (PKU), are pregnant, or have experienced any adverse side effects when consuming the sweetener. Infants and children also should avoid products containing artificial sweeteners. Other people who choose to include aspartame in their diet should consume moderate amounts of it and pay attention to the number of foods they eat that contain the sweetener. For the weight manager, an occasional diet soft drink can temporarily satisfy a sweet tooth, but it probably won't help you lose weight, and it certainly won't boost your mood.

Eat and Be Merry

The diet and mood puzzle is far from complete; many questions remain to be answered. Are a person's responses to diet and carbohydrates ingrained in the genetic code, or developed in infancy or even in the womb? Why do some people react to small amounts of sugar while other people can eat cups of sugar with no apparent side effects? And what are the other, nonchemical causes for cravings? These are still important questions with no clear answers.

It's in Our Genes

The number one reason we choose a food is because it tastes good, and few foods taste as good as sweets do. That's because of the four types of taste buds (sweet, sour, bitter, and salty), sweet holds the most prestigious spot: on the tip of the tongue.

Since Paleolithic times, our preference for sweets as a species has been an important survival mechanism: Sweet foods tend to be nourishing (high in calories) and safe, while many bitter foods are toxic or poisonous. The taste preference allowed our ancient ancestors to easily identify and gather sweet-tasting foods such as fruits, which are rich in vitamins, minerals, and calories. These foods were limited in quantity and to the time of year they were available. However, our cave-dweller bodies now live in affluent societies where easy and unlimited access to highly processed and concentrated sugar has resulted in each American eating his/her weight in sugar each year. Our genetically programmed taste buds have collided with this glut of sugar always within reach.

Besides a taste for sugar, it is likely that each of us inherits a unique balance of appetite-control chemicals that, combined with habits, memories, and culture, determine our individual food preferences. Studies show, for example, that preferences for sweet-and-creamy foods precede weight gain, and are probably regulated in part by genetics in overweight people. On the other hand, genetics is no excuse for out-of-control appetites. Keep in mind that a craving is only a feeling—it is not a command. And it's a command that can have a negative impact on your health and waistline if it leads you to eat all the wrong foods. Even though the initial relief of satisfying a craving might appear to end the urge to eat, in the long run it encourages stronger and more frequent temptations and leaves you more vulnerable to the next snack attack. Your best bet is to work with these cravings, genetic or not, by following the guidelines outlined on page 54.

Deconditioning a Conditioned Response

It is likely that some cravings are merely habits. Much as Pavlov's dog learned to salivate in anticipation of food when a bell rang, humans seek rewards. If a midafternoon sweet snack makes you feel good, you are likely to have it again. Repeating this behavior over and over results in a habit or even a craving.

Controlling cravings in these situations is a simple matter of changing your behavior. You can substitute a more nutritious food when you snack, for example, replacing the midmorning doughnut with a whole wheat bagel or exchanging the afternoon candy bar for a piece of fresh fruit or a custard-style, nonfat yogurt. Or it can mean developing a new habit to replace the old one. You can take a walk during your high-crave time of the day or ride an exercise bicycle rather than eat potato chips while you watch television in the evening. Try these alternatives, and the craving should subside within two weeks.

Cravings, Old Tapes, and Other Memorabilia

Layered over our appetite-control chemistry are complex emotional, psychological, and cultural influences. Childhood food associations, memories, cultural beliefs and traditions, and other powerful emotional cues urge us to eat and to crave certain foods, and shape each of our food preferences. For example, women who regularly experience food cravings also report more frequent bouts of boredom and anxiety than do women who are less prone to cravings. In these "chicken-or-the-egg" cases it is difficult to determine whether the craving is mediated by nerve chemistry or is a conditioned response to an uncomfortable situation.

Keeping the Food & Mood Journal in chapter 12—where you record when, what, and how much you eat, and how you felt before and after eating—can help you pinpoint the internal signals that cause your cravings. Information from the journal helps you plan strategies for making healthier food choices or finding a non-food alternative to inappropriate eating, such as exercising, visiting a friend, or gardening. (See chapters 10 and 11 for more information on how to identify and avoid emotional eating.)

Listen to Your Body—It's Trying to Tell You Something

Food cravings sometimes are the body's way of correcting a deficiency. People who are protein-deficient crave protein-rich foods, and people who are well-nourished self-select diets that contain a modest 15 percent of total calories as protein. Pica, or the craving for nonfoods such as dirt (a source of iron), is common in people who are iron-deficient. Glycogen stores (the short-term supply of sugar stockpiled in the liver and muscles) depleted by dieting, intense aerobic exercise, or meal skipping can lead to hunger and to cravings for carbohydrates as the body attempts to restock drained fuel stores.

Unfortunately, most of the time the body doesn't provide such clear signals of its nutrient needs. The prevalence of nutrient deficiencies and the glut of bad food choices in this country attest to the fact that we don't instinctively choose the foods our bodies need most. We often are better off using our heads (and common sense), not our instincts, when it comes to nourishing our moods and bodies.

The Basics of Craving Control

You can subdue your cravings and stay on track, even when faced with a battle between your willpower or good intentions and a stew of appetite-triggering chemicals at work on your body and mind (see Table 2.3, "Carbohydrate Cravings Control Guidelines," on page 54).

- If you are a carbohydrate craver, realize you can't "will away" your cravings, so work with them instead. Make sure every meal contains some foods rich in carbohydrates, such as whole-grain bread, cereals, crackers, or starchy vegetables. Plan a complex carbohydrate–rich snack during that time of the day when you are most vulnerable to snack attacks.

- Pinpoint your true craving. Is it for something cold and sweet? Crunchy? Chewy? Once you have identified exactly what you want, then find a low-fat food that will satisfy that craving. Keep in mind that by following the Feeling Good Diet guidelines, your cravings for fatty or overly sweet foods will slowly dwindle. (See "Cravers Versus Noncravers," on page 64.)

- Try "urge surfing." G. Alan Marlatt, Ph.D., professor of psychology at the University of Washington, suggests in his book *Relapse Prevention* that cravings are similar to a wave that builds, then breaks on the beach. Overcoming the temptation to indulge is much like riding the wave as it builds, crests, breaks, and subsides. Most cravings fade within five to fifteen minutes. The temptation to give in to a craving becomes less frequent and progressively weaker when you outlast the urge. Visualize yourself riding any urge you have like a wave until it crashes on the shore. (See chapter 12 for information on how emotions affect cravings, and what to do about it.)

- Limit sweets. People who know they are sensitive to sugar should avoid sweets or eat them in small doses and always with other, more nutritious foods. Most people know that cakes, cookies, candy, sweetened cereals, and soda pop are high in sugar. However, many people are surprised to find sugar listed on the labels of catsup, salad dressings, commercial spaghetti sauce, and even frozen entrées. Table 2.4, "Sweet Surprises: The Sugar Content of Certain Foods," on page 65, provides a partial list of commonly used foods and their added sugar content.

- Nibble, don't gorge: You can ward off a 1,000-calorie binge by consuming several small meals and snacks throughout the day, which maintains steady blood-sugar and neurotransmitter levels.

- Don't diet, at least not in the traditional sense of the word. Drastic diets and diet pills that radically alter normal eating patterns don't work in the long run and they also interfere with brain chemicals. Also steer clear of low-carbohydrate weight-loss diets that upset brain chemistry and aggravate cravings. Instead, develop a

Box 2.1   Cravers Versus Noncravers

Cravers are energized by carbohydrates, while a plate of pasta will put a noncraver to sleep. Consequently, these foods should be carefully planned into the day's food pattern to enhance energy and work performance.

CARBOHYDRATE CRAVER'S EATING PATTERN	STANDARD EATING PATTERN
BREAKFAST	
Whole wheat waffle topped with fresh berries and fat-free sour cream. Nonfat milk	Omelette made with egg substitute, grilled vegetables, low-fat cheese. Whole wheat toast, orange juice
SNACK	
1/2 whole wheat bagel with 2 slices fat-free luncheon meat, sliced tomato, and sprouts. Nonfat milk	Strawberry-kiwi low-fat yogurt mixed with peeled and chopped kiwi fruit
LUNCH	
Bowl of Curried Squash Soup* Tossed salad with 1/2 cup kidney beans Sourdough French bread Orange juice	Cold Curried Chicken Salad with Cranberries* Sourdough French bread Nonfat milk
SNACK	
Air-popped popcorn, oatmeal cookie, pretzels, bagel, or other all-carbohydrate snack	2 slices fat-free luncheon meat, whole wheat crackers, fruit
DINNER	
If you want to relax: 3 ounces grilled chicken or fish, brown rice, steamed vegetable, and low-fat milk	Linguini with Fresh Tomatoes, Capers, and Lemon,* tossed salad, fruit
If you want to exercise or work: Fettuccine à la Tomato and Basil,* tossed salad, fruit, low-fat milk	3 ounces grilled chicken or fish, brown rice, steamed vegetables, fruit

* See "Recipes for Feeling Your Best" at the back of this book.

weight-management plan, based on the Feeling Good Diet and daily exercise, with a goal to lose no more than two pounds per week. A gradual shift in eating and a slow-and-steady approach to weight loss helps "down regulate" your body's appetite-control chemicals. Gradual weight loss also helps burn body fat and keep the weight off (see Table 2.5, "A Weight-Loss Plan for Carbohydrate Cravers," on pages 66–67, and "A Sample Weight-Loss Diet for the Carbohydrate Craver," on pages 67–68).

- Exercise at least five times a week. Daily movement, especially aerobic activity such as walking, jogging, swimming, or bicycling, helps regulate blood-sugar levels and other nerve chemicals, and provides an endorphin rush without the calories. This is not an option—you must exercise if you want to control your cravings!

- Learn to cope. Effective coping skills, a strong social support system, and limited or no alcohol, cigarettes, and medications that compound an emotional problem also are important considerations for controlling your cravings.

- Diet is not shaped by food cravings alone; it also takes an attitude of acceptance and an accommodating environment. You can offset unhealthy cravings by tailoring your home and work environments to support healthful eating. For example, plan ahead how you will handle risk-prone situations, eliminate tempting foods from the environment, or encourage support from friends and family.

Table 2.4   Sweet Surprises: The Sugar Content of Certain Foods

Most people know candy bars, desserts, and honey are sweet treats. But did you know sugar is also in the following foods?

FOOD	SERVING SIZE	TEASPOONS OF ADDED SUGAR
Fast-food chocolate malt	1 medium (20 ounces)	29.0
French vanilla low-fat yogurt with raspberries	1 cup	13.0
Commercial light cheesecake	1 slice or 7.5 ounces	11.6
Coca-Cola	12 ounces	9.3
Fat-free ice cream	1 cup	9.3

FOOD	SERVING SIZE	TEASPOONS OF ADDED SUGAR
Low-fat fruited-yogurt	1 cup	8.8
Commercial blueberry muffin	1 (4.5 ounces)	8.0
Cranberry juice cocktail	1 cup	6.4
Sherbet	1/2 cup	6.7
Applesauce, sweetened	1/2 cup	4.3
Instant oatmeal (cinnamon/spice)	1.5 ounce packet	4.3
Peaches, in heavy syrup	1/2 cup	4.0
Canned ravioli	1 cup	4.0
Canned spaghetti sauce	1/2 cup	4.0
Gatorade	1 cup	3.5
Beans and franks	3/4 cup	3.3
Dessert wine	3.5 ounces	3.0
Barbecue sauce	2 tablespoons	3.0
Peaches, in light syrup	1/2 cup	2.3
Granola bar	1	1.8
Chewing gum	1 stick	1.5–0.6
Cream-style corn	1/2 cup	1.5

Table 2.5   A Weight-Loss Plan for Carbohydrate Cravers

1. Identify the amount of calories required to maintain your desired weight and that will allow no more than a 2-pound weight loss each week. A rule of thumb for estimating your calorie needs is to multiply your desirable weight by 12. For example, if you want to weigh 130 pounds, then $130 \times 12 = 1,560$ calories. Strive for no less than 1,500 calories if you are short or relatively inactive (add an additional 500 calories if you are tall and/or active). You should increase exercise, not cut calories further, if you can't lose weight on this low-calorie plan.

2. Based on this calorie allotment, plan four to six small meals balanced in protein and starch and low in fat.

3. As part of your calorie allotment, plan a small carbohydrate-rich snack for the time of day when cravings are most likely to occur.

4. Plan an aerobic exercise break during your high-risk time of day to divert attention away from snacking and help change body chemistry so you will be less prone to snacking

later in the day. Even if you have no time for a regular workout, a walk around the block will help.

5. Monitor your weight loss. If you are losing more than 2 pounds a week, increase calories by 100 to 200 calories a day. If you are not losing at least 1 pound a week, reduce your daily calorie intake by 100 to 200 calories (but not below 1,500 calories) and increase your daily exercise.

Box 2.2   A Sample Weight-Loss Diet for the Carbohydrate Craver

This menu supplies approximately 1,500 calories. Optimal levels of all vitamins and minerals cannot be guaranteed when calorie intake is this low, so choose a moderate-dose multiple vitamin and mineral supplement when following any low-calorie diet.

BREAKFAST

1/2 cup oatmeal cooked in 2/3 cup nonfat milk and topped with:
   2 tablespoons toasted wheat germ
   2 tablespoons raisins

6 ounces orange juice
Herb or green tea

MIDMORNING SNACK

1 cup nonfat, plain yogurt mixed with:
   2 tablespoons chopped dates

Iced green tea or water

LUNCH

Thai Tofu Salad (serve hot or cold):

Cut into cubes 3 ounces of firm tofu and heat in a nonstick pan for five minutes. Add 2 cups preshredded cabbage mix and 1 tablespoon peanut sauce. Cook over medium heat for 2 minutes (or until heated through, but still crunchy). Top with 1/4 cup chopped fresh cilantro.

1 whole wheat pita bread, toasted
2 medium tomatoes, sliced and topped with:
   2 minced cloves of garlic, 2 tablespoons chopped fresh basil, 1 teaspoon balsamic vinegar
Herb tea or sparkling water with lemon

DINNER

4 ounces roast chicken breast (stuff chicken with fresh rosemary and onions before roasting)

Glazed Carrots:

Peel and slice 2 carrots into $1/4$" diagonals; cook in 1 teaspoon olive oil and $1/3$ cup orange juice until tender. In a small bowl, mix until smooth $1/2$ teaspoon cornstarch, $1/4$ teaspoon ground ginger, a pinch of nutmeg, and 3 tablespoons water. Add ginger mixture to carrots and stir over medium heat until sauce thickens. Sprinkle with 2 teaspoons chopped chives and a pinch of red pepper flakes (optional).

1 cup mashed parsnips topped with $1/4$ teaspoon ground nutmeg

Sparkling water with lime juice

SNACKS (MIDAFTERNOON AND EVENING): PICK ONE SELECTION FOR EACH SNACK FROM THE FOLLOWING

1 cup Cheerios with 2 tablespoons dried apricots

2 graham crackers and $1/2$ cup orange juice mixed with 1 cup sparkling water

2 fig bars

1 slice raisin toast topped with 1 tablespoon fat-free cream cheese and 3 slices apple

50 thin-stick pretzels

$1/2$ whole wheat English muffin topped with 1 tablespoon raspberry jam

1 bread stick

$31/2$ cups air-popped popcorn

6 vanilla wafers

15 low-fat tortilla chips and 2 tablespoons salsa

2 small oatmeal cookies

1 medium sweet potato, baked

1 cup vegetable soup with 3 saltine crackers

Nutritional information:
1,530 calories; 18 percent fat (30.6 grams),
60 percent carbohydrate, 22 percent protein.

CHAPTER THREE

Other Food Cravings: Sweet-and-Creamy, Chocolate, and Salt

- Do you check to see if anyone is paying attention, then sneak into the kitchen to graze on the half gallon of ice cream?
- Do you plan to have just one of the cookies your mother made, only to nibble away the entire tin?
- At parties, do you hover around the dessert section of the buffet?
- Can you eat an entire medium cheese pizza and not feel stuffed?
- Do you swear chocolate has a voice? Do chocolate brownies beckon, and does a dark-chocolate-with-almonds candy bar cry out for you to have a taste?

No one can explain exactly why we crave foods high in fat or salt. Yet with just about every aspect of life triggering appetite, from your body's chemistry and basic instincts to seductive television commercials and the aroma of warm cinnamon rolls from a local bakery, it is amazing that these cravings aren't more frequent. Our cravings have little to do with willpower and much to do with evolution, chemistry, emotions, easy access, and enticing advertising. Your best defense is a well-developed plan to work with these cravings rather than against them.

Your "Fat Tooth"

Although many people assume they crave sweets and claim they have a sweet tooth, in reality they probably are searching for fat. Adam Drewnowski, Ph.D., director of the Nutritional Sciences Program at the University of Washington, disagrees with the theory that people crave carbohydrates only because of the effect these foods have on brain levels of serotonin, a neurotransmitter that has a calming effect (see chapters 1 and 2). Drewnowski's research shows that it also is a desire for fat—or more specifically, sweetened fat—that leads some people to indulge in chocolate, ice cream, and cookies.

"These so-called carbohydrate-rich foods derive as much, if not more, of their calories from fat than from sugar; the sugar just makes the fat taste better," says Dr. Drewnowski. For example, 54 percent of the calories in some ice cream comes from fat; a chocolate chip cookie is up to 40 percent fat calories; and a Hershey's special dark chocolate bar is 51 percent fat calories.

Fat alone is unpalatable. But add even a little sugar and you have a sweet-and-creamy combination that brings out the craving in even the most ardent dieter. Dr. Drewnowski's studies on food preferences using varying amounts of sugar and fat showed that people are least likely to choose a high-sweet, low-fat food such as jelly beans or popsicles, and they are most likely to choose a sweet-and-creamy food with a taste and texture similar to sweetened whipped cream.

Sugar masks the fat in foods. When people are asked to taste foods containing various amounts of sugar and fat, their perception of the fat content decreases as the sugar content increases. For example, commercial cake icing contains 70 percent sugar and 15 to 20 percent fat, which is too sweet for most adults. However, this icing gains in appeal if the fat content is increased to 25 percent or more. In other studies, few adults place sweetened nonfat milk (high-sugar, low-fat) or unsweetened cream (low-sugar, high-fat) at the top of their list of cravings. Yet the majority of adults responded favorably to sweetened heavy cream (high-sugar, high-fat). So, sweet-and-creamy is the dynamic duo: Fat makes the food desirable, and sugar makes the fat invisible. Consequently, people who are not really carbohydrate cravers have no idea how much fat they are eating, and accuse the sugar of prompting the uncontrollable urge to eat.

A Matter of Texture, Aroma, and Taste

Granted, few people drool at the thought of greasy foods. The craving for fat is mostly unconscious and has a lot to do with texture, flavor, and aroma of foods; fat makes foods mouthwatering, delectable, tantalizing, and palatable. For instance, the butterfat in ice cream makes it creamy and smooth. The marbling in meat makes it tender. The fats used in deep-frying make French fries and onion rings crispy and crunchy.

Don't underestimate the importance of aroma! If something smells good, we are most likely to eat it. Because fat carries many of the best aromas in food, we are drawn to the sizzling steak, the roast turkey, the smell of chocolate, and the whiff of bread baking. The more turned on you are by the smell of foods, the more likely you are to battle food cravings. According to scientists at the Monell Chemical Senses Center in Philadelphia, as people age they lose their smell sensitivity and also report fewer cravings than they did when they were younger. Although only a few studies have investigated the effects of aroma on brain chemistry, it is very likely that the complex smells of food trigger jumps in serotonin, endorphins, or other brain chemicals, just as the anticipation of a meal releases insulin into the blood (see chapter 10 for more on the importance of smell on taste and appetite).

The pleasurable qualities of foods—that is, how they feel in the mouth, their aromas, and flavors—determine which foods we will eat and how much we love them, and even help shape our memories. For example, take a moment to relax, then note the first one or two words that come to mind to describe each of the following foods:

a croissant	a fresh orange
chocolate pudding	potato chips
a carrot stick	peanut butter

If words such as *flaky*, *smooth*, *creamy*, *rich*, *crunchy*, *juicy*, *crisp*, *gooey*, or *sticky* came to mind, you are not alone. When asked to describe foods, most people use texture terms rather than terms to describe color (did *brown* come to mind when you thought of chocolate?) or flavor (did *citrusy* come to mind when you thought of oranges?). Our connection with aroma is so strong that we remember special holidays by the smell of a turkey roasting, and the smell of brownies baking can trigger the memory of a conversation you thought was long forgotten. More often than not, it is fat in the food that brings us these appealing sensations.

People rank taste as the number one factor influencing which foods they eat. And "creamy" foods taste great. In one study at Duke University, normal-weight, nondieting women were given several different meals that varied in taste, including a bland-fat meal, a tasty-fat meal, a bland-carbohydrate meal, and a tasty-carbohydrate meal. The tasty versions of both the carbohydrate and the fatty meals were more satisfying and reduced hunger more than either of the bland meals. (See chapter 10 for more on taste and satiety.)

Ya Gotta Love 'Em

Our bodies evolved to love fat. This super-dense source of calories helped our ancient ancestors survive famines, plagues, and hardship. Day in and day out, generation after generation for almost 4 million years, our hunter-gatherer ancestors ate what they could find or kill. Most of the time it was roots and berries, complemented occasionally with wild game. "Fruits, roots, legumes, nuts, and other plants comprised about 60 percent to 65 percent of the diet, with very lean wild game and eggs making up the difference," says S. Boyd Eaton, M.D., adjunct associate professor of anthropology at Emory University in Atlanta. Our ancient ancestors had limited access to fatty foods, and over millions of years evolved a complicated appetite-control chemistry to make sure they ate lots of fat when it was around. Combined with vigorous lifestyles, these nutrient-packed diets explain why the average cave person was as fit, lean, tall, and strong as today's well-trained athlete.

Today, machines do our work; we sit more than we gather; and we depend on cars, not legs. Foods are processed more than they are fresh; refined grains are staples, not novelties; our meat sources are domesticated, not wild; and vegetables are a side dish, not the main course. "For one hundred thousand generations people had been hunter-gatherers. Compare that to the five hundred generations [that] people have been farmers, the ten generations since the Industrial Age, and the one generation since computers and you see that there have been major changes in how we live and eat in a very short period of time," says Dr. Eaton.

Therein lies the problem. It takes tens of thousands of years for the body to adapt to even small changes in the environment. Our biochemistry and physiology remain fine-tuned to low-fat diets and high-intensity activity. Escalating obesity rates are one result of genetics and lifestyle colliding. "Our ancestors who stored body fat efficiently resisted starvation during famines and lived to reproduce," says George Armelagos, Ph.D., professor of anthropology at Emory University. "Our bodies weren't designed for today's never-ending abundance of easily digested carbohydrates and fat, along with no activity."

Here's a quick look at how your body entices you to eat those greasy chips or creamy ice cream. More importantly, we'll also take a look at how you can work with your chemistry and satisfy your cravings without sacrificing your waistline or your health.

Fat for Survival

It is no coincidence that our brain's craving center is next door to our reproduction center. Sarah Leibowitz, Ph.D., a professor of neurobiology at Rockefeller University who has pioneered research on the body's control center for food cravings, believes that our fundamental drive to survive (to reproduce) rests on the body's ensuring that it receives enough calories to meet energy demands today and to store for future famines. Dr. Leibowitz's research found the body has a built-in appetite system for fat, the long-term storage fuel. This appetite is regulated by a brain chemical called galanin, which rises as the day progresses and triggers a desire for fatty foods such as meats, creamed sauces, and salad dressing for lunch, or a chocolate truffle or bowl of ice cream for a midafternoon or late-night snack. The connection between fat cravings and galanin has been clearly identified in laboratory animals. In an experiment where galanin was injected into the hypothalamus—the appetite-control center of the brain—animals self-selected fat-rich diets.

Galanin is also closely connected to the pleasure response triggered by the endorphins. "Galanin and the endorphins coexist in the same nerve cells and work together," says Dr. Leibowitz. So, while galanin is triggering a craving for ice cream, the endorphins are making the experience pleasurable. Another neurotransmitter called enterostatin also interacts with galanin as a shutoff switch for fat cravings. Inject this neurotransmitter into the brains of animals, and they lose their desire for fatty foods. Researchers suspect the balance between enterostatin, the endorphins, galanin, and possibly serotonin is critical for appetite control. In contrast, no studies have shown that any over-the-counter diet pills, such as pyruvate or hydroxycitric acid (HCA), are effective in burning fat and reducing cravings for fatty foods.

Galanin works with other hormones to convert dietary fat into body fat. As galanin levels go up, so does body fat, while metabolism slows. Weight gain results.

In laboratory animals, the more galanin produced, the more weight an animal is likely to gain in the future. Perhaps this is one reason obese people prefer fattier foods and, although they consume the same amount of calories as do lean people, more of those calories come from fat. Combined with a disturbance in the hormone-like compounds that usually turn off appetite—such as insulin from the pancreas and cholecystokinin (CCK) from the digestive tract—Dr. Leibowitz speculates that an excess of galanin could escalate a craving into a weight problem.

What turns on the galanin system? As mentioned in chapter 1, galanin levels rise naturally as the day progresses; therefore, they are lowest in the morning and highest from afternoon until bedtime, which corresponds to the time when most people experience cravings for fatty foods. Galanin levels also rise when estrogen levels are high, which might explain the cravings for sweet-and-creamy foods associated with premenstrual syndrome (PMS). In essence, estrogen, by way of galanin, makes a woman want to eat and deposit fat in preparation for childbearing. Fad diets also play havoc on galanin levels. Strict diets or a quick weight loss generate a flood of metabolic debris that signal the appetite-control center in the brain to raise galanin levels. This triggers a fat craving—probably as a survival mechanism to safeguard the body's fuel stores.

Stress also adds to the food cravings. Everything from boredom to anxiety can set off a craving. Interestingly, the stress hormones, such as norepinephrine (a cousin to adrenalin) and corticosterone, both secreted from the adrenal glands during stress, raise galanin levels, which increase cravings for fatty foods, overeating, and weight gain. Women with high levels of these stress hormones are more apt to favor high-fat foods like potato chips, according to a study from Yale University. However, rather than stewing in their own juices during times of stress, this group would be better off exercising daily, which boosts endorphins and helps eliminate the stress hormones.

In short, some cravings stem from the root of your being, originating in your genetic code. Trying to override these cravings can lead to a binge. Restrictive diets, erratic eating habits, or even very low-fat diets are the worst thing you can do if you crave fat, because they disrupt this natural cycle of nerve chemicals. Researchers already are investigating the next generation of diet pills that will turn off galanin production, thereby short-circuiting our cravings for cheeseburgers, fudge brownies, and doughnuts without interfering with healthy appetites. But until a safe drug is developed that can do this, the only way to curb a fat tooth is to work with it (see "Cravings Finale," later in this chapter).

More on Endorphins and
Fat Cravings

According to Dr. Drewnowski, endorphins—the natural morphinelike substances in the brain that produce euphoric or pleasurable feelings—might be the culprit in sweet-fat cravings. "Few theories on food cravings take into account the importance of the pleasure response," says Dr. Drewnowski. Both sugar and fat are suspected to release endorphins in the brain and produce a natural euphoric feeling.

These suspicions are supported by several studies, including those conducted by Elliot Blass, Ph.D., at Cornell University. Dr. Blass found a similar link between the endorphins and cravings for sweet-and-creamy foods. People eat more food when endorphin levels are high, which explains why you can't eat just one potato chip or one slice of pizza. He speculates that when people go on restrictive diets or drastically reduce fat intake, they set up a rebound effect, where they swing from abstinence to binge eating. In contrast, avoiding very restrictive weight-loss diets and slowly lowering dietary fat—perhaps taking even a year or more to reach your goal of 30 percent or less calories from fat—is the most effective way to work with endorphin levels and avoid the rebound effect.

On the other hand, some high-fat foods, such as chocolate, could become addicting if consumed too often or in too great a quantity. Some people are especially sensitive to the pleasurable experience of eating creamy foods and show a heightened response to both the aroma and taste for foods like chocolate, French fries, or chips. Eating these foods daily could desensitize their appetite-control chemicals. As a result, they eat more of the food to get the same pleasurable feeling and fullness. If eating a sweet-and-creamy (cookies or chocolate) or crunchy-and-greasy food (potato chips) leads to wanting more of that food, you could be one of these people. If you eat a particular fatty food to feel better, to be more energetic or alert, or to improve your feelings of well-being, you could be suffering from a mild food addiction. In this case, you can stop the addiction by eliminating the food from your diet. The addiction should subside within three weeks. Don't be surprised, however, if the craving comes back in full force when you eat that food again. That's because even one bite can trigger the addiction.

The Fat Thermostat

Leptin—a hormone that plays a key role in our preferences for fatty foods—regulates body fat so impressively that obese laboratory animals injected with leptin shed a third of their weight (all of it fat) in two weeks. Mice born with a genetic defect resulting in lower leptin levels overeat and become obese; inject them with leptin, and they eat normally, move more, and lose weight. The same goes for people. People with low leptin levels typically are tempted by a plate of fudge or a bag of chips. Leptin sends messages to the brain about the body's fat stores. When elevated, it serves as a stop-eating signal possibly by turning off NPY or galanin, but sends a start-eating signal when low by turning on NPY, galanin, or other neurotransmitters. Severe dieting lowers body fat stores too rapidly, which lowers leptin levels and turns on fat cravings. This might explain why most people inevitably regain the weight they have lost on fad diets.

Even if people are born with a leptin deficiency, that doesn't mean they are fated to overeat and be overweight. In a study on identical twins where one twin from each pair ran daily, all the couch potatoes and none of the runners were overweight. So even if there is a genetic predisposition to weight gain, it can be overcome with exercise.

Leptin also might be influenced by what we eat—in particular, zinc-rich foods. Researchers at Harvard Medical School found that low zinc intake reduced leptin levels. When the same people were given zinc supplements, blood leptin levels increased, which should reduce appetite and enhance weight regulation. In other studies, animals fed zinc-poor diets switched their preference from carbohydrate-rich foods to fatty, high-calorie foods.

While further studies are needed to clarify the link between zinc and food cravings, one interesting connection is with aging and taste. Even a moderate zinc deficiency reduces a person's taste sensitivity. As people age, they eat fewer zinc-rich foods such as meat, lose their sense of taste, and report fewer cravings for specific foods. Theoretically, if the loss of taste and altered leptin levels are caused, at least in part, by poor zinc intake, then sweet-and-creamy foods won't taste as good to an older person. This would explain why people's interest in fatty foods such as chocolate diminishes as they age. The solution here is clear: Increase your daily intake of zinc-rich foods, such as extra-lean meat, oysters, whole-grain breads, or cooked dried beans and peas, and/or take a moderate-dose multiple vitamin and mineral supplement that contains at least 15 to 20 milligrams of zinc.

A Calorie Is Not Just a Calorie

There is more to fat than taste and texture. An ounce of fat is more than twice as calorie dense as an ounce of pure carbohydrate or protein. Often, removing fat from the diet means more food can be eaten for fewer calories. Substituting half a baked chicken breast for half a fried chicken breast saves almost 100 calories, with no loss of taste or amount of food. Replacing regular cream cheese with fat-free cream cheese saves 75 calories per ounce. A half-cup serving of nonfat, frozen yogurt instead of the same size serving of ice cream saves you 175 calories and more than a tablespoon of fat. (See Table 3.1, "Ways to Trim the Fat," below.)

But the fat issue is more than just calories. Calories from fat are more fattening than calories from either protein or carbohydrates. One reason for this is that fat is built to be stored, requiring only about 3 percent of its calories to convert it into hip and belly fat. In contrast, the body uses up almost 25 percent of their calories converting excess carbohydrates and protein into body fat. Even then, you must

---

Table 3.1   Ways to Trim the Fat

Cutting the fat means you can eat as much or more food and maintain or even lose weight—not to mention the benefits to your health!

INSTEAD OF	CHOOSE	CALORIES SAVED	FAT (TSP) SAVED
1 ounce of cubed cheddar cheese in a salad	1 teaspoon grated Parmesan cheese	105	2
2 tablespoons walnuts in cookie dough	2 tablespoons nuggetlike cereal	47	2
1/2 cup cream and 2 tablespoons butter to thicken cream sauces and soups	1/2 cup pureed vegetable	216	8
Fish baked in 1 tablespoon butter	Fish baked in wine, garlic, and herbs	100	2 1/2
1 ounce of croutons in a salad	1 ounce chopped celery	128	more than 1

INSTEAD OF	CHOOSE	CALORIES SAVED	FAT (TSP) SAVED
2 tablespoons oil in a muffin mix	2 tablespoons pureed prunes	172	6
1 piece of coffee cake	1/2 whole wheat bagel with 1 teaspoon fat-free cream cheese	127	1 1/2
3 ounces regular bacon	3 ounces Canadian bacon	331	8
1 cup granola	1 cup Cheerios	506	7
2 pork sausage patties	2 turkey sausage patties	69	2
1 tablespoon mayonnaise on a sandwich	1 tablespoon fat-free mayonnaise	88	2 1/2
1 ounce of potato chips	1 ounce of pretzels	44	2
1 slice garlic bread	1 slice French bread	69	1 1/2
1/2 cup stuffing mix	1/2 cup no-butter stuffing mix	65	2
4 ounces snack pudding	4 ounces instant sugar-free pudding	90	1
1/2 cup premium frozen yogurt	fat-free frozen fruit or gelatin bar	120	1
1/4 cup peanuts	1/4 cup toasted garbanzo beans	38	3 1/3
1 serving apple pie	1 serving Apple-Cranberry Upside-down Pie*	153	3
1 regular brownie	1 To-Die-For Low-Fat Brownie*	103	3
1 tablespoon margarine	1 tablespoon reduced-fat margarine	50	1
1 ounce American cheese	1 ounce reduced-fat cheese	33	1
2 ounces bologna	2 ounces fat-free bologna	140	17
1 tablespoon mayonnaise	1 tablespoon reduced-fat mayonnaise	50	6
1 tablespoon salad dressing	1 tablespoon reduced-fat salad dressing	34	4

* See "Recipes for Feeling Your Best" at the back of this book.

consume an excessive amount of calories as carbohydrates before the body will convert those calories to fat. Consequently, the more fat people consume, regardless of calories, the more likely they are to be overweight. According to a study conducted at the University of Tennessee, the most consistent predictor of body weight in women is the amount of fat in the diet. Of course, most fat-laden foods are calorie dense, so eating more fat usually means eating more calories (see "America's Big Secret," below).

America's Big Secret

As Americans, we're fatter than ever, yet we say we're eating less fat. What's going on? Well, contrary to the latest fad-diet books, our love of pasta and cookies isn't why we're gaining weight. According to a study from Yale University School of Medicine in New Haven, Connecticut, we're fatter because we're guzzling more calories and not much less fat, which lowers the percentage of calories from fat, not the actual fat grams.

Of course, part of the problem could be that no one admits to what's on the plate. Women underestimate their calorie intake by up to 17 percent, saying they eat 1,635 calories, when in fact they consume closer to 1,925 calories daily, report researchers at the University of Washington in Seattle. The more overweight people are, the more they underestimate their food intakes, state researchers from both the University of Vermont in Burlington and the Institute for Nutrition Research at the University of Oslo in Norway. Finally, we are moving less, which means more calories are stored rather than used.

These and other findings suggest that fat cravings sustain a vicious cycle. Whatever makes people fat also contributes to cravings for fatty foods, and the fatty foods make people fatter. The good news is that as you lower your fat intake, your fat cravings should subside. Researchers at the Cancer Research Center in Seattle surveyed 448 women who had participated in nutrition classes to lower their fat intake; 56 percent reported that being on low-fat diets made them dislike the taste of fat. More than 60 percent said they actually felt physical discomfort after eating high-fat foods. Thus, following a low-fat diet can reprogram the body's chemistry, reeducate your palate, and help you maintain a more desirable weight.

Why We Crave Fat: A Simple
Explanation

Restrictive fad diets catapult most people to the edge of desire for forbidden fatty foods. Dieters can eat diet-friendly foods such as raw vegetables, diet soda, skinless baked chicken, and fruit for just so long before the sensory deficit entices them to indulge. Although this doesn't mean they have to eat fatty foods, since flavorful low-fat fare can tantalize taste buds just as easily, they turn to salty, high-fat foods because they are readily accessible.

Cravings also are triggered by their positive rewarding nature. Cookies are an example of how well-established patterns of food and good times (positive reinforcers) lead to future cravings. People who remember the smell of baking cookies from when they were children, who were rewarded with cookies when their report cards were good, and who have snuck away from work with a friend to have a cookie and coffee break are likely to associate these sweet treats with life's most cherished moments. Subsequent cravings for a cookie are intertwined with feelings of love, peace of mind, refreshment, and escape. (See chapters 10 and 11 for a detailed look at the psychology behind food choices.)

Fake Fats: There's No Such Thing as
a Free Lunch

Imagine eating French fries, doughnuts, double-dipped cones, and fudge without a worry about your heart or your waistline. Fat substitutes—such as Simplesse, Olean (Olestra), Oatrim-10, Z-Trim, and Salatrim—have made this dream come true. These fake fats are promising breakthroughs for sweet-and-creamy cravings since they mimic the feel of fat without the calories.

- Simplesse is made with egg and milk protein and can be used in any food not baked or fried.
- Olean (Olestra) is derived from edible oils and sugars but is calorie-free because it is made from molecules too big to digest.
- Oatrim-10 is a derivative of oat bran that has some cholesterol-lowering effects.
- Z-Trim is a fiberlike substance made from soybeans, rice, peas, corn, and wheat or oats that also has a slight cholesterol-lowering ability.

- Salatrim is made from processed vegetable oils and is used in some fat-free chocolate items, such as semisweet baking chips.

Olestra: Hero or Villain?

Olestra is one of the most controversial of the fake fats. It makes great-tasting, low-fat junk food; however, by passing through the digestive tract unabsorbed, it causes diarrhealike symptoms and intestinal gas in some who eat it. It also binds to fats in the digestive tract, including the fat-soluble nutrients, such as vitamins A, D, E, and K. While some of these vitamins are added to Olestra-laden products to offset a deficiency, other fat-soluble compounds, such as the carotenes (including beta carotene, lycopene, and lutein), are not. Consequently, people who regularly eat Olestra-cooked foods have up to a 50 percent drop in blood levels of these health-enhancing nutrients. The carotenes help fight cancer, but most Americans already consume too few of them: Aggravating poor intake by eating even an 8-ounce pack of Olestra-laden potato chips could tip the scale from a marginal to a serious deficiency. Only decades of Olestra use will determine if the need to satisfy a fat tooth by using this fake fat leads to a higher incidence of cancer, heart disease, cataracts, or even premature aging.

The Scoop on Orlistat

Orlistat is an enzyme-blocking drug that reduces fat absorption by up to 30 percent, which means even if you eat a high-fat food, only approximately two-thirds of the fat is absorbed. However, like Olestra, Orlistat has its side effects. It probably can't be consumed in doses large enough to have a significant effect on fat intake, since excessive unabsorbed fat in the digestive tract causes an unpleasant condition called steatorrhea, which is characterized by abdominal bloating, fatty diarrhea, and gas. It also reduces beta carotene absorption by one-third and vitamin E by up to 60 percent, according to the findings of researchers at the Hoffman-La Roche laboratories in Nutley, New Jersey.

Are Fake Fats the Answer to Dieting?

The big question is: Will these fake fats soothe your fat tooth and help you in weight management? Don't get your hopes up. Theoretically, fat substitutes should help solve our cravings for fat. However, the reality is when people eat foods containing fake fats, they eat less fat but they compensate by eating more calories either at the same meal or later in the day. In fact, calorie consumption has increased in the past decade even though there are more reduced-fat items on supermarket shelves than ever before. The only way reduced-fat foods will help people lose weight is if people choose reduced-fat foods that are also reduced-calorie, and stick to reasonable portions.

Of course it doesn't take a scientist to realize that chowing down on more highly processed, nutrient-bleak foodlike products laced with fake fats or fake sugars is a far cry from eating more fresh fruits and vegetables. Reduced-fat potato chips are not healthful foods; it's just that they are less unhealthful than their full-fat counterpart. You are still eating empty calories, which promotes weight gain. Fake fats won't magically make anyone slim; the only way to do that is to eat a healthful diet and exercise daily. On the other hand, some fat-free versions of staple foods, such as sour cream or whole wheat crackers, are a great alternative for people trying to cut back on empty calories. When adding reduced-fat items to your diet, it's a matter of being selective and using a little common sense.

Chocoholics: Can't Live With It, Can't Live Without It

Chocolate is America's favorite flavor. Chocolate has been described as irresistible, wicked, naughty, an essential food, and divine. Some people can't get through the day without it. Others indulge their cravings in secret. In a study conducted at the University of Pennsylvania, researchers found that chocolate was liked by everyone, but women were by far its biggest advocates. One in every two women reports having cravings for chocolate; most craved chocolate more than any other food and were more likely to crave chocolate when they were premenstrual. In fact, the more severe the PMS symptoms, the more likely a woman is to crave chocolate. Chocolate cravings in women and men usually start midday, with half of the chocolate in the United States consumed as snacks between lunch and bedtime.

Our obsession with chocolate could be partially cultural. While a man receives a bottle of whiskey as a gift, a woman receives chocolates, possibly to sweeten her heart to love. Valentine's Day has become an annual tribute to chocolate and love. Chocolate also is closely associated with indulgence and pleasure. It is not a member of any food group and is rarely part of the steak-and-potatoes main course, so it is not a part of our daily routines or any of their obligations, responsibilities, or commitments. Conse-

Saving Graces

What could be better than to hear that chocolate is good for you! Well, life just got a little bit better.

- *Hearty news:* Recent research shows that chocolate is chock-full of antioxidants that protect arteries and the heart from damage that leads to atherosclerosis and heart disease. A small candy bar (1 to 2 ounces) has the same amount of these antioxidants, called phenols, as you'd get in a five-ounce glass of red wine. Even a cup of hot chocolate made with 2 tablespoons of cocoa powder contains 146 milligrams of phenols. Dark chocolate has the most phenolics, while white chocolate has none. Better yet, the antioxidants in chocolate appear more potent than those in wine.
- *A good fat:* Isn't chocolate high in saturated fat? Yes. Cocoa butter, the fat in chocolate, is high in saturated fat, but it is a type of fat called stearic acid, which is converted to oleic acid, a heart-healthy monounsaturated fat also found in olive oil. So chocolate doesn't raise blood cholesterol levels or your risk for heart disease—that is, as long as you don't mix it with butter, cream, eggs, or shortening.
- *Face-off:* In the past, eating chocolate was thought to cause or aggravate acne. Recent studies have dispelled this claim.
- *Mineral makeover:* Chocolate is a good source of several minerals, including copper, magnesium, and calcium (if it's milk chocolate).
- *Misquoted:* Chocolate contains caffeine, but not that much. In fact, one ounce has only 6 milligrams, compared to 130 to 180 milligrams in a cup of coffee.
- *A matter of portion:* Chocolate also isn't high in calories. A Kiss contains only 25 calories. Of course, there is the issue of eating the whole bag!
- *Dental friendly:* Chocolate does not promote dental caries, primarily because the fat helps protect the teeth from the acids otherwise formed from sugar. Chocolate also might contain an antibacterial agent that helps fight plaque formation.
- *Oops:* On the downside, chocolate is not recommended for people susceptible to migraine headaches.

quently, chocolate symbolizes an escape from day-to-day drudgery. Gourmet chocolates are touted as "sinfully delicious" and "wickedly rich." Most people can't resist the little legal "sin" that chocolate provides now and again (see "Saving Graces," above).

Chocolate's pleasantness might extend beyond indulgence to strike at the tip of your taste buds and the heart of your cravings. The cocoa butter in real chocolate gives it a rich texture. Cocoa butter is solid at room temperature but melts in your mouth at body temperature, providing what has been termed "a moment of ecstasy." While unsweetened chocolate is bitter, it becomes the queen of the sweet-and-creamy desserts when mixed with sugar.

Chocolate has the perfect mix of sugar and fat to turn on almost every appetite-triggering neurotransmitter. The sugar in chocolate sparks serotonin release and soothes NPY levels, contributing to the sense of well-being. The sweet taste it has also releases endorphins in the brain, giving us an immediate rush. The fat in chocolate enhances its rich flavor and aroma and satisfies galanin levels. The endorphin rush alone that is set in motion with a bite of chocolate produces a powerful pleasure sensation that is likely to be habit-forming, which might explain why some people say they are addicted to chocolate.

Then there are all the other chemicals in chocolate that make us feel good. Chocolate contains theobromine and caffeine, compounds that provide a mental lift. A compound called phenylethylamine (PEA) found in chocolate stimulates the nervous system, increases blood pressure and heart rate, and is suspected to produce feelings similar to those experienced when a person is "in love." PEA also is linked to the endorphins and, thus, the pleasure response. Finally, a study from the Neuroscience Institute of San Diego reported that chocolate contains a substance called anandamide, which mimics the effects of marijuana and boosts the pleasure you get when you eat chocolate. Although the amounts of anandamide and PEA in chocolate are probably too low to have a significant effect, these compounds remind us that there's a lot more to chocolate than just a heartthrob aroma and melt-in-your-mouth texture.

Even the aroma of chocolate could affect brain chemistry. Researchers at the University of Pennsylvania found that when chocolate cravers were given chocolate, white chocolate, or capsules of cocoa powder, only eating the real chocolate curbed cravings, which implies that the aroma of chocolate plays a part in the craving and pleasure of the chocolate experience.

Others argue that a craving for chocolate is really the body's craving for its nutrients, such as magnesium. If this is the case, why don't people crave other magnesium-rich foods such as soybeans, peanuts, and beet greens? In fact, chocolate cravings usually can be satisfied only by chocolate or something that mimics its texture, taste, and aroma. Since cocoa contains more than four hundred distinct flavor compounds—more than twice as many as any other food—it is likely there are yet unexplored elements in it that trigger cravings, passions, and euphoria.

In short, no one knows why we love chocolate, but few will deny the cravings are

Some Chocolate Tricks

Here are a few ideas for chocolate snacks that fit the low-fat guidelines outlined in the Feeling Good Diet. Keep in mind that *low fat* does not mean *low calorie*, and that many of these selections are still high in sugar.

1. Fight chocolate with chocolate. Use cocoa powder: It has only 30 percent fat calories compared to 50 percent fat calories in whole-milk hot chocolate, 60 percent fat calories in some chocolates, and 76 percent fat calories in unsweetened chocolate. Use it in muffins, cookies, or blender drinks for a rich chocolate flavor with less fat. It's the ingredient in the three low-fat chocolate recipes in the "Recipes for Feeling Your Best" section at the back of this book: To-Die-For Low-Fat Brownies, Civilized S'Mores, and Chocolate Chip Cupcakes.

2. A fat-free chocolate glaze for desserts and fruits can be made by combining 2 tablespoons cold nonfat milk, 1 cup sifted confectioners' sugar, and 1 teaspoon unsweetened cocoa.

3. An extra-rich chocolate angel food cake can be made with one package of angel food cake mix prepared according to directions, combined with 1/3 cup unsweetened cocoa; the cake will have only 7 percent fat calories and less than 160 calories per serving.

4. Cut the fat by half in a brownie or chocolate recipe by using low-fat vanilla yogurt; cut it even more by replacing all the fat with baby-food prunes and/or applesauce.

5. Use chocolate-flavored syrup with 3 percent fat calories. Spoon it over nonfat vanilla yogurt, fresh strawberries, or orange slices, or use it as a dip for frozen grapes and bananas.

6. Eat chocolate with meals. At the end of a meal you are less likely to overindulge and more likely to choose small portions.

7. Buy chocolate in small quantities. Avoid the five-pound box of chocolates, the oversized candy bar, or the half gallon of ice cream. Instead, one or two chocolate Kisses (25 calories each), a Tootsie Roll, or two Dove Promises can satisfy the craving without going overboard.

8. Keep chocolate Kisses, Dove Promises, and other small chocolate treats in the freezer. It's easier to eat less when they're frozen.

9. Warm fat-free fudge in the microwave and spread it thinly on graham crackers for a reduced-fat snack, or melt a Hershey's Kiss on a rice cake in the microwave, then spread it and let it chill.

10. Try a low-fat chocolate slushie. Combine a cup of nonfat milk, 1/4 cup sugar, 3 tablespoons

cocoa powder, and 2 teaspoons vanilla extract in a saucepan over medium heat, stirring constantly until mixture comes to a low boil and all ingredients are blended. Let simmer for three minutes, stirring occasionally. Remove from heat and cool. Transfer to a covered container and freeze. Once frozen, transfer to a blender and whip. Pour into a glass and enjoy!

11. Some people report that taking a daily magnesium supplement (350 to 500 milligrams) helps curb their chocolate cravings.

12. Switch to nonfat: Cut the calories by 31 percent and the fat from 8 to 1.2 grams by switching from whole to nonfat chocolate milk. Cut calories in half and fat to nothing by switching from chocolate ice cream to nonfat chocolate frozen yogurt. A slice of low-fat chocolate cream pie has half the calories and 64 percent less fat than the full-fat traditional pie if the chocolate pudding is made with nonfat milk, the graham cracker crust is fat-free, and the whipped cream is reduced-fat.

13. Try any of the following: Cocoamint Velamints; a Fudgsicle (only 70 calories and 13 percent fat); sugarless hot cocoa; an Alba 77 chocolate shake (whip in a blender with ice for a 70-calorie milk shake); Cocoa Krispies cereal (high in sugar, but less than 1 gram of fat in a 1-cup serving); sugar-free chocolate pudding made with nonfat milk; add 3 tablespoons of sugar-free hot chocolate mix to nonfat plain yogurt (tastes like pudding); Weight Watchers Chocolate Mousse pops (45 calories and less than 1 gram of fat); or blend a can of diet chocolate soda with nonfat milk and ice for a chocolate soda.

14. Want a chocolate snack for less than 100 calories? Try any of these: an Andes Creme de Menthe Thin mint (4); Oreo Cookies (2); chocolate pudding made with 1 percent low-fat milk ($2/3$ cup); plain M & Ms (23); miniature chocolate bars (2 pieces or $1/2$ ounce); chocolate-covered raisins (24); chocolate chips (1 tablespoon); a York peppermint patty (2); chocolate sprinkles (2 tablespoons); or chocolate syrup (2 tablespoons).

15. Cut out caffeinated coffee for three weeks and see if your chocolate cravings also subside.

16. Try low-fat, low-calorie versions of traditional desserts. Sara Lee Lights—Double Chocolate Cake and other varieties—have less than 200 calories per serving. Pepperidge Farm offers several varieties in their frozen-dessert line that contain no more than 190 calories per serving. Low-fat Hostess cupcakes that are jam-filled rather than cream-filled have reduced the fat from 24 percent to 7 percent. Finally, Entenmann's fat-free chocolate cake is a low-fat version of the original.

17. Melt chocolate chips in a double-boiler, then dip dried apricots, minipretzels, or mini–rice cakes in it. Set on a tray lined with waxed paper (approximately 25 calories each).

18. If the smell of chocolate is your downfall, try a little perfume or aftershave applied under your nose.

real. Because chocolate urges, more than other cravings, are not likely to "just go away," the best tactic is to include a small chocolate snack in your eating plan and give it a low-fat face-lift (see "Some Chocolate Tricks," on pages 85–86).

That Craving for Salt

A craving for something salty is the most elusive of all the urges to eat. No one really knows why some people crave salty potato chips, French fries, salted nuts or popcorn, or pizza instead of ice cream or chocolate. Some people even combine cravings, such as ice cream and chips, pretzels dunked in chocolate, or other sweet-and-salty snacks. Although there is nothing inherently wrong in satisfying a craving for salt, the salty foods that we tend to eat often are major contributors to fat in the diet, which can add unwanted pounds.

One theory for the increased cravings for salty foods in women, especially during the two weeks prior to their periods, could be the effect of the female hormone estrogen on the antidiuretic hormones, vasopressin and aldosterone, which cause fluid retention. Some women gain up to ten pounds of added water weight during this time of the month, which turns on their salt cravings to help maintain the normal salt concentration in the body.

Salt cravings could stem from low calcium intake as well. Researchers at the Monell Chemical Senses Center in Philadelphia report that people with low calcium intakes also are most prone to cravings for salty foods. This link is supported by studies on laboratory animals that don't crave salt but become salt lovers when fed calcium-poor diets. Add calcium to their diets, and their salt cravings subside. More than half of the people in the United States consume suboptimal amounts of calcium, which could contribute to our insatiable salt appetites. The same researchers also report that low-protein diets trigger salt cravings, at least in animals.

Salt cravings might result from the body's memory of very early experiences, dating back even as early as conception. People are most likely to report cravings for salty foods if their mothers experienced serious morning sickness during pregnancy, or if they were given diuretics or fed sodium- or chloride-deficient diets as infants or children. Finally, the crunchy textures of many salted snack foods could satisfy our need to bite down on something to relieve stress or anger. Although there are no studies as yet to support this theory, the crunchy textures of chips or pretzels do provide a cathartic outlet for tension held in the jaw.

We know the taste for salt is innately appealing to people. However, most people consume much more salt than they need, which means at least a portion of our salt cravings is habit. We can reprogram our taste buds by either cutting back or by trying one or more of the following suggestions to soothe that salt craving without the fat and calories:

- Substitute lemon juice for salt in cooking or in salads.
- Use Papa Dash Lite Lite Lite Low-Sodium seasoning or Salt-Sense to flavor foods.
- Snack on nonsalty crunchy foods, such as baby carrots, jicama strips, or celery.
- Drink a tall glass of ice water and wait fifteen minutes; the craving might subside.
- Experiment with other spices and flavors; you might be craving taste, not salt (see chapter 10 for additional ways to add flavor to your diet).

Cravings Finale

The Feeling Good Diet helps you appease and curb your cravings and balance those cravings with nutritional good sense. Within a few weeks of following the guidelines in chapter 12, you should note a drop in your cravings and improved feelings of well-being, energy, and general mental health. The longer you stick with this eating plan, the better you will feel.

Your first step is to develop a plan to curb your cravings or schedule them into your eating plan. That means keeping a journal, such as the one on page 89. Look for patterns and times of the day you are most prone to a craving for something sweet, creamy, chocolaty, or salty. Then devise solutions. (Use Worksheet 3.1, "Your Cravings Control Plan," on page 90, to chart your progress.) For example, if you feel overwhelmed whenever you pass by a doughnut shop or the bakery, you can:

- Avoid the situation by driving a different route to work.
- Plan a new response by selecting a low-fat alternative such as a bagel rather than the higher-fat doughnut.
- Eat beforehand to eliminate hunger and your vulnerability to the tempting food.

Cravings Control Record

Write down everything you eat and drink and how you felt before and after the meal or snack. At the end of two weeks, review your records to identify your craving-prone times of the day or situations, how you use food to improve your mood or energy level, and the types of foods you are most likely to crave. Then develop a plan to curb your cravings or schedule them into your eating plan. Use this sheet as a master copy.

DATE: _____

WHEN?	WHAT?	HOW MUCH?	WHERE?	THOUGHTS/FEELINGS BEFORE	THOUGHTS/FEELINGS AFTER

Worksheet 3.1   Your Cravings Control Plan

Use the following worksheet to plan and monitor your cravings control progress. Customize the form, using check marks, bar graphs, or written notes to best suit your needs. Keep in mind you want to take small steps toward long-range goals. Use this worksheet as a master copy.

Long-term goal for managing my fat tooth: _____

Short-term goal for this week is (include details, such as when, where, and how often): _____

_____

MONTH/DAY   **WHAT PROGRESS DID I MAKE TOWARD MY GOAL?**

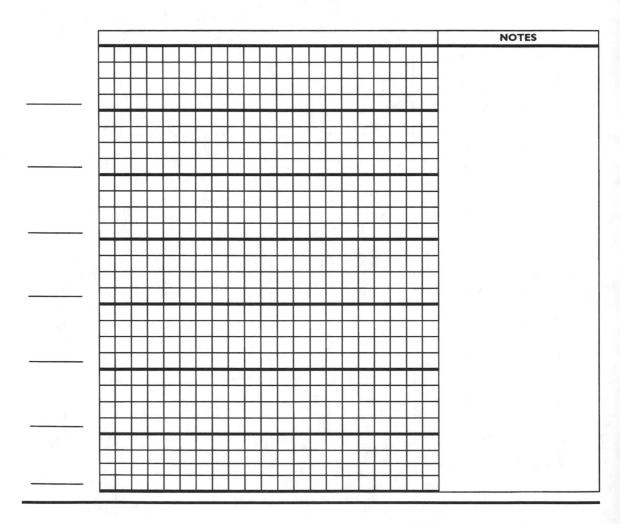

If your cravings come during your energy lull in the day, such as midmorning or midafternoon, you can:

- Bring a nutritious and pleasurable food with you to work so you are not at the mercy of office vending machines or the snack cart.
- Select nonfat foods that will give similar satisfaction to their high-fat counterparts: If you crave something sweet and creamy, try a creamy yogurt; fat-free cream cheese and jam on crackers; or a piece of Lemon Chiffon Pie.*

Late-night cravings for sweet-and-creamy or salty-and-greasy foods are most common when you skip meals or snack during the day, avoid eating breakfast, or eat too many sugary foods throughout the day. These cravings are a conditioned response; the more often you snack at night, the stronger your body's cravings will be in the future. Often, just two weeks of following the Feeling Good Diet is all it takes to put an end to late-night cravings. Of course there is nothing wrong with a small snack at night if it fits your eating plan and is chosen from nutrient-packed foods. You may even use this time for an indulgence, such as a small serving of ice cream.

In addition, try the following suggestions to curb any cravings you have for fatty foods:

- Do something else: If you feel a craving coming on, go outside for some fresh air, chat with a friend, take a walk, go for a bike ride, or hold a baby. . . . Do anything that removes you from the cues to eat and takes your mind off the food.
- Exercise. You get an even bigger endorphin boost from regular exercise than you do from chocolate and other sweet-and-creamy foods. The more you exercise, the greater your endorphin high will be and the longer it will last after the exercise session. This might explain why most people report a drop in cravings and either a decline or at least no increase in hunger when they exercise regularly. So, plan your exercise to match the time of day you are most prone to food cravings.

* See "Recipes for Feeling Your Best" at the back of this book.

- Focus on fiber: Fruits, vegetables, whole grains, and legumes are fiber-packed foods that are filling without being fattening. The soluble fibers found in these foods are especially effective in curbing erratic swings in blood-sugar levels, which ultimately helps reduce food cravings. Fiber-rich, unprocessed foods are usually low in fat, so you can eat larger quantities of them, chew more, and feel more satisfied. For example, a tablespoon of salad dressing or peanut butter has the same number of calories (100) as more than three cups of salad or air-popped popcorn. For meals and snacks, include at least two fruits and/or vegetables and at least one serving of whole-grain breads and cereals or legumes, such as kidney beans, chickpeas, or black beans.

- Drink water: A glass of water consumed fifteen minutes before a meal helps curb hunger and results in lower calorie intakes.

- Slowly reduce dietary fat: Granted, the study was on rats, not people, but researchers at Health Canada in Ontario found that it takes several weeks for the body to switch metabolic gears when converting from a high-fat to a low-fat diet. So, take your time when rebalancing brain chemistry and cutting back on fat. For example, if your body is accustomed to a large serving of something sweet and creamy late at night, reduce the serving size and slowly substitute more nutritious foods so that eventually you are either not eating after dinner or are choosing only nutrient-packed snacks.

- Think creamy, without the fat: Include stews and creamy soups, such as Curried Squash Soup,* in your weekly meal plan. Have a creamy fruit-and-yogurt smoothie for a snack (such as Pumpkin Pie Smoothie* or Zinger Smoothie*). Snack on custard-style low-fat yogurt. These soups, smoothies, and snacks provide the creamy feel of fat and are filling without being fattening. Thicken soups with pureed potato, winter squash, or cornstarch; thicken a smoothie with a banana.

- Choose fat-free alternatives to traditional staples: Choose fat-free sour cream, cream cheese, yogurt, cheese, luncheon meats, and whole wheat crackers (such as the Savory Cilantro Dip with Baked Tortilla Chips*). Use reduced-fat alternatives to other staples, such as peanut

* See "Recipes for Feeling Your Best" at the back of this book.

butter. Carefully read labels on fat-free desserts; they are likely to be just as calorie-dense as original versions since they compensate for the fat by adding more sugar. Try not to fall into the mental trap of eating more because the food is low in fat.

- Keep portions in perspective. A serving of a brownie or a cupcake is 1 to 2 ounces, about the size of a Ping-Pong ball. Two to four chocolate kisses or ten potato chips is a serving.

- Savor the taste: Since fat carries the aroma and many taste sensations in food, a craving for something sweet and creamy could be fueled by a desire for something tasty. If this is the case, adding other noncaloric spices such as cinnamon, vanilla, or nutmeg to nonfat yogurt, low-fat cereals, or angel food cake recipes can sometimes appease the fat tooth without adding unwanted calories. (See chapter 10 for more information on flavor and appetite.)

- Have your salad dressing on the side and dip your fork lightly into the dressing before packing the lettuce onto your fork. You'll get the same taste of dressing but will cut your fat intake to a fraction.

- Eat slowly: Put down your fork between bites, chew slowly, taste and enjoy each mouthful, stop to enjoy the company, and take your time when eating. While rapid eating is the hallmark of a food addict, eating slowly to let your body work with the endorphins maximizes the pleasurability of the meal while countering the endorphins' message to wolf down too much food.

- Throw it out: If you can't resist eating too much of a fatty food, don't buy or order it. If someone else brings it into the house, put it down the garbage disposal or toss it in the garbage can (under something so disgusting, you won't be tempted to dig it out).

- Make changes gradually: Don't fool yourself that you can abruptly replace a double cheeseburger and large fries with lentil soup and be pleased. Instead, reeducate your taste buds gently; order the cheeseburger, but bring raw vegetables from home. Next month replace the cheeseburger with a grilled chicken sandwich along with vegetables and orange juice. Or plan a small chocolate snack instead of finishing that entire half gallon of chocolate ice cream.

- Don't grocery shop when you're hungry: You'll be much more likely to give in to cravings when your appetite-control chemicals are raging. Eat first, then shop.

- Chew sugarless gum while cooking: You'll be less tempted to snack on fatty snack items or taste the cream sauce!
- Keep tempting foods out of sight: The sight of food can trigger a craving.
- Schedule a snack time. Plan a small amount of a tempting food into your menu so you won't feel deprived.
- Change your habits: Many cravings are merely habits that can be relearned. Find a different, healthier, or lower-fat food for your midafternoon snack. Eat it regularly, and within three weeks you might find you've reeducated your taste buds.
- View no food as forbidden: We are most likely to crave a food if we feel we shouldn't have it. You might find that the craving subsides when you no longer deprive yourself.

CHAPTER FOUR

No Energy? Could Be Your Diet

- Has your energy level taken a hike?
- Do you need a cup of coffee in the morning to jump-start your day, and another cup midmorning?
- Do you have trouble concentrating after lunch or do you often skip socializing in the evening because you're "too worn out"?
- Do you get faint on the stair climber or get a side-stitch when you jog?
- Do you blame your lack of "oomph" on your busy schedule or do you assume you were born this way?

Think again. Fatigue can be a result of a variety of problems, ranging from stress, a lack of sleep, or too much wine last night to serious conditions like heart disease, clinical depression, or anemia. However, the answer to waning energy could be as simple as your diet. Lagging energy levels create a catch-22, where you are too tired to eat well, which only prolongs and aggravates the fatigue. Want to break the cycle? Take Quiz 4.1, "Reading Your Vital Signs," on page 96, then read on.

If your vim and vigor are gone, the first place to check is your body's fuel tank. You wouldn't expect your car to run on bad gas, so why assume that the much more complicated body machine can keep going on anything but a quality fuel mix? "The biggest mistake people make is they eat too little early in the day, start craving sweets by midafternoon, and end up eating anything in sight," says Nancy Clark, M.S., R.D., author of *Nancy Clark's Sports Nutrition Guidebook: Eating to Fuel Your Active Lifestyle, Second Edition* (Human Kinetics, 1997).

Quiz 4.1   Reading Your Vital Signs

How do your energy boosters stack up to your energy busters? Rate how often you practice the following dietary habits, then total your score for a quick check of how your diet stacks up. Score as follows: 3—always; 2—often; 1—seldom; 0—never.

	SCORE
1. Do you eat four or more meals and snacks in a day?	_____
2. Do you eat breakfast?	_____
3. Do you limit sugar intake?	_____
4. Do you eat sugary foods alone?	_____
5. Do you limit caffeinated beverages to three 5-ounce servings or fewer each day?	_____
6. Do you consume at least 2,500 calories each day of fresh fruits and vegetables, whole grains, low-fat milk products, nuts, and protein-rich foods?	_____
7. Do you take iron supplements when your iron intake is marginal?	_____
8. Do you avoid severe calorie-restricted diets?	_____
9. Do you snack lightly or not at all in the evening?	_____
10. Do you avoid eating large meals?	_____
11. Do you drink at least six glasses of water each day?	_____
12. Do you avoid tobacco?	_____
13. Do you limit alcohol intake to five drinks or fewer each week?	_____
14. Do you get at least seven hours of restful sleep each night?	_____
15. Do you take time each day to relax?	_____
16. Do you exercise daily?	_____

Scoring:

More than 40: Your diet and lifestyle support high energy. If you still suffer chronic fatigue, consult your physician and ask for a serum ferritin test to assess iron status.

30 to 39: Your diet and lifestyle might be contributing to fatigue. Select two changes from the preceding list that you will make to energize your diet.

Less than 30: Your diet and lifestyle are major contributors to waning energy levels. Select four or more changes, based on the above list, to get yourself back on track. After you have successfully implemented the dietary and/or lifestyle changes, expect to wait at least three weeks before your energy level improves.

Any eating habit that interferes with a steady supply of carbohydrates to the body—from erratic eating to skipping meals—will undermine your energy level. Blood-sugar levels begin to drop within four hours of eating, so frequent small meals and snacks rather than two or three big meals are best for maintaining a constant energy supply and avoiding fatigue. Complex carbohydrates in whole grains and starchy vegetables—from breads, rice, and pasta to lima beans and yams—are the fuel of choice, since these fuels are digested gradually, maintain an even blood-sugar level, and provide a constant fuel supply for the body and the brain.

Quick-weight-loss diets cause fatigue. "Cutting calories early in the day to lose weight is likely to leave most people in an energy drain that interferes with the daily routine, exercise, or even enjoying life," says Ms. Clark. For example, a 120-pound woman needs between 1,800 and 2,200 calories daily (men and larger or more active women need even more), but the average intake for young women in the United States is 1,667 calories (women after age 55 average only 1,360 calories a day). That means many people force their bodies to function on fumes. While excess body weight contributes to fatigue, drastically cutting calories to maintain a desirable weight also undermines energy. A better approach to eating is to diet less and exercise more, which burns calories, helps boost energy levels, and decreases fatigue-related moods such as depression and despondency. How do you maintain a desirable weight and stay energized? Eat regularly, cook light, and mix a little protein with fiber-rich carbohydrates.

Your Mother Was Right

One out of four people start every day without breakfast; 50 percent eat breakfast only occasionally. That's far fewer breakfast eaters today than thirty years ago. Of course, life was more relaxed then; more moms were home to cook leisurely breakfasts, and fewer people dieted. Today, cutting calories to lose weight is one of the main reasons people skip the first meal of the day, along with not having enough time for a meal and not feeling like eating. But the modern-day breakfast-skipping habit is likely to backfire.

Breakfast is the most important meal. This is the only time during the day that eight, and perhaps ten or more, hours have gone by between meals. "By sunrise, the body is essentially fasting and that first meal of the day literally breaks the fast," says Gretchen Hill, Ph.D., associate professor in the department of animal science at Michigan State University. During the hours since dinner, and even while sleeping, the body still needs fuel to keep its millions of metabolic processes functioning. Much of that fuel comes from readily available stores of glucose; more than half of your glucose reserves are drained by morning and need a jump-start that only comes from eating a carbohydrate-rich meal. Allow even four hours to pass between meals, and blood-sugar levels drop, resulting in fatigue, poor concentration, irritability, and lethargy. Double that time, and you can imagine the energy-draining effects of failing to stop and refuel!

Skip breakfast and you still might feel fine, full of energy, and raring to go for the first few hours after you wake up. That counterfeit burst of energy comes from a mind and body revved from a good night's sleep. This initial energy glow wears off as the morning's demands stress a body already running on fumes. "While breakfast increases the metabolic rate by 25 percent, which is one of the reasons why people report they feel better after eating in the morning, skipping breakfast slows the metabolic rate and leaves a person feeling tired, sluggish, even cold," says C. Wayne Callaway, M.D., associate clinical professor of medicine at George Washington University. By afternoon, even if you eat a relatively good lunch in an effort to boost lagging energy levels, you never will regain the daylong energy you would have had if you'd taken five minutes to eat breakfast. In fact, don't think you can find a quick-fix snack to end midday doldrums after skipping breakfast; the best you can hope for energy-wise is to quit for the day and start over tomorrow by eating breakfast. Use the Food & Mood Journal in chapter 12 to monitor how you feel when you skip breakfast and when you eat breakfast. Don't forget to record coffee! Look for subtle differences in how your breakfast habits affect your energy and mood, such as drinking more coffee midafternoon or going to bed earlier on those days when you didn't eat breakfast.

Breakfast—A Basic Instinct

At an even deeper level, skipping breakfast undermines your basic instincts. While investigating the effects of brain chemicals on appetite, Sarah Leibowitz, Ph.D., professor of psychology at Rockefeller University, found that levels of neuropeptide Y (NPY) were highest in the morning and jump-started the day's eating cycle by dictating a preference for carbohydrates. This theory is true in animals, who eat more carbohydrates when NPY levels are high or when NPY is injected into their brains.

NPY is a nerve chemical that ensures we replenish the fuel stores depleted since dinner, so it's no wonder breakfast foods are typically high-carbohydrate ones, such as waffles, toast, pancakes, oatmeal, cereal, and fruit. NPY is a very powerful nerve chemical. However, it doesn't go away just because you skip breakfast. Instead, NPY levels remain on until the cravings lead to overeating later in the day.

Stress adds to the problem, since it amplifies NPY levels. Skip breakfast, then venture into a day filled with time demands, deadlines at work, overbooked schedules, even boredom, and raging NPY levels are boosted even higher by the stress hormones norepinephrine (a cousin to adrenalin) and corticosterone, both secreted from the adrenal glands. The result is, a day without breakfast can lead to an even greater likelihood of increased food cravings, overeating, and weight gain (see "Two Dozen Quick, Easy, and Energizing Breakfasts," on pages 100–101).

Breakfast Rules

If you are a seasoned breakfast avoider, start eating breakfast, even if you're not hungry. "It takes two to three weeks to reset the appetite clock," says Dr. Callaway. After that you should notice a gain in energy and mental power—if you're choosing the correct foods.

Avoid high-sugar breakfasts, such as doughnuts and coffee, that provide an initial energy boost but leave you drowsy within a few hours. The best energy-boosting breakfasts are ones that are light, low-fat, healthful, and that mix a little protein, such as yogurt or peanut butter, with even more carbohydrates, such as cereal, toast, or low-fat waffles. Why the mix of protein and carbs? Researchers at the Institute of Food Research in Reading, the United Kingdom, report that eating breakfast helps you feel more upbeat if that breakfast is mostly grains and fruit. In their study, sixteen people answered questionnaires about their moods and took tests measuring their memories before and after eating either low-fat, high-carbohydrate or high-fat, low-carbohydrate breakfasts. Those people who ate the low-fat, high carbohydrate breakfasts reported feeling more cheerful and more energetic for at least two and a half hours. In contrast, high-fat or big breakfasts slow you down and muddle thinking.

Box 4.1   Two Dozen Quick, Easy, and Energizing Breakfasts

Along with these quick-fix suggestions, try setting the breakfast table the night before, portioning out foods at night to save time in the morning, or fixing a brown bag breakfast to take with you in the morning.

1. Yogurt-blueberry-cereal sundae: Layer nonfat vanilla or lemon yogurt, fresh blueberries (or any fresh berry), and low-fat granola in a parfait glass. Serve with orange juice.
2. Fruit smoothie: In a blender, combine one 6-ounce carton nonfat plain yogurt, 3 tablespoons orange juice concentrate, $1/2$ can apricots canned in light syrup, 1 banana, and 2 tablespoons toasted wheat germ (optional). Blend until smooth.
3. Pancake roll-ups: Make pancakes using low-fat pancake mix, nonfat milk, and 2 tablespoons wheat germ. Place sliced bananas along the middle of each pancake and roll into a "burrito." Top with apricot sauce or jam and a dollop of fat-free whipped cream. Serve with nonfat milk or orange juice.
4. A $1/2$ cantaloupe filled with nonfat lemon yogurt and sprinkled with granola.
5. A bowl of your favorite cereal topped with sliced bananas and nonfat or 1 percent low-fat milk. Serve with 100 percent fruit juice.
6. $1/2$ cup egg substitute scrambled with sliced red bell pepper, onion, and 1 ounce cheddar cheese. Serve with whole wheat toast and fruit juice.
7. Instant oatmeal cooked in nonfat or 1 percent low-fat milk and topped with wheat germ, dried fruit, brown sugar, and extra milk if desired. Serve with fresh fruit or juice.
8. Breakfast burrito: Fill a heated flour tortilla with chopped and lightly sautéed green bell pepper, onion, and pimiento; scrambled egg substitute; and grated cheese. Top with salsa and serve with nonfat milk or fruit juice.
9. Top fat-free cottage cheese with sliced kiwi, fresh strawberries, fresh blueberries, and other fruit. Drizzle with honey and serve with fruit juice or a slice of whole wheat toast.
10. Cinnamon-raisin bread dunked in low-fat cinnamon-apple yogurt. Serve with a large glass of 100 percent fruit juice.
11. French toast made with nonfat or 1 percent low-fat milk and topped with fat-free cottage cheese and pineapple. Serve with fruit juice.
12. Veggie melt: Steam broccoli and cauliflower pieces, sliced mushrooms and carrots, and stuff into a whole wheat pita with melted smoked, low-fat mozzarella and honey dijon mustard. Serve with grapefruit juice.
13. Prepare hot cereal the night before: Place dry cereal (quick-cooking oats, Wheatena, multigrain cereals, etc.) in a preheated, wide-mouth thermos. Add steaming milk and

close tightly. The cereal will be ready and warm by morning. Serve with fresh fruit and orange juice.

14. Breakfast sandwich: Toast whole wheat, pumpernickel, or rye bread and top with a slice of Muenster or farmer cheese mixed with dried fruit. Serve with fresh fruit or juice.

15. Eat-on-the-run breakfast: A muffin (preferably whole wheat, oat, carrot, or bran), a minibox of raisins, and a box of orange juice or 6 ounces of low-fat yogurt.

16. Leftover breakfast: Have a little something from the night before, such as a slice of pizza, a reheated baked potato filled with vegetables and cheese, a piece of chicken with toast and some fruit, or a bowl of tomato soup with crackers.

17. Breakfast crepes. Heat a store-bought crepe and fill with fat-free ricotta cheese and fresh fruit. Serve with fruit juice.

18. Peanut butter candy: Mix equal parts peanut butter, toasted wheat germ, and honey. Spread it on a slice of whole wheat bread. Serve with nonfat milk and fruit.

19. Fast-food breakfast: McDonald's Apple Bran Muffin, two pieces of fruit (brought from home), and a carton of low-fat milk.

20. Trail-mix breakfast: Mix your favorite ready-to-eat cereal with almonds, dried fruit, pumpkin seeds, and/or sunflower seeds (in a ratio of two parts cereal to one part everything else). Serve with fruit, nonfat milk, or juice.

21. Pocket breakfast: Scramble 1/2 cup egg substitute with 1/2 cup fresh, chopped spinach; 1 tablespoon grated cheddar cheese; and salt and pepper to taste. Fill a whole wheat pita bread with egg mixture. Serve with orange juice.

22. Peel and slice one kiwi and mix it into low-fat strawberry-kiwi yogurt. Serve with a slice of whole wheat toast and a glass of orange juice.

23. Fill 1/2 papaya with low-fat lemon yogurt and sprinkle with nutmeg. Serve with graham crackers and a glass of orange juice.

24. The gourmet coffee shop special: At your local gourmet coffee shop, order a bran muffin, a bottle of orange juice, and a Grande Coffee Latte made with 1 cup skim milk and sweetened with NutraSweet (optional).

Combining a little protein with the carbohydrates at breakfast helps keep you full and energized throughout the morning hours. However, according to researchers at the Massachusetts Institute of Technology (MIT), too much protein at breakfast also leads to fatigue and sleepiness that can linger into the evening hours. These findings were verified in another study from The Wageningen Agricultural University in The Netherlands, where researchers found that planning breakfast around carbohydrates with small amounts of protein reduced hunger throughout the morning, while high-fat, protein-laden breakfasts, such as eggs and

---

Box 4.2   How to Choose a Breakfast Cereal

Ready-to-eat cereal is one of the best fast foods around. It takes less than five minutes to prepare and, if chosen well, is one of the most nutritious breakfasts you can eat. When researchers at Michigan State University surveyed eleven thousand men and women about their breakfast habits, the ones who ate cereal consumed more vitamins, minerals, and fiber and less fat than those who ate nothing or ate higher-fat breakfasts. Why? Cereal is a great source of carbohydrates and usually is low in fat. More importantly, people who feast on bowls of flakes in the morning also pour milk on top and are more likely to include fruit with the meal than people who order sausage and eggs at a restaurant. But, there are more than two hundred cereals on market shelves, and not all of those are worthwhile choices. Look for a cereal that supplies:

- 3+ grams of protein.
- 3+ grams of fiber.
- Less than 200 calories.
- No more than 2 grams of fat.
- Less than 4 grams of sugar.

It is difficult to identify the amount of sugar in a packaged food, since labels seldom separate carbohydrates into sugar and starch. Instead, check the ingredients list to get an idea of the sugar content; choose only those cereals that do not list sugar in the first three ingredients. Be careful: Sugar comes disguised as many names, including corn syrup, high-fructose corn syrup, dextrose, honey, and brown sugar. Many cereals meet the preceding criteria, including: Shredded Wheat, Grape-Nuts, Nutri-Grain Flakes, Nutri-Grain Nuggets, Cheerios, Wheaties, Fiber One, and Wheat and Raisin Chex.

---

bacon, led to overeating at lunchtime (see "How to Choose a Breakfast Cereal," above).

Healthful, light breakfasts are easy to prepare. It shouldn't take more than five minutes to fix everything you need to fuel yourself through the morning hours. Just follow the three basic guidelines in "Breakfast Rules," on page 103. Breakfast also can be as individual as the person eating it. It needn't be fancy or traditional. A slice of vegetable pizza with a large glass of orange juice will boost energy just as well as a bowl of cereal. Just make sure to limit sugar and fat and focus more on carbohydrates from fiber-rich, whole-grain sources.

Box 4.3   Breakfast Rules

Three simple guidelines are all you need for an energy-boosting breakfast:

1. Include two servings of fruits (or vegetables) from the following list:

- 6 ounces 100 percent fruit or vegetable juice (avoid all juices made with "pure grape" or "pure apple juice concentrate," since these "all-natural" fruit beverages are actually primarily sugar water. Instead, choose 100 percent orange juice, grapefruit juice, orange-pineapple juice, tomato juice, or fresh squeeze your own juices if you have time.)
- a piece of fruit, such as a plum, pear, apple, banana, orange, tangerine, grapefruit, kiwi, cantaloupe or other melon ($^{1}/_{2}$), papaya ($^{1}/_{2}$), or peach
- $^{1}/_{2}$ cup fruit canned in its own juice
- dried fruit, 2 tablespoons or more

2. Select one to three servings of a high-carbohydrate, high-fiber food from the following list:

- one slice whole wheat bread, $^{1}/_{2}$ whole wheat bagel or English muffin, one whole wheat flour tortilla, or one low-fat whole wheat scone
- one low-fat muffin, preferably whole wheat, bran, carrot, or fruit-filled
- one slice of corn bread
- 1 to 2 ounces of ready-to-eat cereal
- $^{1}/_{2}$ cup cooked whole-grain hot cereal, such as oatmeal, multigrain cereal, or wheat germ

3. Select 1 serving of a protein-rich food from the following list:

- fat-free or low-fat milk or yogurt (1 cup), cottage cheese (2 cups), cheese (1 ounce), or ricotta cheese (2 ounces)
- one thin slice of meat, such as turkey, chicken, or beef (1 to 3 ounces)
- cooked dried beans and peas, such as peanut or almond butter (2 tablespoons) or tofu (3 to 4 ounces)
- $^{1}/_{4}$ to $^{1}/_{2}$ cup egg substitute, 1 whole egg, or 2 egg whites

Wake Up and Smell the Coffee

Coffee's welcoming aroma and promise of instant energy have made it the number one mind-altering drug and the second most popular beverage in this country, just behind soft drinks. Americans consume half of the world's coffee, or more than one thousand cups per person per year.

Caffeine is what makes coffee the morning cup of ambition. Caffeine blocks a nerve chemical called adenosine that otherwise blocks other energy-boosting brain chemicals. Thus, caffeine helps the alertness chemicals do their job. Virtually all of the caffeine in coffee is absorbed and is quickly distributed to all parts of the body. Within half an hour, caffeine's stimulating effects can be felt, leaving you less tired, more alert, better able to concentrate, and faster to react. You type faster and with more accuracy, drive better in rush-hour traffic, and show improved short-term memory. A person feels better after a cup of coffee, and this improved mood adds to the likelihood of going back for more.

It's this "more" that is a double-edged sword. The initial high from caffeine is followed by mild withdrawal symptoms, one of which is fatigue. A vicious cycle can result as you drink more coffee to prevent the inevitable letdown. The fatigue, an irritable or depressed mood, and reduced work performance associated with caffeine withdrawal can begin within hours of the last cup and can last up to a week or more. People's tolerance to caffeine varies widely. Withdrawal symptoms are reported in some people even with small amounts of daily caffeine, such as one to two cups, while other people can tolerate higher doses with no problems.

Caffeine also lingers in the body for hours. As a consequence, coffee drinkers take longer to fall asleep, sleep less soundly, wake up more often, and greet the morning groggier than nonusers. A restless night is likely to leave you dragging the next day. Substituting a cup of tea or a cola for an evening cup of coffee will not avoid insomnia, since both the tea and the cola contain the same amount of caffeine as a cup of instant coffee. Instead, try herbal tea. Finally, coffee acts as a diuretic, contributing to dehydration, which causes fatigue. The irony is that people report having more energy within weeks of giving up caffeine.

Coffee Basics

There is no need to give up coffee; just cut back. One to three 5-ounce cups, or the equivalent of 300 milligrams of caffeine or less, in the morning or early afternoon appears to be safe and, except for the most sensitive people, should not contribute to fatigue.

You should pay close attention to your serving size and the caffeine content of the beverage you choose. Scientific studies use the 5-ounce cup, while a typical mug could contain twice that amount. Caffeine intake also should be compared to body weight; short or young people should scale down their caffeine intake to two servings or less. For example, one 12-ounce cola to a 30-pound child is equivalent to five cups of instant coffee to a 150-pound adult. Read the labels of our favorite beverages: Even some bottled waters advertised as quick-pick-me-ups contain hefty amounts of caffeine.

People struggling with fatigue who drink a lot of coffee should gradually reduce their intake by one or two cups a day, with a goal of limiting coffee to no more than three daily cups. You are most likely to feel tired or experience other symptoms of coffee withdrawal, such as headaches, if coffee intake is reduced too quickly. Or, try switching to instant or an instant blended with chicory or grain. These coffees contain half the caffeine of regular brews. You also might try blending regular with decaffeinated coffee before brewing, or have your local coffee shop prepare a blend of regular and decaffeinated. Grain-based beverages such as Pero, Postum, and Cafix are coffee substitutes that contain no caffeine and have only 7 to 12 calories per serving. You also can satisfy your taste for coffee by blending fat-free vanilla or chocolate frozen yogurt with decaffeinated espresso. These are robust alternatives to the second or third cup of coffee. (See Table 4.1, "The Caffeine Scoreboard," on page 106).

How you blend your coffee can affect its content. Most coffee in the United States is not boiled and is brewed using filters. However, a coffee pot variously called the *cafetière*, the French press, or the plunger pot makes what is essentially boiled, unfiltered coffee. This type of brew is rich in two oil compounds called cafestrol and kahweol, which researchers suspect elevate heart-disease risk.

Brewed Dessert

Americans spend $1.9 billion on specialty coffee blends and flavored beans each year, and that figure is expected to soar to $3 billion by the turn of the century. A robust brew is one of the few pleasures that remains calorie-free, as long as it's ordered black. Add whipped cream, whole milk, chocolate syrups, and other goodies and you chalk up more fat and calories than some desserts. For example, top any gourmet coffee drink with whipped cream and you've added 110 calories of fat. If

Table 4.1   The Caffeine Scoreboard

ITEM	CAFFEINE (MILLIGRAMS)
COFFEE (5-ounce cup)*	
Brewed, drip method	60–180
Instant	30–120
Decaffeinated	1–5
CAFE LATTE, CAFE MOCHA,	51–57
CAPPUCCINO (8 ounces)	
(16 ounces)	102–130
ESPRESSO (2.7 ounces)	51–130
TEA (5-ounce cup)*	
Brewed	20–110
Instant	25–50
Iced (12-ounce glass)	67–76
COCOA BEVERAGE (5-ounce cup)	2–20
CHOCOLATE MILK (8 ounces)	2–7
DARK CHOCOLATE, SEMI-SWEET (1 ounce)	5–35
SOFT DRINKS—COLAS (12-ounce serving)	
Sugar-Free Mr. Pibb	59
Mountain Dew	54
Tab, Coca-Cola/Diet Cola	46–47
Dr Pepper, Colas, Diet Colas	36–40
Canada Dry Diet Cola	1
NONPRESCRIPTION DRUGS	
Dexatrim/Dex-a-Diet II/Dietac, Vivarin	200
Prolamine	140
Aqua-Ban diuretic, No-Doz, Appedrine	100
Excedrin	65
Anacin, Midol, Vanquish, Dristan	30–33
PRESCRIPTION DRUGS	
Cafergot (migraine headaches)	100
Norgesic Forte (muscle relaxant)	60
Fiorinal (tension headache)	40
Pain medications, such as Darvon	30–32

* Caffeine content will vary depending on the strength of the brew.

consumed daily over and above your needed calories, that's just enough to produce a 1-pound weight gain each month.

Take that large cappuccino or latte made with a shot of espresso and 2 percent milk; they pack in 150 to 200 calories and 1 to 2 teaspoons of fat. If your gourmet coffee drink is made with whole milk, the calories can jump to 250, with up to 3 teaspoons of fat. Top your latte with whipped cream and grated milk chocolate and you're sipping more calories and fat than is in a half cup of butter pecan ice cream (or about 350 calories and 20 grams of fat). A café mocha made with whole milk contains up to 400 calories and almost 7 teaspoons of fat—that beats out chocolate fudge cake by 150 calories! Add a dollop of whipped cream and the calories jump to more than 500; now you've used up 60 percent of your daily allotment for fat, or more than 40 grams.

What about those gourmet cold coffee drinks? These drinks are usually a combination of coffee, sweetened milk, ice, and syrups. They range in calories from 120 calories to 315, depending on the quantity of chocolate and flavored syrups, the type of milk, and how big they are. For example, an iced grande mocha has 190 calories and 3 grams of fat if it's made with nonfat milk, but more than 260 calories if it's made with whole milk. Add another 110 calories if there is whipped cream on top. Even at 200 calories, that's the calorie equivalent of a fudge brownie, a piece of devil's food cake, or four oatmeal raisin cookies.

You can have your latte and drink it, too—just make a few simple changes in the ingredients.

- At the coffeehouse, request that your coffee drink be made with skim, not whole or even 2 percent, milk. (It's called a "skinny.") That cuts the calories in half and sidesteps the fat in any coffee beverage.
- Cut out the 2 teaspoons of sugar and use a sugar substitute and you've saved another 40 calories.
- Top your mochas with cinnamon and cocoa powder sprinkled lightly for low-fat flavor, and "just say no" to the whipped cream and chocolate shavings.
- Order an espresso with a twist of lemon for a no-calorie jolt.
- Home brews fare better when it comes to fat and calories. A cup of cappuccino made from powder averages only 75 calories and 2 grams of fat.
- View gourmet coffees as your dessert for the day and have the whipped cream and chocolate shavings, then "just say no" to the ice cream that night.

Sugarcoated Sleeping Pill

Do you grab a candy bar when you feel tired, or soothe your weary mind with a doughnut? These quick fixes are temporary highs that could be fueling your fatigue. A sugary snack can send some people on a blood-sugar roller coaster. Researchers at Kansas State University measured mood in 120 college women who drank 12 ounces of water or beverages sweetened with either aspartame or sugar. Within thirty minutes, the women who drank the sugar-sweetened beverage were the drowsiest. Some people are so sensitive to sugar or caffeine that they feel tired, irritable, or depressed within an hour of eating even two cookies or drinking one cup of coffee. Others can tolerate larger sugar doses before symptoms develop.

According to Larry Christensen, Ph.D., chairman of the department of psychology at the University of South Alabama, 50 percent of the people suffering from depression in his studies report improvements in energy levels within a week of eliminating sugar and caffeine. "At first, we noted a link between depression and caffeine or sugar. However, we redirected our focus when we realized that mood changes were mediated by an energy component; people who stopped using sugar and caffeine first felt more energetic and then their mood improved." Christensen adds that most people on antidepressant medications don't benefit from the dietary change.

Sugar is a good source of carbohydrates—the energy fuel—so why do sweets bring you down? Unlike starch, which slowly releases carbohydrate units called glucose into the blood, sugar rapidly enters the bloodstream, causing a dramatic rise in blood sugar. To counteract this rise, the pancreas quickly releases the hormone insulin, which shuttles excess sugar from the blood into the cells. Consequently, blood sugar drops, often to levels lower than before the snack.

Sugar also increases tryptophan levels in the brain and triggers the release of the brain chemical serotonin, which in turn slows you down. Harris R. Lieberman, Ph.D., research scientist, and Bonnie Spring, Ph.D., professor of psychology at Massachusetts Institute of Technology, report that people feel sleepier and have "less vigor" for up to three and a half hours after eating highly refined carbohydrate snacks as compared to snacks that contain more whole grains or a little protein.

Finally, people who frequently snack on sweets are likely to consume inadequate amounts of the energizing nutrients. Researchers at the Division of Human Nutrition in Adulate, Australia, report that the more sugar people consume, the higher their calorie intakes and the lower their intakes of vitamins and minerals—in particular vitamin C, beta carotene, the B vitamins, magnesium, potassium, and zinc.

Using sugar as a quick fix for dwindling energy results in a temporary high. In the long run, it could create a vicious cycle. "The person suffering from chronic tiredness and depression who turns to sugary foods may relieve the fatigue and feel better for a short while, but the depression and fatigue return," says Dr. Christensen. The person then must either reach for another sugar fix or seek help elsewhere. As opposed to the temporary sugar high, eliminating sugar and caffeine from the diet is a permanent solution. "Ninety percent of our patients went cold turkey [eliminated all sugar and caffeine from the diet]. They felt worse at first, but an overwhelming number of them felt better and had more energy within a week," says Dr. Christensen.

In short, snack defensively, rather than feed your fatigue. Choose nutrient-packed time-released carbohydrates, such as whole-grain bread sticks, fresh fruit, and crunchy vegetables, low-fat granola, a soft pretzel, or a fruit-filled crepe (prepackaged crepes are in the produce section) for between-meal snacks. Include at least two food groups at each snack and make at least one fresh fruit, vegetable, or grain. (See Table 4.2, "Snack Right," on pages 110–111, for healthful snack ideas.) Your best bet is to combine fruit with another nutrient-packed food, such as low-fat yogurt, whole grain crackers, or cereal, that delivers a steady stream of carbohydrates and maintains a constant blood-sugar level.

Is Hypoglycemia to Blame?

Every condition, from fatigue to personality disorders, has been blamed on hypoglycemia, or low blood sugar. Hypoglycemia is not a disease but a symptom of abnormal blood-sugar regulation. It is common in those suffering from diabetes and is typically characterized by blood-sugar levels below 50 milligrams/100 dl of blood. Documented symptoms of hypoglycemia include pallor, fatigue, irritability, inability to concentrate, headaches, palpitations, perspiration, anxiety, hunger, and shakiness or internal trembling. However, many more people believe they have hypoglycemia than actually test positive when given blood-sugar tests.

Dr. Callaway suspects that people can experience pharmacological effects from sugar, even if blood-sugar levels remain within the normal range. People's responses to fluctuating blood-sugar levels vary greatly. Some people experience symptoms when blood-sugar levels are well within the normal range, while others report no

Table 4.2   Snack Right

Energizing snacks include the following:

- One mango, peeled and sliced, and topped with fresh lime juice. Serve with nonfat milk.
- One pita pocket sandwich made with one whole wheat pita pocket bread filled with 1 ounce of grated jalapeño cheese, one diced fresh tomato, 3 tablespoons grated zucchini, and $1/2$ cup drained, canned kidney beans.
- 1 cup frozen seedless grapes or blueberries. Serve with 1 cup 1 percent low-fat milk, heated and flavored with almond extract.
- One whole-grain muffin with raisins and nuts, topped with 1 tablespoon cashew butter. Serve with 1 cup fresh pineapple chunks.
- A serving of Zucchini Torte.* Serve with one sliced tomato.
- Fruit fondue: 2 cups fresh fruit (such as strawberries, bananas, oranges, and/or kiwi) cut into large chunks and dipped into $1/4$ cup fat-free chocolate syrup. Serve with nonfat milk.
- Large prawns, steamed and dipped in tomato-based cocktail sauce. Serve with fat-free crackers and grapefruit juice.
- Cooked large white beans (fava) marinated in lemon juice, garlic, fresh sage, and wine. Serve with French bread.
- One soft pretzel, served with 6 ounces low-fat strawberry-kiwi yogurt with one peeled and chopped kiwi fruit.
- One slice cheese pizza, piled high with grilled vegetables, such as green or red bell pepper, red onions, mushrooms, eggplant, and zucchini. Serve with fruit juice.
- Three fig bars and 1 cup warmed nonfat milk flavored with almond extract and sprinkled with nutmeg.
- $1/2$ cantaloupe filled with 6 ounces low-fat lemon yogurt and topped with 1 tablespoon lemon zest.
- Two slices extra-lean ham lunch meat, 12 fat-free whole wheat crackers, and 1 cup fresh-squeezed orange juice.
- Fruit parfait: In a parfait glass, mix the following with 1 tablespoon orange juice concentrate, layer, and top with 1 tablespoon light whipped cream: one orange, peeled and sectioned; $1/2$ cup fresh strawberries; $1/2$ banana sliced.
- Candied-ginger fruit salad: In a bowl, mix one peeled and sectioned orange, $1/2$ peeled and sliced banana, $1/2$ peeled and diced mango or papaya, and one sliced plum. Toss fruit with

* See "Recipes for Feeling Your Best" at the back of this book.

1 tablespoon orange juice concentrate, 1 teaspoon lemon peel, and 1 tablespoon crumbled candied ginger. Place in parfait glass and serve with one ladyfinger cookie.

- Garlicky eggplant and tomato spread with pita bread: Bake whole eggplant at 400 degrees for one hour. Scoop out insides of eggplant and mix with 3 tablespoons minced sun-dried tomatoes, two minced garlic cloves, 1 teaspoon lemon juice, 1 teaspoon olive oil, and salt and pepper to taste. (A pinch of red pepper flakes give this dip a little zing!) Refrigerate overnight. Dunk one whole wheat pita bread broken into wedges into 1/2 cup of this dip.
- Pita spread: 1/2 whole wheat pita bread filled with 1 ounce feta cheese, 1 tablespoon chopped olives, 1/4 cup chopped cucumber, and 2 tablespoons chopped tomato. Serve with 1 cup orange pekoe tea.
- 1 cup nonfat plain yogurt mixed with 2 tablespoons chopped dates and 1 tablespoon chopped almonds. Serve with fresh fruit.
- One baked apple, stuffed with 2 tablespoons chopped walnuts, 1/2 teaspoon ground cinnamon, and 2 teaspoons honey. Serve with steamed 1 percent low-fat milk flavored with almond extract.
- Late-night sweet treat: Mix one sliced banana, three apricot halves (canned in juice and drained), and 2 teaspoons honey. Serve with nonfat milk.
- Revitalize smoothie: In a blender, 1 cup nonfat milk, 2 tablespoons orange juice concentrate, 2 tablespoons wheat germ, one banana, four apricot halves (canned in juice and drained), and ice cube (optional). Whip until thoroughly blended.
- Tropical fruit salad: one sliced papaya, 1 cup pineapple chunks, 3 tablespoons mandarin orange slices (canned and drained), 1/3 cup sliced avocado, 1 tablespoon orange zest, and 2 tablespoons low-fat bottled lime salad dressing. Serve with 1/2 cup nonfat cottage cheese.
- One Thai Wrap.*
- Veggie sandwich: Romaine, red cabbage, radicchio, cucumber, plum tomato slices, and grated carrots with hummus tahini dressing stuffed into a whole wheat pocket bread.
- Grilled chicken breast slices, sun-dried tomatoes, shredded romaine lettuce, and pesto sauce in a whole wheat pocket bread.
- Grilled eggplant sandwich: Marinate eggplant slices in balsamic vinegar, then grill. Serve on whole wheat bun with smoked low-fat mozzarella cheese, roasted red peppers, and Dijon-style mustard.
- California burrito: Fill a 10-inch flour tortilla with roasted zucchini, green onions, fresh tomatoes, brown rice, grilled red peppers, and fat-free ricotta cheese.

* See "Recipes for Feeling Your Best" at the back of this book.

symptoms even when blood-sugar levels have dropped substantially. It is likely that each person has a unique blood-sugar range, with fatigue or mood changes occurring when levels fluctuate above or below these levels. The best dietary advice for sugar-sensitive people is to:

- Consume several small meals throughout the day, rather than the feast-and-famine scenario of a few large meals.
- Consume fiber-rich carbohydrates with protein at each meal and snack. The soluble fibers found in oranges, apples, legumes, and oats are particularly effective in slowing the absorption of sugar. They allow a slow, steady release of sugar into the blood and help avoid the rapid rise in blood sugar associated with sugary or highly refined snacks.

Bypassing the Midday Doldrums

Even if you eat a nutritious breakfast and snack right during the morning, your energy could diminish as the day progresses if you don't stop to refuel. In short, what and how much you eat for lunch could determine how you feel midafternoon. Here are the two rules to follow:

- *Keep lunch light.* A low-fat midday meal that contains approximately 500 calories maintains afternoon alertness and boosts energy levels, while fasting or overindulging in high-fat, high-calorie lunches of 1,000 calories or more can leave you yawning and unable to concentrate. A fatty meal also increases blood tryptophan levels (and, therefore, brain serotonin levels), thus lowering your fatigue threshold.
- *Mix protein with carbohydrates.* Carbohydrate-rich foods—from bread to dessert—elevate serotonin levels and make you drowsy in the afternoon and evening. In contrast, protein-rich foods increase brain levels of the amino acid tyrosine, a primary building block for the energizing chemicals dopamine and norepinephrine; consequently, people feel more alert, vigilant, and better able to concentrate. Women are more susceptible than men to this carbohydrate-induced drowsiness. But anyone is likely to be less alert and to make more

mistakes after a carbohydrate-rich lunch, such as pasta, as compared to a protein-packed turkey sandwich.

Plan your carbohydrates so they work with your energy level, not against it. For example, you may feel relaxed after a carbohydrate-rich dinner of spaghetti, but the same meal at lunch could make you sluggish. Light lunches, such as a tuna sandwich, fruit, and low-fat milk, or a salad, French bread, and yogurt are most likely to keep you going throughout the afternoon. Other "brain-power" foods include a small amount of fish, veal, skinless chicken, or legumes, combined with grains and vegetables.

As discussed in chapter 2, carbohydrate cravers are an exception to the rule. According to researchers at the Massachusetts Institute of Technology (MIT) in Cambridge, people who crave sweet or starchy foods in the afternoon might have extra-low levels of serotonin. While other people feel drowsy, carbohydrate cravers are energized and more alert after they eat carbohydrates, especially if they are complex carbohydrates, such as cereals, breads, pasta, or starchy vegetables.

Ironing Out Fatigue

Iron deficiency is epidemic and could be the leading cause of fatigue in women. While as few as 5 percent of women are anemic, as many as 80 percent of exercising women and 39 percent of premenopausal women in general are iron deficient. Iron deficiency usually goes unnoticed, since routine blood tests for iron status, such as the hemoglobin and hematocrit tests, reflect only a person's risk for anemia, the final stage of iron deficiency. Long before the onset of anemia, the tissue stores of iron have slowly drained, leaving a person feeling tired and irritable. Concentration and exercise ability is "not up to par," work performance suffers, and the immune system is affected, placing a person at higher risk for developing and fighting colds and infections.

The Truth Behind Iron-Poor Blood

Iron is a component of hemoglobin in red blood cells and myoglobin within the muscles and other tissues. These iron-dependent molecules are responsible for transporting oxygen from the lungs to all of the cells and within the cells. When dietary intake of iron is inadequate or when iron absorption is poor, iron in the tissues is released to make up deficits in the blood. The cells slowly suffocate from lack of oxygen, and you feel sluggish, can't concentrate, or are exhausted after even minimal effort, such as walking up a flight of stairs. Symptoms worsen as the deficiency progresses to anemia. Women—especially those who exercise, have been pregnant within the past two years, consume little or no red meat, or consume diets of less than 2,500 calories—are at particular risk for iron deficiency.

A menstruating, moderately active woman should consume at least 18 milligrams of iron daily (more if her menstrual flow is heavy or if she uses intrauterine devices for birth control). According to Fergus Clydesdale, Ph.D., professor and head of the department of food science at the University of Massachusetts in Amherst, a well-balanced diet supplies approximately 6 milligrams of iron for every 1,000 calories. Based on this ratio, women must increase their average intakes from 2,000 calories to at least 3,000 calories daily to meet their daily requirements. But women consume much less than that, which explains why iron intake is closer to 8 to 10 milligrams a day.

Women also consume most of their total day's iron intakes from vegetables, fruits, and grains, where only 2 to 7 percent of the iron is absorbed, while the well-absorbed iron in red meat (with 20 to 30 percent absorption) is limited. If a woman also drinks tea or coffee with her meals, iron absorption could fall even further.

Jan Johnson-Shane, Ph.D., R.D., an associate professor of nutrition at Illinois State University, has studied the beneficial effect of red meat on iron status. Her research found that small amounts (3 ounces a day) of red meat was all it took to improve iron status. Dr. Johnson-Shane says, "It's important to look at the total fat intake, with red meat being only one source of fat in the diet. If the serving is small, say three ounces, and extra-lean cuts are used as a side dish, rather than the main course, then red meat is an excellent source of iron while still falling within the guidelines of a low-fat diet."

Iron Basics

Everyone, especially premenopausal women, should monitor their iron status. Serum ferritin is the most sensitive indicator of iron status, but physicians don't routinely measure it, so be your own health advocate and request more sensitive tests than the typical hemoglobin and hematocrit tests for tissue iron levels, including serum ferritin, transferrin saturation, and total iron binding capacity (TIBC). A serum ferritin value below 20 micrograms/liter or a TIBC value greater than 450 micrograms/liter are red flags for iron deficiency.

Also, increase your dietary intake of iron-rich foods, such as extra-lean meat, legumes, tofu, green leafy vegetables, and prune juice. In addition, a moderate-dose iron supplement (18 milligrams daily) should improve iron status, mental function, and energy level within three weeks. Severe iron deficiency requires a higher-dose prescription supplement.

Since iron buildup in the body is possibly linked to an increased risk for cancer, there is no reason for postmenopausal women or men to supplement with iron unless a serum ferritin test shows they are iron deficient, and then only with physician approval and monitoring. (See Table 4.3, "Ironclad Rules," on page 116).

Vitamins and Minerals in Short Supply

Cutting corners on almost any vitamin or mineral will cause fatigue. For example, suboptimal intake of one of the eight B vitamins results in fatigue, poor concentration, apathy, and being out of breath after minor physical effort. Even a low intake of vitamin C has been linked to an increased risk for fatigue. A short supply of minerals also can drag you down, since many of these nutrients maintain and regulate the nervous system and energy metabolism. For example, a magnesium deficiency causes muscle weakness and fatigue, probably because of the mineral's role in converting carbohydrates, protein, and fat into energy. To guarantee optimal vitamin and mineral intake, follow the Feeling Good Diet and the guidelines in chapter 14 for choosing supplements.

Can Food Allergies Cause Fatigue?

While symptoms of a food allergy usually show up as skin rashes, digestive tract problems, and breathing difficulties, vague symptoms such as fatigue and headaches also have been attributed to food allergies, albeit with some controversy. For example, people are more likely to experience fatigue when they consume capsules of chocolate than when they take inert capsules (placebos) they think contain chocolate. (The suspicion that a food craving is a symptom of a food allergy has not been supported by the research.)

The problem with identifying a link between food allergies and fatigue is that nine times out of ten, a person who reports an adverse reaction to a particular food

---

Table 4.3   Ironclad Rules

There's more to consuming enough iron than just eating iron-rich foods or taking a supplement. Iron status, in fact, is more a balance of iron-inhibitors versus iron-enhancers in the diet. To tip the scale in your favor:

1. Consume small amounts of extra-lean meat—9 percent fat or less—with large amounts of iron-rich grains, vegetables, and beans (for example, spaghetti and meatballs).
2. Always eat a vitamin C–rich food with an iron-rich food, such as orange juice with a bowl of iron-fortified cereal.
3. Cook acidic foods, such as tomato-based sauces, in cast-iron cookware.
4. Take iron supplements on an empty stomach (unless it causes nausea) and avoid taking calcium or zinc at the same time you take iron.
5. Drink tea and coffee between meals, since these beverages contain compounds called tannins that can reduce iron absorption by 80 percent or more.
6. Limit your consumption of unleavened whole-grain breads, such as whole wheat biscuits or tortillas, since they contain a substance called phytate that inhibits iron absorption. This effect is reduced when vitamin C–rich foods are eaten with these foods—for example, a bean burrito made with a whole wheat tortilla (an unleavened whole-grain product) combined with vitamin C–rich cilantro and tomatoes.

---

does not show any symptoms when that food is consumed under "controlled" situations, i.e., in a double-blind situation where neither the scientist nor the person know who is consuming the food and who is consuming an inert substance called a placebo. Consequently, while many people say they are allergic or intolerant to a food, in reality very few people actually test positive for a true food allergy.

A true food allergy is any negative reaction to a food or food component that involves an immune response. The reaction can be immediate or delayed up to twenty-four hours and always includes skin, respiratory, or digestive tract problems. The symptoms can range from mild to life-threatening, depending on a person's tolerance level and the dose ingested. Any food can cause an allergic reaction; however, the following foods are most frequently implicated in allergic reactions:

cow's milk	soy	eggs
peanuts	wheat	corn
peas	fish	crustaceans

shellfish	tomatoes	nuts
chocolate	strawberries	oranges

The diagnosis of food allergies requires an array of different tests, including a patient history, physical examination, special immune-function tests, a trial "elimination" diet, and a "food challenge," where suspected foods are systematically added to the person's diet with physician monitoring of symptoms. Never does the result of one test determine a conclusive diagnosis of food allergy.

You can do some sleuthing on your own to identify the foods you can and can't tolerate. For example, a home-version of the Elimination Diet begins by systematically eliminating all beef, pork, poultry, milk, rye, and corn from the diet for two weeks. If your symptoms improve on this diet, you might be sensitive to one of the foods eliminated. To identify the exact offending food(s), start adding back one food at a time every two to three days. If no symptoms occur after eating a food for at least three days, then cross that food off your "trouble-prone" food list. (It helps to keep a journal during this process.) In phase two of the Elimination Diet, remove all beef, lamb, milk, and rice from the diet for two weeks. The same procedure holds true here as it did in phase one. In phase three, you can test for allergic reactions to lamb, fowl, rice, corn, rye, and milk by eating only vegetables, fruit, beef, potatoes, soybeans, lima beans, coffee, and olive oil for two weeks.

You might not be allergic to food, per se, but to molds growing on some foods. Mold allergies often produce subtle symptoms such as headaches, fatigue, or nasal congestion. It is best to consult a physician to confirm a mold allergy. The following foods are possible mold accumulators:

cheese	yogurt	canned tomatoes	dried fruits
beer	mushrooms	vinegar-containing	sour breads such
wine	tomato products	foods such as	as pumpernickel
sour cream	such as paste	mayonnaise	and rye breads
buttermilk	and catsup	and relishes	

The Intolerance Factor

More likely than not, a person's reaction to a food is caused by an intolerance, not an allergy. These reactions are caused by some biological idiosyncrasy, a digestive tract disorder, an enzyme deficiency, or even psychological factors. The symptoms might mimic an allergic response, such as a rash or abdominal discomfort, but also include headaches, mood swings, fatigue, or even sleep problems. Almost any food or food ingredient can produce a reaction, including chocolate, wine, legumes, coffee, pork, food additives, peas, nuts, or canned tuna. However, the most well-known intolerance is to milk products, caused by a deficiency in the enzyme lactase that breaks down milk sugar (lactose).

While milk allergy is very rare (the 1 to 2 percent of children who are allergic to milk usually outgrow the problem by the time they are two years old), lactose intolerance is relatively common. But it's not an all-or-nothing affair. In all but the most severe cases, a person can consume small quantities of milk products. The smaller the serving size, the less likely a person will experience symptoms. Fat slows the transit of food through the digestive tract, thus making it easier for bacteria to handle the lactose load. Therefore, whole or chocolate milk might be better tolerated than skim or unflavored milk.

Fermented dairy products, including cheese and yogurt, are another solution. Half of the lactose is removed when milk is processed into cheese; aged hard cheeses, such as Swiss and Cheddar, have the lowest lactose content. Bacteria called *Lactobacillus bulgarius* and *Lactobacillus acidophilus*, contained in some commercial yogurts, digest lactose when yogurt is fermented and stored. They also continue to digest more lactose in the small intestine after a person eats the yogurt. Consequently, many people can handle yogurt even if they can't drink milk. Even if you suffer from all the symptoms linked to lactose intolerance, beware of diagnosing yourself. Similar symptoms also are signs of other, more serious conditions and should be checked by a physician.

Additives, Preservatives, and Fatigue

In the past one hundred years, more new compounds have been added to the food supply than had been introduced in all the prior millions of years combined. Are additives at the root of food allergies or fatigue? Yes and no.

Most additives appear to be as safe as any naturally occurring chemical in foods, at least based on science's limited understanding of how additives might affect health in the short- and long-term. However, some additives, such as monosodium glutamate (MSG), produce mild discomfort in some people, while other additives, such as the sulfites used as a preservative in some wines, shrimp, and processed potatoes, have been deadly to a few highly sensitive people.

If you suspect you might react to MSG or some other additive or preservative, check with an allergist or test yourself by eliminating all foods that contain that substance (MSG can be listed on a label as "monosodium glutamate"; "hydrolyzed vegetable protein or HVP"; or "flavoring") for at least two weeks. If symptoms disappear, then slowly add back one food at a time and monitor your mood, physical health, and emotions. Adverse reactions usually develop within minutes to an hour of ingesting MSG, which helps in the diagnosis.

Chronic Fatigue Syndrome: A Dietary Approach

Chronic fatigue syndrome (CFS) affects four to ten out of every one hundred thousand adults. It shares similar symptoms with fibromyalgia, a chronic disorder of soft tissue, and is characterized by debilitating fatigue that does not subside with bed rest and that reduces daily activity below 50 percent of normal for at least six months. Common symptoms include mild fever, sore throat, painful and swollen lymph nodes, muscle aches and weakness, prolonged fatigue after exercising, headaches, mood swings, joint pain, and sleep disorders. People suffering from CFS also can struggle with depression and poor concentration. There is no foolproof test for CFS, which makes diagnosis difficult.

Unfortunately, there are no clearly defined dietary guidelines for the prevention and treatment of CFS. The outdated theory that the illness can be treated by avoiding all funguslike foods, such as mushrooms and yeast breads, and using antifungal medications has been rejected since there is no connection between CFS and yeast. Preliminary evidence shows that serotonin levels might be too high in CFS sufferers. If that is the case, then reducing your carbohydrate intake and increasing protein intake might help rebalance brain chemistry. Your best bet is to follow the Feeling Good Diet, which contains all the nutrients known to strengthen the immune system and maintain optimal health. Follow the guidelines in chapter 14 for choosing a multiple vitamin and mineral supplement, as well as extra magnesium and antioxidants. In addition, avoid sugar, caffeine, and alcohol, which only add more stress to the body. Moderate, daily exercise also can help maintain muscle, metabolism, and even boost energy in many people battling chronic fatigue.

The Energizing Lifestyle

Whether you are a lark and accomplish your best work in the morning or an owl who comes alive after dark, what and how much you eat can affect how energized you feel. The Feeling Good Diet forms the foundation for fighting fatigue. In addition, the following rules are important energy boosters:

- Eat a breakfast that includes some protein and some carbohydrates. Select at least one serving of protein-rich foods, such as legumes, meats, or low-fat dairy, and at least two to three servings of fruits, vegetables, and grains.
- Limit caffeinated beverages to three servings or less and don't drink tea and coffee with meals, since compounds called tannins in these beverages significantly reduce iron absorption.
- Never eat sugar by itself and limit the day's intake to less than 10 percent of total calories.
- Eat several small meals and snacks throughout the day, so that you eat approximately every four hours.
- Eat a moderate-sized, low-fat lunch that contains a mixture of protein and carbohydrates. Select at least one serving of protein-rich foods, such as legumes, meats, or low-fat dairy, and at least three servings of fruits, vegetables, and grains. Carbohydrate cravers should select even more grain and starchy vegetable servings.
- If you are a carbohydrate craver, plan a carbohydrate-rich snack for your low-energy period of the day. (See page 52 for a list of carbohydrate-rich snacks.)
- Eat a light meal in the evening and avoid excessive snacking after dinner.
- Consume ample amounts of iron-rich foods and take an iron supplement if your serum ferritin levels are below 20 micrograms/L.
- Avoid severe calorie-restricted diets. Too few calories means too little

fuel and nutrients, which can leave you drowsy. Long-term food restriction also results in lethargy, fatigue, depression, poor mental functioning, and greatly decreased feelings of energy.

- Drink water. Chronic low fluid intake is a common, but often overlooked, cause of mild dehydration and fatigue. Water helps rid the body of waste compounds that contribute to fatigue. Thirst is a poor indicator of water needs. A general rule of thumb is to drink twice as much water as it takes to quench your thirst, or at least six to eight glasses a day.
- Avoid or limit alcohol to no more than five drinks a week. Alcohol dehydrates the cells and suppresses the nervous system, causing poor attention, inability to concentrate, and fatigue. Alcohol also interferes with a good night's sleep.

Exercise is one of the best antidotes for fatigue. The link is clear: People who exercise also feel more energetic, while the sedentary get drowsier. Exercise increases blood flow to the muscles and brain, releases energizing hormones, and stimulates the nervous system to produce chemicals, called endorphins, that elevate mood and produce feelings of well-being. According to Dr. C. W. Smith, at the University of Arkansas for Medical Sciences in Little Rock, "Exercise should be part of everyone's lifestyle, but may be a particularly important part of the treatment of patients with depression and chronic fatigue. It will reliably and consistently decrease feelings of tiredness and despondency . . ."

In one study, eighteen people rated their energy levels after twelve days of either eating a candy bar or walking briskly for ten minutes. Results indicated that walking increased energy levels and lowered tension, while the sugary snack increased feelings of tension and only temporarily raised energy levels, followed by an increase in fatigue and reduced energy. It's likely that along with enhancing body chemistry and reducing stress hormones, exercise lowers blood pressure, fills the lungs and tissues with oxygen, and increases levels of adenosine triphosphate (ATP), the high-energy substances generated in our body cells. Stretching also relieves muscle tension that comes from fatigue-producing stresses and helps move blood throughout the body, as well as oxygenates the brain.

Finally, you don't have to take feeling tired lying down. Holly Atkinson, M.D., in her book *Women and Fatigue*, recommends keeping a journal to identify when you are most energized (i.e., are you a lark or an owl?), tired, or in the best and worst moods. Find out what precedes your high and low energy, including sleep, stress, diet, or exercise habits. Once you have identified the source of your fatigue, you can develop a plan to combat the blahs and rev up your engine. Keep in mind that there is no magic bullet for becoming more energetic. Energy is a complicated blend of stamina and vitality, ambition and curiosity, an upbeat attitude and a focused mind. However, take good care of your health and work with your body's natural energy and you stack the deck in favor of more energy. (See Table 4.4, "Herbs and Supplements to Fight Fatigue: What Works, What Doesn't, and Why," below.)

Table 4.4   Herbs and Supplements to Fight Fatigue: What Works, What Doesn't, and Why

Carnitine: This vitaminlike substance is supplied in ample amounts from milk, poultry, fish, and meat, yet a deficiency could cause fatigue. Carnitine helps transport fat across cell membranes and into the energy-producing centers of the cells, called the mitochondria. There is no evidence that healthy people benefit from carnitine supplements.

Coenzyme Q10: Also called ubiquinone, coenzyme Q10 (CoQ10) helps convert food and oxygen into energy. Produced in the body and obtained from the diet, CoQ10 might improve heart function, boost immunity, and function as an antioxidant, much like vitamin E and selenium, in protecting the blood vessels, heart, brain, and other tissues from free-radical damage. No optimal dose has been established.

Colloidal minerals: These "tonics," comprised of tiny particles of minerals suspended in liquid, are promoted as energy boosters. There is no scientific evidence that this form of minerals is any better than any other form; even the term *colloidal minerals* is without meaning. Colloidal minerals also might contain dangerous heavy metals such as arsenic, which can build up to toxic levels in the body.

Creatine: Does this amino acid mix really boost strength and energy during exercise? Possibly, but only in athletic events that require short bursts of energy, such as basketball, soccer, and track and field. No one knows the best and safest dose, but studies have used 20 to 30 grams of supplemental creatine a day during the first five to six days to "load" the muscles, then have dropped that dose to 2 to 5 grams a day as maintenance. Theoretically, creatine supplements could suppress the body's natural ability to manufacture this compound or could lead to kidney damage. There is no guarantee that a creatine supplement is pure, since there's little or no government regulation.

DHEA (dehydroepiandrosterone): DHEA is a key energy hormone. Studies show it lowers heart-disease risk; increases muscle mass, strength, and immune function; and improves mood, energy, libido, physical well-being, mental capacity, and memory. DHEA levels drop as a person ages, while supplements raise dwindling levels and might boost energy. Side effects range from mild problems such as acne and facial hair in women to more serious risks for breast and uterine cancer in women, prostate cancer and aggressiveness in men, birth defects in pregnant women, and liver damage. The biggest risk is that no one knows the long-term consequences.

Energy in a can: Several canned shakes are advertised as energy-restoring drinks. Save your money and snack on minimally processed foods, which have all the vitamins, minerals, and protein found in the fabricated shakes but also contain phytochemicals and fiber, which boost health naturally.

Ginseng: Many good studies on ginseng have been conducted on humans in recent years with very encouraging results. There appears to be a definite improvement in quality of life when consuming ginseng, especially in combination with vitamins. However, there is no scientific evidence to support claims that ginseng boosts energy or endurance.

Superoxygenated water: Oxygen-enriched water is advertised as an energy elixir. But where's the research? There is none. This one is a gimmick. You don't get oxygen through the digestive tract; you get it via the lungs into the blood. And, you get more than your red blood cells can carry by just breathing at sea level.

Vitamin B_{12}: Even a mild deficiency of this B vitamin results in fatigue, depression, and poor mental function. A deficiency is unlikely when a person is young and consumes ample amounts of B_{12}-rich foods, such as meat, milk, and other foods of animal origin. However, absorption decreases and requirements increase with age, making a deficiency more likely. Physicians can detect deficiencies by measuring serum B_{12} levels (the outdated Schilling test is not a sensitive indicator of vitamin B_{12} status). If low, B_{12} shots or supplements might be required.

CHAPTER FIVE

PMS and SAD

- Do you crave chocolate and doughnuts during the winter months or the week before your period? At the same time, do you feel clumsy or bloated?
- Do you snap at your friends or hope you make it through the day without crying in public?
- Are you confident, clearheaded, and physically fit throughout the month, then suddenly tearful, muddled, and uncoordinated the week before your period?
- From November to March or for a few days every month, are you unable to control your anger or do you just want to be left alone?
- Do you sleep too much, yet feel tired all day long?

Don't worry, you're not crazy. You probably have premenstrual syndrome (PMS), Seasonal Affective Disorder (SAD), or both. PMS is the moodiness, anxiety, depression, food cravings, and bloated feeling many women experience the week to ten days before their periods. The symptoms subside once their menstrual periods begin, and are followed by a symptom-free phase that lasts until after ovulation of the next cycle. People with SAD dread the autumn and winter, when they battle depression, increased appetite and weight gain, lethargy, and an insatiable need to sleep.

PMS and SAD have a lot in common. PMS symptoms worsen during the winter months for people with SAD. Many of the symptoms of both PMS and SAD, once thought to be all in a person's head, are now suspected to be triggered by brain chemicals such as serotonin (which regulates mood and appetite); enkephalins and endorphins (which are responsible for a sense of well-being); and gamma-aminobutyric acid (GABA), which stimulates the central nervous system. A few changes in diet might work wonders for people with either PMS or SAD.

Premenstrual Syndrome: The Period
Before Your Period

Menstruation might be a slight inconvenience, but the mild to severe mood shifts and physical changes that accompany PMS can be the true test of a woman's courage. Some women describe the shift in personality as a Dr. Jekyll and Ms. Hyde phenomenon: They feel and act fine for three weeks out of the month, then are "possessed" by a flood of emotional and physical feelings for the few days before their periods.

Somewhere between 20 and 90 percent of all women are affected by PMS, although only about 5 percent suffer symptoms severe enough to warrant medical attention. Despite its pervasiveness, PMS has been difficult to isolate and define. Consequently, PMS is a catchall for any unexplained problem and is blamed for everything from moodiness to murder. What makes PMS so elusive is its complexity. Up to 150 different symptoms have been documented, from headaches, fatigue, forgetfulness, and mood swings to weight gain, breast tenderness, anxiety, and food cravings. A woman might have any one or a combination of symptoms, and the symptoms can vary each month.

For years women were told their symptoms were "all in your head." Granted, many women say they felt better after taking a placebo they thought was medication, suggesting a psychological component. However, current research also shows that PMS results from a complex of factors, including fluctuations in hormones, hormonelike substances called prostaglandins, and nerve chemicals such as serotonin; fluid and sodium retention; and low blood sugar. In addition, blood fat levels such as cholesterol also rise and fall in rhythm with the menstrual cycle. Many of these factors might be influenced by nutritional deficiencies or excesses, and can be at least partially improved with changes in diet.

Keep in mind that these hormonal shifts are part of a woman's natural monthly rhythm. They signal that something very important is happening in her body: She is preparing for conception and motherhood. Therefore, PMS can be viewed either as a disorder or as a time of awareness and celebration. In cultures where people honor the female cycle, PMS symptoms often are nonexistent. For example, Italian women who never have heard of PMS report feeling a sense of well-being and happiness before their periods.

Who Is a Candidate for PMS?

Since many PMS symptoms result from the natural and normal fluctuation in female hormones, any menstruating woman is a likely candidate for PMS. This monthly problem crosses all boundaries, affecting married and unmarried women, women with and without children, working and unemployed women. Although PMS is most often found in women between the ages of twenty-five and forty-four, exceptions always exist, including reports of PMS in young girls before menarche and in some women perimenopausally.

A variety of lifestyle factors seem to aggravate symptoms, including stress, an inadequate amount of outdoor physical activity, and a diet that is high in sugar and refined carbohydrates, salt, saturated fat, alcohol, and caffeine. Keeping a diary of body and mood changes is the best way to determine if the symptoms you experience are related to PMS. You are a likely candidate for PMS if your symptoms cluster during the second half of your monthly cycle (see Worksheet 5.1, "The PMS Calendar," on page 127).

The What and Why of PMS

Four categories of PMS symptoms have been identified. A woman might experience symptoms from one or more of these categories, or the pattern of symptoms might change each month:

1. *Tension symptoms:* nervous tension, teariness, mood swings, irritability, and anxiety.
2. *Hyperhydration symptoms:* weight gain, swelling in the hands and feet, breast tenderness, and bloating.
3. *Craving symptoms:* increased hunger, gastrointestinal problems, cravings for sweet or salty foods, headaches, dizziness, and a pounding heart.
4. *Depression symptoms:* fatigue, poor concentration and memory, frequent crying, insomnia, depression, and confusion.

Worksheet 5.1 The PMS Calendar

Check symptoms daily on the following calendar, starting on day one of your menstrual cycle (the first day of bleeding). Indicate the severity of the symptoms by using 0 (no symptom), 1 (minor symptom), 2 (interferes with normal activities), and 3 (severe). Keep this calendar for three months, then answer the questions in "Do I Have PMS?" on pages 128–129. Use this sheet as a master to make copies.

CYCLE DAY	1	2	3	4	5	6	7	8	9	10	11	12	13	14	15	16	17	18	19	20	21	22	23	24	25	26	27	28	29	30	31
Date																															
Bleeding																															
Angry outbursts																															
Anxiety																															
Bloating/Swelling																															
Breast tenderness																															
Concentration/Memory problems																															
Cravings for sweets																															
Cravings for salty foods																															
Depression/Hopelessness																															
Dizziness																															
Fatigue																															
Forgetfulness																															
Headaches																															
Heart Palpitations																															
Hot Flashes																															
Hungry all the time																															
Insomnia																															
Mood Swings																															
Nausea/diarrhea/constipation																															
Overly sensitive																															
Teariness																															
Wish to be alone																															

Elevated levels of the female hormones—estrogen and progesterone—might be a contributing factor in PMS symptoms. Women with severe PMS symptoms report they feel much better when they are given medications that block these hormonal rises, while women who do not suffer from PMS show no differences in mood or physical well-being after taking the same medications. This suggests that women with PMS are more sensitive to fluctuations in hormone levels, in the same way that some people can't tolerate alcohol. However, fluctuations in other chemicals, such as serotonin, also contribute to PMS symptoms. (See Quiz 5.1, "Do I Have PMS?" below.)

Quiz 5.1   Do I Have PMS?

The only way you will know whether or not you have PMS is to keep a symptoms diary for three months and record your mood, health, and food intake every day. You probably have PMS if you notice changes for the worse—depression or irritability, breast tenderness or abdominal bloating, or poor eating habits—during the ten days prior to the onset of menstruation for at least two of the three months recorded. Review your symptoms diary and answer the following questions to determine your PMS status. Answer yes or no to the following questions.

During the week to ten days prior to your period:

_____ **1.** Does your mood take a turn for the worse—do you feel more depressed, tearful, irritable, angry, hopeless, or insecure?

_____ **2.** Are you more uptight, on edge, tense, anxious, or stressed?

_____ **3.** Do you have trouble concentrating, problem solving, or remembering details?

_____ **4.** Are you less interested in hobbies, friends, work, or life?

_____ **5.** Are you easily fatigued or do you experience a low energy level?

_____ **6.** Do you notice an obvious change in your eating habits—overeating, food cravings, or food aversions?

_____ **7.** Do you have trouble sleeping?

_____ **8.** Do you notice any physical changes, such as breast tenderness, abdominal bloating, joint or muscle pain, weight gain, or headaches that do not occur during other times of the month?

If you answered yes to any of the above questions:

_____ **9.** Are these symptoms independent of other health conditions, such as illness, stress, long-term medication use, or a diagnosed personality disorder?

_____ **10.** Have these symptoms been identified by keeping a symptoms diary for at least three months?

_____ **11.** Do these symptoms interfere with your work, social life, or family obligations?

_____ **12.** Would you estimate that these symptoms are at least a third worse than any symptoms you experience during and for the two weeks following your period?

Scoring:

If you answered yes three or more times to questions 1 through 10, you probably experience some degree of PMS. The more yes answers, the more extensive are your symptoms. If you answered yes to questions 11 and/or 12, you could be suffering from moderate to serious PMS problems that will benefit from diet and exercise changes as well as discussing your symptoms with a physician.

PMS, Calories, and Cravings

PMS triggers food cravings: One out of every three women experiences increased hunger and food cravings during the two weeks before her period and can consume up to 87 percent more calories than at any other time during the month. PMS and sweets also go hand in hand. Women who are depressed and battle food cravings during the premenstrual phase also are most likely to turn to chocolate and other sweets, with sugar increasing by up to 20 teaspoons daily.

Researchers at the Massachusetts Institute of Technology (MIT) have found that the most frequently reported symptoms of PMS, including cravings for carbohydrate-rich foods, sleep disturbances, and depression, coincide with dwindling serotonin levels. When comparing PMS sufferers with women who did not experience PMS symptoms, the researchers found that the daily energy intake of the PMS women increased from 1,892 calories to 2,395 calories, and carbohydrate intake increased 24 percent during meals and went up 43 percent during snacks. After eating a high-carbohydrate snack, the women showed some relief from depression, tension, anger, confusion, sadness, and fatigue, and they felt more alert and calm. The researchers concluded that premenstrual women overeat carbohydrates in an attempt to raise serotonin levels and improve their negative moods. See chapters 1 and 2 for more information on how carbohydrates affect serotonin levels and mood.

Low levels of endorphins also might influence PMS symptoms. A surge in the pleasure-producing endorphins coincides with ovulation, but levels drop off during the premenstrual phase, possibly contributing to the depression, hunger, irritability, food cravings, and other mood changes associated with PMS. C. James Chuong, M.D., and colleagues at the Mayo Clinic report that endorphin levels are lower during the premenstrual phase (the two weeks before the onset of menstruation) in women with PMS than in the same women during the rest of the month or in PMS-free women. The researchers conclude that the endorphin deprivation might contribute to the onset of symptoms. The low endorphin levels also might set off cravings for sweet-and-creamy foods that possibly elevate endorphin levels and mood.

But eating sweets only aggravates PMS. Research conducted at Texas A&M University shows that depression and fatigue often vanish when sugar (and caffeine) are removed from the diet. Some women are so sensitive to sugar that even one doughnut could affect their mood. This sugar sensitivity might be aggravated during PMS, intensifying the emotional highs and lows, escalating a minor food craving into a binge, and magnifying PMS symptoms.

As opposed to the temporary sugar high, eliminating sugar and caffeine from the diet and consuming more complex carbohydrates, such as sweet potatoes, corn, or whole-grain pastas and breads, might be a permanent solution. In one study, PMS sufferers reported they were less tense, angry, confused, and tired when they ate a bowl of cornflakes rather than a candy bar. They also felt more alert. When is as important as what, when it comes to carbohydrates. Many women report they feel much better if they include a snack midmorning that contains approximately 40 grams of complex carbohydrates (such as a small whole wheat bagel). Lunch can contain some protein and carbohydrates, such as a turkey sandwich, a bowl of soup, and a piece of fruit. To curb the mood and hunger swings that peak from midafternoon to bedtime, plan an all-carbohydrate snack midafternoon and a high-carbohydrate meal, such as pasta, for dinner.

Tinkering with Estrogen, the Natural Way

Several recent studies also suggest that increasing whole-grain carbohydrates might help balance estrogen swells, not only lowering breast cancer risk but also possibly curbing PMS symptoms. One study found that blood levels of estrogen and progesterone decreased in women who consumed low-fat, high-fiber diets, which enhance estrogen excretion and, thus, might improve hormonal balance and PMS symptoms. Increasing fiber, however, takes determination. To meet the recommended 25 to 30 grams, you need to follow the Feeling Good Diet's guidelines of at least five fresh fruits or vegetables, several whole grains, and a serving of legumes every day.

On the other hand, soybeans and soy products contain estrogenlike compounds, called phytoestrogens, that help offset fluctuations in a woman's natural estrogen. While not exactly like estrogen, phytoestrogens act much like the female hormone, binding to the body's estrogen receptors and supplementing the effects of estrogen without the discomfort. According to Mark Messina, Ph.D., associate professor at Loma Linda University and an expert on soy, women need two to three daily servings of traditional soy foods, which provide 60 to 90 milligrams of phytoestrogens (1 serving = $^1/_2$ cup tofu or 1 cup soy milk).

PMS Pills, Potions, and Powders

Rather than give in to the tears, moodiness, and chocolate cravings the two weeks before their periods, PMS sufferers are offered a variety of dietary supplements, foods, and bars that claim to boost serotonin levels, curb mood swings, and tame cravings. Some are even promoted by scientists at prestigious universities. All of them are pricey—up to $2.50 a day! To get such a bang for your buck, these miracle powders, pills, and potions must contain something pretty sensational, right? Only if you consider sugar and starch a scientific breakthrough. Granted, carbohydrates raise dwindling serotonin levels and ease PMS symptoms. But, you get the same amount of carbs and the same mood boost from an English muffin with honey, or four graham crackers with jam. "Most of these products are the equivalent of eating a handful of jelly beans," says Adam Drewnowski, Ph.D., director of the Nutritional Sciences Program at the University of Washington. A better PMS cure costs only pennies and can be found on most aisles of any supermarket: whole-grain breads, cereals, pasta, and crackers.

What You Can Do About PMS:
From Fat and Coffee to Supplements

PMS might have come out of the closet, but its treatment is still in the dark ages. There is much more to be learned about this syndrome, so in the meantime it is wise to err on the side of moderation.

Fat: Fact and Fallacy

While adding more fibrous vegetables, fruits, whole grains, and legumes to your diet, cut back on saturated fat. The fats in meat and fatty dairy products raise blood levels of estrogen, which might aggravate PMS symptoms. Substituting more fillet of sole (or, better yet, legumes and tofu) for less filet mignon would help cut back on your saturated fat intake. The added benefit of switching to a low-fat diet is that it also lowers your risk for hormone-related cancers, such as breast cancer.

On the other hand, including a small amount of safflower oil in the daily diet might help reduce PMS symptoms. Although poorly understood, a special fat found in abundance in safflower oil called linoleic acid might help regulate prostaglandins, which are hormonelike compounds that cause some of the abdominal bloating and breast discomfort associated with PMS. One or two tablespoons of safflower oil in the daily diet (in salad dressing, cooking, or baking) would supply enough of the linoleic acid to meet the body's needs without jeopardizing your low-fat dietary goals.

One study on evening primrose oil, which contains vitamin E and a fat called gamma linolenic acid (GLA), reported that the oil might help regulate the production of prostaglandins that affect breast tenderness, irritability, and depression. However, one study does not a conclusion make. In addition, most commercial primrose oil supplements contain mostly linoleic acid, not GLA. Other sources of GLA include borage oil and black currant seed oil. Borage seed oil can contain harmful compounds called pyrrolizidine alkaloids (UPAs). Select only products that state they are certified free of UPAs. Safety on long-term usage of these oils is unknown.

Caffeine, Alcohol, and Other Drinks

Some of the beverages women choose during the PMS phase only aggravate the problem. Coffee and other caffeinated beverages are a case in point. Women who consume caffeine-containing beverages each day, including coffee, tea, and colas, or even caffeine-containing medications, also might be more likely to have PMS and to suffer from severe mood and physical changes, such as fatigue, irritability, anxiety, headache, breast tenderness, food cravings, constipation, and acne, than women who consume less or no caffeine. The effect might be dose-dependent—that is, the more caffeine a woman consumes, the greater is her risk for PMS and the more severe are her symptoms. However, because PMS symptoms are unique to each woman, some women can tolerate caffeine, while caffeine aggravates symptoms in other women.

How caffeine aggravates PMS symptoms is unclear, although caffeine's effects on the nervous system are well-known and probably contribute to PMS symptoms, especially headaches, irritability, and anxiety. Women with PMS should consider eliminating all caffeine from their diets to test whether or not the coffee, tea, chocolate, and colas are contributing to their symptoms. Changes should be evaluated after several months, since results might not show up immediately.

PMS sufferers are more likely than other women to drink more alcohol during the premenstrual phase. Although the increased alcohol intake might slightly reduce the pain and discomfort associated with PMS, it also aggravates antisocial behavior, hostility, and anger. Worse yet, alcohol raises blood levels of the stress hormone cortisol and increases the permeability of cell membranes, affecting how well nerve cells function, and possibly contributing to mood swings, depression, and other emotional problems. Alcohol intake during the menstrual cycle also is associated with other harmful behaviors, such as increased tobacco use. Women with PMS, especially those women with moderate to severe symptoms, should avoid alcohol or limit intake to no more than five drinks a week (one drink equaling one 6-ounce glass of wine, one 12-ounce beer, or one shot of alcohol).

On the other hand, PMS sufferers should drink more water. A study from the University of Alberta found that women with PMS drink much less water than do other women, possibly because they mistakenly believe that drinking water causes fluid retention. In fact, just the opposite is true. Drinking more water and consuming less salty snack foods help the body rid itself of excess fluid, which might reduce swelling, breast tenderness, and bloating associated with PMS.

Supplements: Will They Do the Trick?

PMS sufferers consume more calories and fewer vitamins and minerals than do other women. PMS symptoms often improve when these women switch from their highly refined and processed diets to nutrient-packed diets with or without supplements.

Researchers at the U.S.D.A. Forks Human Nutrition Research Center in Grand Forks, North Dakota, report that many of the physiological, psychological, and behavioral symptoms related to the menstrual cycle might be associated with nutrition. In their study, menstrual symptoms were compared to blood levels of different vitamins and minerals in PMS sufferers. Results showed that low blood iron levels were most common in women suffering from depression, mood swings, and breast pain. Mood swings and poor concentration also were associated with low intakes of vitamins A, B_2 and B_6, folate, calcium, copper, and zinc. Even carotenes, such as lycopene and lutein, fluctuate throughout the menstrual cycle, possibly contributing to symptoms. Here are a few more examples:

Vitamin B₆: Some women report they feel less depressed, irritable, and dizzy, and have fewer headaches and less bloating, weight gain, and fatigue when they supplement with vitamin B_6. One study at St. Thomas's Hospital in London reported that vitamin B_6 supplements improved breast pain, called mastalgia, in women suffering from PMS who were unresponsive to hormonal therapy. However, in another study, 70 percent of the women taking "sugar" pills, who were told the pills were vitamin B_6, reported improvements in symptoms, which suggests that at least some women respond to any therapy they believe will work.

How vitamin B_6 might help treat PMS is controversial. Some researchers theorize that pharmacological doses of this vitamin (200 to 800 milligrams) reduce blood estrogen levels and increase progesterone levels, thus improving the balance between these two female hormones. Other researchers speculate that the vitamin aids in the manufacture and release of serotonin, which in turn regulates appetite, pain, sleep, and mood. Another theory is that a suboptimal level of vitamin B_6 produces a domino effect on the body's hormones: It decreases the release of dopamine, which increases levels of a hormone called prolactin, which triggers PMS symptoms. In short, disagreement prevails over if, why, or how vitamin B_6 is useful in the treatment of PMS.

Even if vitamin B_6 is effective, no one should self-medicate with this water-soluble vitamin in doses greater than 150 milligrams without physician supervision. Vitamin B_6 can be toxic when consumed in large amounts for extended periods of time. In one study, twenty-three of fifty-eight women taking large supplemental doses of vitamin B_6 for PMS developed numbness and tingling in their hands and feet, burning and shooting pains, clumsiness, and poor coordination. These symptoms subsided when the women discontinued the supplements. Other studies have found no harmful effects from taking vitamin B_6 in doses of up to 150 milligrams for short periods of time.

Vitamin E: Some women report less breast tenderness, bloating, and weight gain when they take large doses of supplemental vitamin E. However, other studies have found no significant improvements regardless of vitamin E intake, so supplementation with this vitamin is considered experimental.

Minerals: "The two most promising dietary links with PMS are calcium and magnesium," says James Penland, Ph.D., a research psychologist with the U.S.D.A.'s Human Nutrition Research Center. Women with PMS typically consume calcium-poor diets. In Dr. Penland's studies, increasing calcium intake to between 1,300 and 1,600 milligrams (the equivalent of four to five cups of milk) reduced PMS symptoms such as mood and concentration problems, pain, and water retention. A second study, from Columbia University in New York, found that women who supplemented with calcium had 48 percent fewer symptoms of PMS. Although the reason why calcium improves PMS symptoms is unknown, researchers speculate the mineral might increase serotonin activity.

A study from the State University of New York in Brooklyn reports that increasing your intake of magnesium also might help curb PMS symptoms. Magnesium levels drop during the last two weeks of the menstrual cycle, which could contribute to constriction of blood vessels, water retention, cramping, headaches, and an oversensitized nervous system that might result in crabbiness and teariness. Increasing your intake of magnesium-rich foods such as nuts, wheat germ, bananas, and green leafy vegetables could help restore magnesium levels and curb these PMS symptoms. "Just increasing dietary intake up to recommended levels often is enough to see an improvement in symptoms," says Dr. Penland.

Dr. Penland and his colleagues also have investigated other vitamins and minerals in relation to PMS sufferers, but the results are inconclusive. In their study, low blood levels of iron, the B vitamins, and zinc were most common in women suffering from depression, mood swings, poor concentration, and breast pain. "These findings indicate that there might be a relationship between diet and PMS, especially with iron, but it is too soon to make recommendations," says Dr. Penland.

Other Means of Relief

The symptoms of PMS can be reduced or even eliminated by following these steps:

- *Step one:* Keep a symptoms diary. Log how you feel each day of the month. Any physical and emotional changes during the two weeks prior to menstruation could be a signal you have PMS. By defining your unique PMS profile, you can tailor your diet to prevent or decrease symptoms (see Table 5.1, "PMS Survival Skills," on page 136).
- *Step two:* Take care of yourself. Treat yourself to a warm bath, a massage, a day off, or a walk in the country on the days when PMS symptoms are raging. Read a good book or watch a favorite television show. Take time to be creative. Pay attention to your eating habits and nourish your body with wholesome, healthful foods and liquids.

Table 5.1   PMS Survival Skills

Follow the basic dietary guidelines outlined in the Feeling Good Diet (chapter 12). In addition:

- Limit all sugars to less than three teaspoons per day. Indulge your sweet tooth with low-sugar sweets, such as The PMS Smoothie or The Pumpkin Pie Smoothie in the "Recipes For Feeling Your Best" section at the back of the book.
- Satisfy chocolate cravings with small amounts of low-fat chocolate foods, such as cocoa made with nonfat milk or chocolate angel food cake with no frosting. Also try the chocolate recipes at the back of this book—Chocolate Chip Cupcakes, Civilized S'Mores, and To-Die-For Low-Fat Brownies.
- Include one to two tablespoons of safflower oil in the daily diet.
- Limit salt to minimize fluid retention and swelling.
- Make sure you consume at least eight servings daily of fiber-rich fruits, vegetables, whole grains, and/or legumes.
- Avoid caffeine, especially when anxiety and breast tenderness are problems.
- When calorie intake is below 2,000 calories, choose a well-balanced, moderate-dose vitamin and mineral supplement that contains 100 percent of the Daily Value for magnesium, zinc, iron, and the B-complex vitamins, and no more than 400 IU of vitamin E.
- Vitamin B_6 supplementation (50 to 150 mg/day) started on day ten of the menstrual cycle and continued through day three of the next cycle has produced positive results in some women.
- Include physical activity in the daily routine. (Active women are less prone to severe PMS symptoms.)
- Consult a physician if symptoms intensify or persist.

- *Step three:* Keep moving. Include some form of mild- to moderate-intensity exercise in the daily routine. Choose an activity that is fun and consider this your playtime. Exercise helps reduce the tidal wave of hormones, increases pleasurable endorphins, curbs hunger, and calms you. Even if you don't feel like moving, do it anyway.
- *Step four:* Avoid stress. Women who regularly suffer from PMS develop much more severe symptoms when they are stressed, including irritability and depression. Choose calming activities and try to avoid high-pressured deadlines and time demands during the premenstrual phase. Delegate assignments at work or at home, cut back on commitments, and let a few responsibilities lag. This is not

the time of the month to be superwoman. It is the time to take care of yourself and avoid stress.

A Final Word

Keep in mind that PMS is so common and so intertwined with normal fluctuations in a woman's hormones that the condition is more a natural biological and emotional experience than a disorder. In some cultures, such as many Native American tribes, women's cycles are viewed as a source of growth and empowerment rather than a curse. However, for those women whose lives are seriously affected by PMS or whose symptoms are caused by unhealthful eating, inactivity, or stress, then diet, regular exercise, and effective coping skills can help curb suffering and improve overall health.

Remember to consult a physician if symptoms intensify or persist, since hormone and/or drug therapy, such as medications that suppress ovarian function, or antidepressants (especially serotonin-reuptake inhibitors such as Prozac), might be indicated. The birth control pill is not as widely and/or as frequently recommended nowadays as a treatment for PMS. Although it curbs the symptoms by blocking the normal ebb and flow of female hormones, many physicians believe this approach is too drastic for garden-variety PMS.

Another reason to check with your physician is that up to three quarters of the women who think they are suffering from PMS actually have another health condition with similar symptoms, including diabetes, hypothyroidism, depression, anxiety disorders, drug or alcohol abuse, anemia, and early menopause. All of these can be effectively treated. (See "Herbs and Supplements for PMS and SAD: What Works, What Doesn't, and Why," below.)

Herbs and Supplements for PMS and SAD: What Works, What Doesn't, and Why

Most over-the-counter remedies, potions, and pills advertised to treat PMS or SAD are based more on hype and very little on science. A few are worth a try:

5-HTP: 5-hydroxytryptophan is the latest natural serotonin booster available over the counter. Used either alone or with pregnenolone or the herb Saint-John's-wort, 5-HTP is suspected to improve mood. However, the research is limited on 5-HTP, and there is no research using this supplement on PMS sufferers.

Black cohosh: This herb is an antispasmodic used for pelvic pain and menstrual cramps. It contains saponins, phytochemicals that are said to stimulate the uterus and increase pelvic blood flow. Black cohosh might be mildly effective, but results can take several weeks to appear. Do not take black cohosh if you suspect you are pregnant, since it might stimulate uterine contractions.

Chaste berry: This herb is supposed to stimulate the pituitary gland in the brain to increase levels of the female hormone luteinizing hormone (LH), and decrease another female hormone, follicle-stimulating hormone (FSH). LH stimulates ovarian secretion of progesterone, so chaste berry might boost levels of this female hormone and help women with irregular periods. This herb also might stimulate the release of dopamine, which might lower levels of another hormone, prolactin, which is elevated in some PMS sufferers. Theoretically, this herb could aggravate PMS symptoms for women sensitive to fluctuations in this hormone.

Cinnamon: Testimonials report that this spice reduces bleeding in women with heavy periods. There is no research to support these claims.

Dong quai: This herb is used to treat menstrual and menopausal symptoms. It contains coumarin (an anticoagulant) and coumestrans (compounds that affect estrogen activity). It also might relax smooth muscles, thus relieving menstrual cramps. However, safety and effectiveness are questionable with this herb, and excessive intake could cause dermatitis. (Smooth muscles are muscles within the body that are distinctively different from skeletal muscles. The fibers in smooth muscles are smaller and shorter. Smooth muscle fibers are found in the gut, the bile ducts, the ureters, the uterus, and so forth. Other smooth muscles are found in the eye muscle, the iris of the eye, and the blood vessels, to name only a few.)

Pregnenolone: A hormone made from cholesterol, pregnenolone is the building block for DHEA, testosterone, and estrogen, hence its nickname "the grandmother of all hormones." Pregnenolone is advertised as boosting energy, relieving stress, and enhancing sex hormones without the dangers of taking too much. But with the possibility of causing liver damage, and with no research on its safety, taking this hormone is like playing Russian roulette with your long-term health. Products provide 10 to 60 milligrams, but warn not to use for more than thirty days without your physician's approval.

Saint-John's-wort: The herb Saint-John's-wort (also called hypericum) curbs the symptoms of depression possibly in a similar way, but to a lesser degree, as some serotonin-raising medications like Prozac. In a study from the University of Salzburg in Austria, 67 percent of people battling SAD felt better after taking Saint-John's-wort, compared to only 28 percent taking placebos. This herb appears to be safe and relatively free from side effects. On the downside, an optimal dose has yet to be identified, and there is no assurance of product quality since herbs in the United States are largely unregulated. For those people interested in trying Saint-John's-wort, suggested doses range from 300 to 900 milligrams daily. Always discuss taking the herb with your physician, especially if you are already taking a mood-elevating medication.

Yarrow: This herb acts as an antispasmodic and an antiinflammatory, which is why some women claim it helps pain and uterine cramps associated with PMS. No well-designed scientific studies have been done to verify these claims.

Are You SAD?

Up to 25 million Americans battle the Winter Blues; an additional 10 million Americans suffer from Seasonal Affective Disorder (SAD). The reasons why our moods slip and our appetites take over by midwinter could be simply that we're cooped up, bored, and restless, or it could have a deeper cause, resulting from a drop in serotonin or melatonin, brain chemicals that regulate sleep, mood, and hunger. "Whatever the reason, most people have some kind of behavior change in the winter," says Norman Rosenthal, M.D., senior researcher at the National Institute of Mental Health in Bethesda and author of *Winter Blues* (Guilford Press, 1998). Children and teens can suffer from the Winter Blues, too, warns Dr. Rosenthal.

Take a good look at your diet. Keep a SAD Food and Symptoms Diary for at least a week (see Worksheet 5.2 on page 140). Write down everything you eat and drink and when, and note whether the meal or snack was high in either carbohydrate or protein. Also record your mood before and after eating (within thirty to sixty minutes). For example, were you tired, lethargic, depressed, enthusiastic, energetic, agitated, tearful, calm, relaxed, alert, refreshed, or optimistic? Also record any differences in what you craved versus what you actually ate. During this one-week trial, avoid drinking any caffeinated or alcoholic beverages, since the effects of these "drugs" might influence how you interpret the way food affects how you feel.

The Winter Blues or SAD: Which Is It?

While other forms of depression strike at any time, the Winter Blues is a seasonal thing; you feel irritable and eat more as the leaves start changing colors in the fall, and you perk up and drop a few pounds come springtime. The seasonal drop in sunlight throws brain chemistry out of whack, making some of us more anxious, depressed, and tired this time of year. We snap at the kids; we sleep more; we crave sweets and, as a result, gain weight.

Worksheet 5.2 The SAD Food and Symptoms Diary

For one week write down everything you eat and drink—whether the meal or snack was high in protein or carbohydrate, the time of day, your mood before and after, and any other notes, such as any differences between what you wanted to eat versus what you actually ate, who you ate it with, what preceded the meal/snack, or what you were doing while you ate. Use this sheet as a master to make copies.

TIME	FOOD	AMOUNT	HIGH PROTEIN OR HIGH CARBOHYDRATE?	MOOD BEFORE	MOOD AFTER	NOTES

Of course, depression, mood swings, and chronic irritability also can be symptoms of other more serious problems, including Seasonal Affective Disorder (SAD). "The Winter Blues and SAD rest on the same continuum, differing only in their degree of severity," says Dr. Rosenthal. People suffering from Winter Blues might feel grumpy and tired, but people with SAD suffer serious depression, with feelings of desperation, anxiety, and exhaustion. They experience intensified PMS symptoms, are not interested in socializing, feel lethargic to the extent that it can interfere with work, sleep more, and report a decreased sex drive. The increased food intake combined with the reduced activity results in weight gain, averaging nine to fourteen pounds or more. During the spring and summer months, the same people can be enthusiastic, energetic (sometimes to the point of being hyperactive), less driven by food cravings, and lose weight. "If your depression interferes with important aspects of your life, such as your job or relationships, or if you have feelings of hopelessness, these are possible symptoms of SAD that should be discussed with a physician," cautions Dr. Rosenthal. The good news is—there is much you can do to maintain your mood and figure while waiting for the hum of bees in the spring. Do you suffer from SAD? Use Worksheet 5.3, "The SAD Calendar," on page 142 to monitor your symptoms.

One in every ten people, including adolescents and adults, develops SAD. Women are four times as likely as men to suffer from this disorder, possibly because of a link to the cyclical secretion of the female hormones—estrogen and progesterone. SAD rates also are high in shift workers who sleep during the day, coal miners who work underground, or submarine crews who live without sunlight for long periods of time. People with histories of mood disorders or alcohol abuse or who have close family members with SAD also are at high risk.

The farther away from the equator you live, the greater is the likelihood you will experience some degree of SAD during the winter months. You might be symptom-free while living in Florida, Southern California, or Italy and then experience SAD after relocating to Oregon, Minnesota, or northern Scotland, while a person living in New Hampshire or Norway who has suffered from SAD for years may suddenly feel "cured" during a winter vacation to the Bahamas.

Worksheet 5.3   The SAD Calendar

Are you unsure whether you suffer from SAD? The first step is to monitor any seasonal changes in mood, energy level, appetite, and sleep patterns. For each month below, color the corresponding box if you answered yes to the question. Use a red pen for those months when the symptom is particularly strong. If you note changes in sleep patterns, increased depression or irritability, or increased appetite and weight gain during winter months and an improvement in these problems in the spring and summer, you could be suffering from the Winter Blues or the more serious SAD. During what months do you:

	JAN.	FEB.	MARCH	APRIL	MAY	JUNE	JULY	AUG.	SEPT.	OCT.	NOV.	DEC.
Sleep more than eight hours a night												
Have difficulty rising in the morning												
Sleep well and awaken rested												
Struggle more with:												
depression												
irritability												
feelings of hopelessness												
reduced self-confidence												
stress, tension, and anxiety												
fatigue												
Feel your best												
Have increased food cravings												
hunger												
Eat more sweets, starches												
Drink more coffee												
Exercise the least												
Exercise the most												
Gain weight												
Lose weight												
Have trouble completing daily tasks												
Avoid socializing												
Become disinterested in normal activities												
Enjoy friends, family, and daily tasks												

SAD and Light

If your mood improves while vacationing down South, it's probably due more to the sunshine than the trip. According to Dr. Rosenthal, dark winter skies are linked to low levels of serotonin, which makes some people drowsy and more prone to depression. Ample sunshine hitting the retinas of our eyes triggers a cascade of events in the brain that lowers a chemical called melatonin and that raises serotonin levels. *Voilà* . . . moods improve!

Dr. Rosenthal and fellow researchers at the National Institute of Mental Health in Bethesda, Maryland, first discovered this link, which led to the successful use of light therapy (also called phototherapy). "Up to 80 percent of SAD and Winter Blues sufferers report at least some relief when exposed for thirty minutes to one and a half hours daily to sunlight or a specialized light box that emits light five to twenty times brighter than typical indoor light," says Dr. Rosenthal. Some people show no improvement after a week of treatment, but do respond when the duration or frequency of light therapy is increased. They report reduced appetite, slowed weight gain, reduced food cravings, elevation in mood, and improved sleep habits (they need up to three hours less sleep and sleep deeper during the night). Symptoms return within days when these people discontinue therapy; consequently, although the length of exposure usually can be reduced after the first few weeks, SAD sufferers usually must continue light therapy throughout the winter months. Apparently, light therapy lowers melatonin levels and rebalances sleep, mood, and appetite. (See the "Resources" section in the back of this book for a list of companies that sell the specialized light fixtures for treating SAD.)

The Serotonin Connection

Approximately 20 percent of SAD patients do not respond to light therapy, and even those who do respond are not completely cured of all symptoms. Serotonin might be the missing piece in the puzzle. The same area of the brain that releases melatonin also regulates serotonin production. In fact, melatonin is manufactured from serotonin. When melatonin levels increase, serotonin levels usually decrease, since more serotonin is converted to melatonin. On the other hand, exposure to light lowers melatonin levels and increases serotonin levels. Consequently, serotonin levels are lower, while melatonin levels are higher, in the winter as compared to the spring and summer, especially in people with SAD.

As discussed in chapter 1, low levels of serotonin are associated with increased carbohydrate cravings, depression, heightened sensitivity to pain, and troubled sleep patterns; when serotonin levels are high, carbohydrate cravings subside, mood is elevated, pain tolerance improves, and sleep is more restful. Since carbohydrate-rich foods stimulate the production of serotonin, SAD sufferers who crave sweets, potatoes, pasta, rice, and bread during the winter months are turning to starchy or sugary foods in an effort to feel better, calmer, and more relaxed, not because they are bored or lack willpower. Their bodies also crave these foods in an effort to fight fatigue. Interestingly, SAD sufferers who eat sweet snacks midday also respond better to light therapy than do people who do not cater to a sweet tooth, which suggests the carbohydrate-induced increase in serotonin combined with the light-induced reduction in melatonin levels is more effective than either therapy alone.

But some SAD sufferers don't respond to carbohydrates. In fact, the more they eat, the more they want. "Some people with SAD crave sweets and starches and can't get enough of them," warns Dr. Rosenthal. If you are one of these people, read on: The solution for you could rest in protein, not carbohydrates.

Protein Power

Some SAD sufferers might be deficient in another nerve chemical called dopamine, which is suspected to decrease with reduced exposure to light. As discussed in chapter 1, dopamine is the brain activator; people are more alert and think more clearly when dopamine levels are high. Consequently, if cloudy winter months lower dopamine levels, this would contribute to the drowsiness, poor concentration, and other mood swings characteristic of SAD.

Fortunately, there is a dietary approach to low dopamine levels. Protein-rich foods, such as extra-lean meat, chicken, fish, and low-fat milk products, raise dopamine levels and help boost energy and mood. "Protein also does not trigger the insulin response that is seen with a high-carbohydrate meal, so blood sugar remains steady," says Dr. Rosenthal. Thus, protein might be the answer to weight problems associated with SAD for some people.

"These people should consume more protein at two of their three main meals," recommends Dr. Rosenthal. That means having scrambled egg substitute with a bowl of fruit for breakfast (instead of oatmeal and toast) and a fish taco or roast beef sandwich at lunch (instead of pasta). The evening meal can supply more carbohydrates from potatoes, pasta, rice, or other grains. (See Table 5.2, "Sample Menu for SAD," on page 145.)

Table 5.2 Sample Menu for SAD

Based on what you learned from keeping the SAD Food and Symptoms Diary, are you sensitive to protein or carbohydrates? Does a protein-rich meal give you an energy boost? Do carbohydrates rev up your motor or leave you drowsy and wanting more to eat? Here are sample menus that will help fuel dwindling energy levels during the day, yet leave you relaxed in the evening, regardless of whether you need protein or carbohydrates.

THE PROTEIN-RICH DIET	THE CARBOHYDRATE-RICH DIET
BREAKFAST	
Omelette made with egg white, low-fat cheese, and spinach; whole wheat toast; cantaloupe; nonfat milk	Oatmeal with wheat germ; whole wheat toast with jam; nonfat milk for cereal; orange juice
SNACK	
Almonds and dried fruit; orange juice	The PMS Smoothie*
LUNCH	
Turkey sandwich on whole wheat; spinach salad with dressing; nonfat milk; nectarine	Curried mixed vegetables and tofu, brown rice, and nectarine
SNACK	
Low-fat cheese and whole-grain crackers; kiwi fruit	Whole wheat bagel with fat-free cream cheese; kiwi fruit
DINNER	
Spaghetti with marinara sauce; steamed green beans; garlic bread; salad with dressing; fruit plate	Broiled salmon; baked potato with fat-free sour cream and chives; steamed green beans; salad with dressing; nonfat milk
SNACK	
1/2 toasted English muffin, with jam	1/2 toasted English muffin, with jam

* See "Recipes for Feeling Your Best" at the back of this book.

The Sunshine Vitamin and SAD

Vitamin D is produced by the body when the skin is exposed to sunlight. Consequently, vitamin D levels drop during the winter months, when sun exposure is at a minimum. Until recently, the only concern with this decline was that it increased a person's risk for developing osteoporosis later in life. Recently, a few studies showed another possible function of vitamin D: A winter-induced reduction in this fat-soluble vitamin might contribute to SAD.

Researchers at Johns Hopkins University showed in one study that people with SAD were more likely than others to have low levels of vitamin D in their blood. Mood improved when these people supplemented their diets with vitamin D. In another study, from the University of Newcastle in Australia, forty-four healthy people reported their moods improved during the winter when they took vitamin D supplements. More research is needed before recommendations can be made. In the meantime, make sure your multiple vitamin and mineral supplement contains 200 to 400 IU of this sunshine vitamin.

SAD Basics

The SAD puzzle is far from complete. What is known, however, suggests that this disorder results from a complex imbalance in several nerve chemicals, hormones, and even in the body's basic cycle of chemicals called the biological clock. Fortunately, there is much a person can do to ease the symptoms and possibly even cure the disorder.

- Try light therapy. It has worked wonders for many SAD sufferers. SAD clinics are scattered around the United States, from San Diego to New York, and offer treatment with medical supervision. There also are clinics in countries around the world, from Australia and Japan to Iceland and Ireland. A second option is to buy your own lighting equipment. There are several options, including the standard model, the window box, and the portable model. Make sure the light is of sufficient intensity and has been adequately tested, and that the bulbs are protected by a screen.
- Take a look at your diet. Use the SAD Food and Symptoms Diary on page 140 or the Food & Mood Journal in chapter 12 for at least a

week. Write down everything you eat and drink and when, and note whether the meal or snack was high in either carbohydrates or protein. Also record your mood before and after eating (within thirty to sixty minutes). Were you tired, lethargic, depressed, enthusiastic, energetic, agitated, tearful, calm, relaxed, alert, refreshed, or optimistic? Also record any differences in what you craved versus what you actually ate. During this one-week trial, avoid drinking any caffeinated or alcoholic beverages, since the effects of these "drugs" might influence your moods and response to foods.

- Analyze your diary. Look for patterns, such as changes in mood that result from eating. For example:
  - How do you feel after a carbohydrate-rich snack?
  - Are you energized or dulled by a protein-rich meal?
  - What times of the day do you eat?
  - Do you eat at regular intervals or do your eating times vary?
  - Do you skip meals and, if so, which ones?
  - Is your food intake evenly distributed throughout the day or is it concentrated into a few big meals?
  - Is there a time of day when your food cravings peak?
  - What foods do you crave?
  - Does the size of your meal affect your mood? Do heavy meals aggravate fatigue, or do light meals help you stay alert?
  - Are snacks and meals planned or impulsive?
  - How hungry are you at meals and at snack time?
  - How fast do you eat? What happens when you eat too fast?
  - Are you taking any medication that might affect your mood or appetite?

Each person will find different patterns and will be affected by the diet in different ways. What is important is that you tailor your food intake to meet your specific needs. For example, if you note from your diary that protein-rich foods are invigorating, then plan a protein-rich meal for breakfast (for example, egg substitute, whole wheat toast, and low-fat milk) and lunch (turkey sandwich, three-bean salad, and fruit; cheese or fish and lots of vegetables; or chili with extra-lean meat and beans, corn bread, and yogurt). Leave the higher-carbohydrate foods, such as pasta, sweet potatoes, rice and vegetable dishes, and breads, for dinner and evening snacks, where they help you relax.

On the other hand, if carbohydrate-rich foods give you an energy boost, then include them in your breakfast (for example, pancakes, waffles, and cereal) and lunch (bean burrito with rice, hot carrots, and vegetables) and leave the higher-protein foods (seafood, chicken, and extra-lean meats) for dinner.

Your diary also provides information on when your body needs nutrients. You might notice that food cravings are highest in the late afternoon and are usually for sweet-and-creamy selections, such as doughnuts, a candy bar, or cookies. Knowing this, you can plan a carbohydrate-rich snack for this time of day. It can be a nutritious, whole-grain bagel, or you can budget your calories to include a sweeter selection, such as a slice of angel food cake or a brownie.

- Do not ignore cravings! Attempts to rid the cupboards and refrigerator of all sweet temptations or to "will away" an urge to eat is likely to backfire, since you are denying your body the very nutrients it needs to self-regulate the nerve chemicals and hormones that affect mood. The need won't go away by removing the food; your cravings will increase. Instead, respond to these cravings, but do so in moderation and with planned, nutritious foods.
- When you sit down to appease a craving, focus on the food. Take small bites and chew them slowly. This way you are likely to eat less, yet feel more satisfied. It might take up to sixty minutes for a meal to affect your mood. So be patient, eat a moderate serving of the craved food, and wait to see if your mood improves. If not, have another small serving.
- Eat breakfast. Even if you aren't hungry, eat something. The protein and carbohydrates in a breakfast meal help regulate the nerve chemicals and hormones that curb the symptoms of SAD.
- Avoid large meals. Meals of more than 1,000 calories, especially if they are high in fat, leave most people feeling drowsy. Lighter meals of approximately 500 calories for breakfast and lunch provide ample fuel without dragging you down. Light meals in the evening are more likely to aid in a good night's sleep.
- Reprogram your body by following the Feeling Good Diet (see chapter 12) and developing a routine that includes several small snacks throughout the day and evening. Include some protein and some carbohydrates at each snack, such as peanuts and raisins, low-fat yogurt and fruit, low-fat cheese melted on an English muffin, or a

bowl of cereal with milk. If you want to nibble in the evening, make it a carbohydrate-rich snack, such as fruit, popcorn, or toast. Keep the snack light and plan it for approximately one hour before bedtime. Plan your snacks so you will not fall prey to impulse eating.

• Don't worry about a little weight gain. Keep in mind that many people gain a few extra pounds in the winter, probably as a natural cycle to increase body temperature and to fuel the body during the cold months. Usually the few pounds gained will drop off come spring.

• Avoid all alcoholic beverages and limit caffeinated beverages to no more than two servings per day. SAD sufferers consume more coffee, tea, and colas during the winter months than during other seasons, probably in an attempt to elevate mood and increase energy. However, the effects caffeine has on the nervous system and the depression and irritability that many people experience during withdrawal from caffeine can aggravate SAD symptoms.

Beyond Light and Diet

Light therapy and diet are the foundation for treating SAD. However, other lifestyle habits and treatments can help curb symptoms. SAD sufferers should practice stress management skills, such as counseling, relaxation techniques, massage, and deep breathing. Exercise has similar benefits to SAD sufferers as it does for women with PMS; it helps balance the tidal wave of nerve chemicals and hormones, increase pleasurable endorphins, curb hunger, relax the body, and improve sleep habits. The added benefit is that if the exercise is outdoors, you get the light exposure you also need. Even moderate exercise, such as a walk at lunchtime, can have noticeable effects on mood and energy levels. A stumbling block to exercise is that many people with either the Winter Blues or SAD don't have the motivation to continue exercising throughout the winter. This is where light therapy comes in handy: It boosts mood enough to help motivate you to get up and move!

If you suspect you suffer from the more serious SAD, your first step is to consult a physician for an accurate diagnosis (there are no tests for SAD, only a personal health history). Once diagnosed, ask your physician about installing UV sunlights in the areas of your house where you spend the most time. Or, take a winter vacation to a sunny climate, regulate your sleep patterns to avoid excessive time spent in bed, and take positive action to reduce depression by replacing negative self-talk with positive thoughts. Your physician might recommend one of several anti-depressant medications, including the tricyclics, the monoamine oxidase inhibitors (MAOIs) such as Phenelzine, the serotonin activating medications such as Prozac, and lithium carbonate, also known as Priadel.

If yours is a mild case of the Winter Blues, try changing your attitude or surroundings. Start by changing how you think or act. The feelings might catch up. Anything becomes a habit if repeated often enough. Research bears this out and shows that when people adopt healthful lifestyles, eat well, exercise regularly, and keep stress at bay, they start feeling better. They also enjoy life more and have a more positive attitude. A good mood is like a snowball rolling downhill. The more you incorporate upbeat qualities into your life, the more vital and enthusiastic you will feel, and the easier it becomes to feel good.

To feel more energetic, start walking as if you are self-confident, self-assured, and energetic. Walk with long, powerful strides, with your head high, your shoulders back, chin up, and your arms swinging freely at your side. Do it every day until it becomes habit. If you want to bring more laughter and humor into your life, surround yourself with people who make you laugh, watch comedy shows on television, rent silly movies, put up a bird feeder in the backyard, volunteer at a day-care center, and/or read funny books. Also, look for people, activities, thoughts, and behaviors that rob you of humor and slowly replace them with more positive experiences. Even laughing, listening to soothing music, and meditation (possibly because they increase mood-elevating nerve chemicals called endorphins) can help offset the Winter Blues. (See "Herbs and Supplements for PMS and SAD: What Works, What Doesn't, and Why," on pages 137–139.)

CHAPTER SIX

Food and the Blues

Have you ever:

- Grazed from the refrigerator at the end of a bad day?
- Found comfort in a gallon of ice cream when alone on a Friday night?
- Wanted to lock yourself away from the world and just eat cookies?
- Soothed midmorning doldrums with a cinnamon roll?
- Reached for a bag of chips when you're feeling down in the dumps?

If you answered "yes" to one or more of these questions, you're not alone. At one time or another, most of us turn to food for solace, comfort, or relaxation when we're feeling down in the dumps. In most cases the indulgence is harmless and comforting. However, some people, in an effort to alleviate depression or loneliness, unknowingly choose foods that make them feel worse and set up a vicious cycle of depression and overeating. If you're using foods to treat depression, then you'd better make sure you're choosing the right ones.

Depression is no laughing matter. Twenty-five percent of all women and 12 percent of all men (or 17 million Americans) experience depression at some point in their lives. Even more people suffer from dysthymia, or sad mind, which is mild, chronic sadness. Suicide is one of the most serious consequences of depression, and even in the best of circumstances, depression undermines every aspect of living. The good news is that according to the American Psychiatric Association, up to 90 percent of people suffering from depression can be treated effectively. Diet and other health habits are the first place to start. (Take Quiz 6.1, "Are You Depressed?," below.)

Quiz 6.1   Are You Depressed?

With the everyday blues, you know you'll get over it and get on with things. With serious depression, you feel like all the energy has drained out of your life and it seems like it's never coming back. Here are a few quick questions to give you an indication whether or not you might be suffering from depression.

1. I'm eating much more (or much less) than usual.
2. I'm sleeping more (or less) than usual.
3. I'm sad most of the time.
4. I feel worthless and often guilty.
5. I often feel tense and irritable.
6. I have no energy, even when I get up in the morning.
7. I have lost interest in most of the activities I used to enjoy.
8. I feel hopeless about the future.
9. I have trouble concentrating, making decisions, or remembering.
10. I cry a lot.
11. I have persistent aches and pains.
12. I think about death or suicide. (If you answer yes, seek immediate help, regardless of your answers to the other questions.)

According to the National Foundation for Depressive Illness, you could be suffering from depression if you have experienced two or more from the preceding list of symptoms for at least two weeks in a row. If so, call your physician or contact any one of the organizations listed under Depression in the "Resources" section at the back of this book.

Stop the Cycle, I Want to Get Off

The same carbohydrate-rich foods that trigger snack attacks (see chapters 2 and 3), make you feel drowsy (see chapter 9), and soothe some symptoms of PMS and Winter Blues (chapter 5) also are the foods you turn to when you are depressed. It's no coincidence that people want pasta, desserts, and other carbohydrate-rich foods when they feel down in the dumps. As mentioned in chapter 1, carbohydrates elevate brain levels of tryptophan and serotonin, which in turn alleviate irritability and elevate mood.

Interestingly, some studies show that carbohydrates elevate serotonin levels, but fail to show any connection with mood as a result. It might be that a certain degree of carbohydrate sensitivity is needed before symptoms are obvious enough to be measured in a scientific study. However, it could be that there is more to the food-mood link than just serotonin.

Chasing the Blues Away

Sugar and starches have different mood-altering effects, even though they both stimulate serotonin production, according to Larry Christensen, Ph.D., chairman of the department of psychology at the University of South Alabama. Dr. Christensen's research shows that depression often vanishes when sugar (and caffeine) are removed from the diet. "We see improvements in mood when sugar is eliminated, even in people who are not depressed; however, these sugar-sensitive people probably would have become depressed in the future." Using sugar to self-regulate mood is a temporary fix. In the long run, it could start a vicious cycle. "The person suffering from depression who turns to sugary foods may relieve the depression and feel better for a short while, but the depression returns," says Dr. Christensen. The person then must either reach for another sugar fix or seek help elsewhere.

Some people are so sensitive to sugar that even small servings of something sweet, such as a cookie or a doughnut, send them on a mood-swing roller coaster. These supersensitive people should eliminate all refined or added sugars from the diet, including hidden sugars in convenience foods such as catsup, canned fruit, fruit "drinks," and fruited yogurt. Other people have higher tolerance levels and experience symptoms only after eating large amounts of sugar, such as a bag of cookies, or after days or weeks of grazing on sweets. They should cut back on concentrated sugars in candy, cakes, and other desserts, but might tolerate the hidden sugars.

A recent study found that some people who are lactose intolerant (unable to digest and absorb milk sugar) also are more prone to depression than people who tolerate milk products. The researchers speculate that high levels of milk sugar in the digestive tract might interfere with tryptophan activity, which would lower serotonin levels and aggravate depression. For these people, avoiding milk sugar by using lactose-free dairy products, adding Lactaid to milk, or avoiding milk products and taking a supplement that contains ample amounts of calcium and vitamin D should alleviate the problem.

Why Does Sugar (or Caffeine) Make You Moody?

How sugar affects mood is poorly understood. "If you ask, 'Does removing sugar or caffeine from the diet improve a person's mood and can they help treat depression?', the answer is 'yes.' But the knowledge base is limited on how these foods exert their effects," says Dr. Christensen. One theory is that concentrated sugars in the diet raise blood glucose above normal levels, which somehow interferes with glucose transport into the cells and tissues. Since glucose is the primary energy source for most body processes, limiting its entry would essentially starve the cells for fuel. Consequently, a person would feel depressed and lethargic after ingesting sugary foods.

A second theory is based on the connection between sugar and the endorphins—those naturally occurring morphinelike compounds in the brain responsible for euphoric feelings. Raising endorphin levels in the brain helps alleviate depression. If sugar does trigger a temporary release of these pleasure-producing chemicals, then turning to sweets is literally a form of unconscious self-medication. Again, the temporary rush in blood sugar and endorphins is usually followed by a more serious crash as blood sugar, endorphins, or other hormones and chemicals drop to lower-than-ever levels.

The sugar-endorphin theory has been tested primarily in animals, but it does provide an interesting link between the cravings for sweets in premenstrual syndrome (PMS), people quitting alcohol or tobacco, and bulimia, and the almost immediate relief from depression, tension, or fatigue when sweets are supplied. These people describe the cravings as, "I need something to make me feel better and calm me down." The sugary snack provides a temporary "quick fix." One more unfortunate consequence of a high-sugar diet is that the more sugar you eat, the more likely your diet will be low in essential vitamins and minerals. It could be that marginal intake of one or more of these nutrients, such as magnesium or vitamin B_6, could be contributing to low energy and depression. (See pages 158–162 for more on these nutrients.)

Caffeine in coffee, tea, and colas, on the other hand, might aggravate depression by lowering serotonin levels. In a study on rats, caffeine was found to raise brain levels of tryptophan, but lower serotonin levels. The researchers concluded that caffeine must decrease the conversion of tryptophan to serotonin, thus precipitating depression. Mood changes that coincide with caffeine withdrawal would last a few days until serotonin production returned to normal levels.

Amino Acid Alchemy

The main reason for snacking on carbohydrates is that these foods raise brain levels of the building block for serotonin—the amino acid tryptophan. Most of the research on tryptophan's effect on serotonin and mood used tryptophan supplements, not food, to get the effect. For example, in a Scandinavian study, tryptophan was as effective as the antidepressant drug imipramine, and had fewer side effects. Other studies report similar results; sometimes the tryptophan was longer lasting than the usual pharmacologic treatment.

But don't go looking for tryptophan tablets, because you won't find them. The Food and Drug Administration (FDA) banned tryptophan supplements from the market in 1989 after an outbreak of a rare disorder called eosinophilia-myalgia syndrome was linked to taking contaminated tryptophan pills. The condition, characterized by severe muscle pain and weakness, mouth ulcers, infection, abdominal pain, fever, and a skin rash, was potentially deadly. A new product called 5-hydroxy-L-tryptophan (5-HTP) is currently available, but its safety also is suspect. Until the FDA lifts the ban on tryptophan, or a safer alternative in pill form is available, the only naturally safe way a person can adjust tryptophan and serotonin levels is by increasing carbohydrate-rich foods.

I'm in the Mood for Fat

If the latest research on dietary fats and depression is true, then our ancient ancestors were probably a lot happier than people are today. The human species evolved on low-fat diets that contained much greater amounts of a group of fats called the omega-3 fatty acids (found in fish, flaxseed, and wild game) and much less of the polyunsaturated fats called omega-6 fatty acids (found in nuts, seeds, and vegetable oils) than we consume today. In the past one thousand years, we have gradually consumed more vegetable oils and less fish oils, and depression rates have gradually increased. Instead of the one to one ratio of fats consumed by our ancient ancestors, today we eat about fifteen to twenty-five times more omega-6 fatty acids than omega-3s, and depression rates have increased one hundred-fold just since the turn of the century.

When researchers monitor eating habits across countries, they find that as fish consumption goes up, depression rates go down. In fact, there is a sixty-fold difference in depression rates across countries from the highest (Japan and Taiwan) to the lowest (North America, Europe, and New Zealand) omega-3 fat consumption. Even postpartum depression decreases as women increase their consumption of fish. Many people also report a drop in mood when they switch too quickly to a low-fat diet.

In addition, serious depression is seen in up to 70 percent of alcoholics. Studies on animals demonstrate that long-term alcohol consumption depletes omega-3 fatty acids in nerve tissue, but this is reversed after prolonged abstinence. In humans, symptoms of depression also increase with prolonged drinking and resolve with sobriety. Upsets in serotonin contribute to these moods, but if the omega-3s are a contributing factor in mood regulation, then abstaining from alcohol and increasing the consumption of serotonin-boosting carbohydrates and omega-3-rich fish might help resolve depression in heavy drinkers. Omega-3 fat levels can drop after as few as two to three drinks, especially if the person consumes an antioxidant-poor diet low in fresh fruits and vegetables.

Omega-3s, in particular one called docosahexaenoic acid (DHA), are highly concentrated in the brain, where they comprise up to 50 percent of the total fats in nerve tissue and might be as critical to the healthy functioning of nerve membranes as they are to arteries, according to Joseph R. Hibbeln, M.D., chief of the Outpatient Clinic, and Norman Salem, Jr., Ph.D., chief of the Laboratory of Membrane Biochemistry and Biophysics at the National Institute on Alcohol Abuse and Alcoholism at the National Institutes of Health. "The high prevalence of depression in patients with coronary artery disease, alcoholism, multiple sclerosis, and postpartum depression might be linked by low concentrations of omega-3 fatty acids in nerve membranes," explains Dr. Hibbeln. "We're suggesting that deficient levels of the omega-3s in the nervous system may increase the vulnerability to depression, just as a deficient level in the circulation may increase vulnerability to heart disease."

It's also possible that fat affects mood by regulating serotonin. Low brain levels of serotonin are linked to increased rates of suicide, depression, impulsive and violent crimes, and alcoholism. While researchers can't measure brain levels of serotonin directly, they can monitor changes in breakdown products of serotonin that show up in cerebrospinal fluid. What they've found is that blood levels of omega-3 fatty acids are predictors of concentrations of these serotonin metabolites. Low blood omega-3 levels and low markers for serotonin appear together. However, eat more fish and you raise both omega-3 levels and the serotonin metabolites, which also improves mood. According to Dr. Hibbeln, "This suggests that dietary intake of these fatty acids might influence the serotonin process and that altering this process may possibly reduce depressive, suicidal, and violent behavior."

While the research is preliminary, it does suggest that lowering the intake of saturated fats in meat, whole milk products, and hydrogenated vegetable oils such as margarine and shortening, as well as cutting back on vegetable oils, while increasing the intake of omega-3 fats in fish could help save your heart and possibly boost your mood. Other good sources of the omega-3s include walnuts, walnut oil, and flaxseed or flaxseed meal. It also means that cutting back on dietary habits that lower omega-3 levels, including alcohol and tobacco, could help improve mood. See Table 6.1, "The Fish That Make You Happy," below.

Table 6.1   The Fish That Make You Happy

Here's where to get the omega-3 fatty acids:

SEAFOOD (3 OUNCES, BEFORE COOKING)	OMEGA-3 FATTY ACIDS CONTENT (GRAMS)
Sardines, in sardine oil	3.3
Mackerel, Atlantic	2.5
Trout, lake	1.6
Anchovy, European	1.4
Bluefish	1.2
Salmon, pink	1.0
Bass, striped	0.8
Oyster, Pacific	0.6
Tuna	0.5
Crab, Alaska King, or Shrimp	0.3
Lobster, Scallops, or Swordfish	0.2

The B₆ Connection

Your mood is affected by more than just amino acids, carbohydrates, and fats. In fact, an equally likely reason for a blue day is inadequate intake of one or more vitamins.

Vitamin B_6 is a case in point. Dietary intake of this B vitamin often is marginal in many segments of the population, including women of childbearing age, children, and seniors. Women typically consume half the recommended amount for vitamin B_6; as many as 15 percent of women consume less than 25 percent of what they need. Pregnant and breast-feeding women often consume only 60 percent of their requirement for vitamin B_6. (Women are more likely to run short on vitamin B_6 than are men because they consume less food in general and fewer vitamin B_6–rich foods such as meat.)

If your diet is short by even 1 milligram of this vital nutrient, you could send your nervous system into a panic. Adequate intake of vitamin B_6 is critical for the development and function of the central nervous system. But how vitamin B_6 affects the nervous system and brain is only partly understood. Even slightly low intakes of the vitamin produce abnormal functioning of several enzymes responsible for the metabolism of a variety of nerve chemicals and nerve modulators, including serotonin, dopamine, and GABA, which regulate behavior. Too little vitamin B_6 also leads to an accumulation of toxic breakdown products from nerve chemicals that irritate the nerves and are linked to many nerve disorders, from depression to seizures (see Quiz 6.2, "Are You Getting Enough Vitamin B_6?," on pages 160–161.)

Confusion and depression are well documented and common, yet vague, symptoms of vitamin B_6 deficiency. In one study conducted at Harvard Medical School and the U.S.D.A. Human Nutrition Research Center at Tufts University, more than one out of every four depressed patients was deficient in vitamins B_6 and B_{12}. In fact, vitamin B_6 deficiency is reported in as many as 79 percent of patients with depression, compared to only 29 percent of other patients. In many cases, giving these patients vitamin B_6 supplements (in doses as low as 10 milligrams a day) raises vitamin B_6 levels in the blood and improves or even alleviates the depression, providing convincing evidence that the deficiency might be the cause, rather than the effect, of the depression.

Granted, overt vitamin B_6 deficiency is rare in the United States; however, even a marginal intake—where a person consumes enough of the vitamin to avoid classic symptoms but not enough to sustain optimal health—could produce subtle changes in personality and mood. In fact, the mood swings and depression that are considered side effects of medications, such as hormone replacement therapy, oral contraceptives, and antituberculosis drugs, might be caused by drug-induced suppression of vitamin B_6 metabolism and the consequent underproduction of serotonin.

To increase dietary intake of this B vitamin, include several servings daily of protein-rich foods such as chicken, nuts, legumes, and fish, as well as bananas, avocados, and dark green leafy vegetables. Whole grains are preferable to refined, enriched grains, since more than 70 percent of the vitamin is lost during processing, while vitamin B_6 is not one of the four nutrients added back during the enrichment stage.

A word of caution about self-medicating with vitamin B_6. Large doses of this water-soluble vitamin can produce nerve damage, including numbness and tingling in the toes, feet, fingers, and hands. Seldom is there a reason to take more than 25 milligrams of vitamin B_6 daily; always consult a physician knowledgeable about nutrition before taking vitamin B_6 supplements in doses greater than 150 mg for long periods of time.

Other Vitamins and Minerals: In the Pink or Feeling Blue?

Getting some, but not enough, of several other vitamins, including vitamin B_1, vitamin B_2, niacin, folic acid, and vitamin B_{12}, and vitamins C and D also might contribute to depression.

Folic acid: A deficiency of folic acid, a B vitamin essential for normal nerve cell growth and maintenance, causes several personality changes, including depression. Poor folic acid intake is found in up to 38 percent of people diagnosed with depression, while some of these people show improvements in mood when they consume more folic acid–rich foods. In contrast, those with high blood levels of folic acid are in the best mood. Some evidence suggests folic acid raises serotonin levels or enhances melatonin production. This B vitamin also is essential for the manufacture of several other nerve chemicals, and helps maintain the nerves and repairs the genetic code within nerve cells. Depressed patients who are folic acid–deficient are less responsive to antidepressant treatment, so they should be supplemented with the vitamin before other treatments are considered.

Vitamin deficiencies might contribute to depression and mood swings common in eating disorders, such as bulimia and anorexia. Researchers at England's

University of Liverpool and the University of Surrey examined the association between folic acid and vitamin B_{12} status, depression, and weight loss in forty-five anorexic girls and compared the vitamin status of this group with the vitamin levels in normal-weight bulimics and normal-weight girls without eating disorders. They found that 37 percent of the anorexics and 14 percent of the bulimics, but only 11 percent of the healthy controls, were deficient in folic acid. The anorexics also were more likely to be vitamin B_{12}–deficient. Anorexics who were depressed were the most likely to be folic acid–deficient, and supplementing with this B vitamin improved their moods.

Quiz 6.2   Are You Getting Enough Vitamin B_6?

Answer yes or no to the following questions:

_____ **1.** Do you consume daily at least 2,000 calories of a variety of minimally processed, wholesome foods?

_____ **2.** Do you consume daily at least six servings of whole-grain breads, cereals (especially oatmeal), pasta, or rice?

_____ **3.** Do you frequently eat bananas, avocados, baked potatoes (including the skin), acorn squash, or spinach?

_____ **4.** Do you frequently eat cooked dried beans and peas, such as lentils, lima beans, navy beans, and white beans?

_____ **5.** Do you choose chicken, fish, and crab rather than red meat, lamb, and lunch meats?

Give yourself 2 points for every yes answer, and deduct 2 points for every no answer to the above questions. Then continue to answer either yes or no to the following questions.

_____ **6.** Are you taking birth control pills, hormone replacement therapy (HRT), anti-Parkinson's drugs such as levodopa, antituberculosis drugs, or anti-Wilson's disease drugs such as D-penacillamine?

_____ **7.** Do you drink more than five alcoholic beverages each week?

_____ **8.** Do you eat a high-fat diet or consume several sweets and desserts daily?

Deduct 1 point for every yes answer, and add 1 point for every no answer to questions 6 through 8. Then total your pluses and minuses for a final score.

Scoring:

10 to 13: Your diet is probably adequate in vitamin B_6. You should consider increasing your dietary intake of vitamin B_6–rich foods or taking a supplement (with physician approval and monitoring) if you suspect larger than normal amounts of this vitamin might help alleviate PMS-related depression.

7 to 9: Your diet might be marginal in vitamin B_6. Increase your intake of this vitamin by adding one or two of the following foods to your daily diet: banana, avocado, chicken without the skin, salmon, potato with the skin, collard greens, brown rice, wheat germ, or oatmeal or cornmeal. If you choose to supplement, find a multiple vitamin and mineral preparation that contains approximately 2 to 5 milligrams of vitamin B_6.

Less than 7: Your diet is likely to be deficient in vitamin B_6. Increase your intake of this vitamin by adding three or more of the vitamin B_6–rich foods listed above to your daily diet. If you choose to supplement, find a multiple vitamin and mineral preparation that contains approximately 2 to 5 mg of vitamin B_6 if you are less than thirty years old, and 2 to 25 milligrams if you are more than thirty years old.

Folic acid deficiency is considered the most common vitamin deficiency in the United States, and intakes approaching half the recommended 400 micrograms are common, especially in women. To compound the problem, folic acid is easily destroyed when foods are stored or cooked too long, reheated, or cooked in large amounts of water, such as boiling spinach in water rather than lightly steaming it. Virtually all of the folic acid is gone when fresh broccoli is stored in the refrigerator for days, cooked until olive green, or allowed to sit under hot lights in a cafeteria. Folic acid–rich foods include dark green leafy vegetables, orange juice, whole grains or folic acid–fortified enriched grains, and legumes.

Vitamin B_{12}: People who consume marginal amounts of vitamin B_{12} also are likely to suffer from depression, memory problems, and even paranoia. Increased dietary or supplemental intake of vitamin B_{12} in these deficient people raises blood levels of the vitamin and elevates mood. You need at least 2 micrograms daily in your early years. The ability to absorb vitamin B_{12} decreases with age, so gradually increase your intake in the middle and later years, from 5 to 25 micrograms daily.

Vitamin D: There might be a connection between plummeting vitamin D levels and an increased risk for depression in the wintertime, according to researchers at the University of Newcastle in Australia. In their study, people battling depression showed marked improvement in mood when they supplemented their daily diets with 400 IU to 800 IU of vitamin D.

Minerals: Low dietary intake of many of the minerals, including calcium, iron, magnesium, selenium, and zinc, can cause depression, irritability, or mood swings. For example:

- Increased intake of calcium might help raise brain levels of the nerve chemical dopamine, which boosts alertness and mood.
- Iron deficiency is common in active women, children, and seniors, and can cause depression associated with fatigue.
- People who are depressed also have low magnesium levels in their blood.
- Selenium supplements (70 to 200 micrograms) have improved mood, while low selenium intake often is reported in people suffering from depression.
- Blood levels of zinc are consistently low in depressed people, which led researchers at the University of Cagliari in Italy to theorize that low zinc status might be a marker for depression.

The Feeling Good Diet is mineral-rich and should supply optimal amounts of all minerals as long as you consume at least 2,000 calories a day. An exception to this rule is iron, which might require a supplement of 10 to 18 milligrams when intake of nutritious foods falls below 2,500 calories. There is little or no evidence that people already optimally nourished will benefit from additional amounts of minerals.

Blues-Free Basics

If food is at the root of your blues, then the Feeling Good Diet in chapter 12 should be the cure. If followed closely and consistently, this eating plan will provide all the vitamins and minerals you need in the right proportion and spaced evenly through-out the day to fuel your spirits and sidestep diet-related mood swings and depression. The seven key points to remember are:

1. Carbohydrate cravers must work with, not against, their cravings. Make sure every meal contains some complex carbohydrate–rich foods, especially whole grains. In addition, plan a carbohydrate-rich snack during that time of the day when you're most vulnerable. (See chapter 2 for details.)
2. Depression and excessive consumption of sugar and/or caffeine don't

mix. People who are fighting depression and who know they are sensitive to sugar should avoid all foods containing sugar, including desserts, sugarcoated cereals, candy, sugar-sweetened beverages, and sugary snack foods such as granola bars. Read labels, since many unsuspected foods contain sugar, including muffins, canned and boxed fruit juices, frozen breakfast foods, and yogurt (see "Sweet Consciousness," on page 164). Eliminate coffee and other caffeinated beverages, foods, and medications. That includes tea, chocolate, cocoa, colas, and medications (see Table 4.1, "The Caffeine Scoreboard," on page 106). Keep in mind that it might take three weeks or more after you have completely eliminated sugar and caffeine from your diet before you notice an improvement in mood.

3. Eat more fish. At least three times a week, substitute seafood for red meat or chicken. Remember to bake, broil, poach, or barbecue, which are low-fat methods that won't add more vegetable oils and saturated fats to the diet.

4. Avoid alcohol or drink in moderation.

5. Pay attention to your intake of vitamins B_6, B_{12}, and folic acid. Take immediate action to improve your diet if you are falling short of your vitamin B_6 needs. Make sure you include at least two folic acid–rich foods in your diet plans—mix spinach with scrambled eggs for breakfast, drink at least one glass of orange juice, steam collard greens and mix into mashed potatoes, or replace iceberg lettuce with romaine lettuce for salads. To maximize your intake of folic acid, purchase vegetables fresh, refrigerate immediately, and use within two days of purchase. Avoid overcooking dark green leafy vegetables; always heat them in a minimum of water; then add the cooking water to soups and stews. Finally, consume the recommended selections of vitamin B_{12}–rich meat, chicken, fish, and/or milk outlined in the Feeling Good Diet.

6. Review your eating habits in the past few months. Have you made dramatic changes in your normal eating patterns? Are you dieting, frequently skipping breakfast, indulging in snack attacks in the evening, eating too many sweets, or limiting the number of times during the day that you eat to less than three snacks and meals? Do you have a food intolerance, allergies, or aversions? Any of these habits will alter brain chemistry and possibly contribute to mood swings.

7. As you adopt the Feeling Good Diet, make changes gradually. The depression people report when cutting back on dietary fat is probably linked to the rapid change in eating habits. Give your brain chemistry and your taste buds time to adapt by selecting two or three small changes and practicing these until they are comfortable.

Sweet Consciousness

Most Americans consume 20 percent of their daily calories as sugar. Although exact recommendations have not been set, it is generally agreed people should cut their intake of added sugar in half. People who consume less than 2,000 calories have little room for "extras" in their diet, so they should consume even less added sugar. Here are some suggestions.

- Cut back on sweets, such as doughnuts, candy, pies, cakes, cookies, and ice cream, since these foods are doubly harmful because of their high sugar and high fat content.
- Limit soft drinks to no more than one serving every two days, since they supply up to nine teaspoons of sugar per serving and are the biggest contributors of sugar in the diet. Colas also contain caffeine.
- Read labels. Although manufacturers are not required to list the percentage of sugar calories, you can get an idea of the sugar content by reading the ingredients list. A food might be too sweet if sugar is one of the first three ingredients or if the list includes several sources of sugar.
- Use more spices. Cinnamon, vanilla, spearmint, and anise provide a sweet taste to foods without adding sugar or calories. Aspartame also can be used in moderation.

Regardless of the name, all added sugar is essentially calories with no redeemable nutrient qualities. A little sugar in the diet adds enjoyment and variety, especially when it comes from natural sources, such as fruit. Going overboard for sweets, however, could undermine your health.

That Exercise Thing You Do

People who stick with an exercise program consistently report they feel good, physically and mentally. Even those who are despondent rave about their better moods once they start exercising. Exercise has proven effective in preventing, reducing, and even curing depression in the young and the old, men and women, people with mild to severe depression, recovering alcoholics, people battling life-threatening illnesses such as cancer, and people recovering from eating disorders.

A daily workout releases brain chemicals, including epinephrine and norepi-nephrine, which boost alertness. Regular exercise also raises serotonin levels, which boost mood in much the same way as mood-elevating medications, such as Prozac. At the same time, exercise destresses the body by lowering blood levels of the "stress hormones," including cortisol, that prepare the body to "fight or flight." Ele-vated cortisol levels are associated with depression and weight gain, while exercise-induced weight loss improves hormone levels and mood. Over time, the body learns to react less intensely to stress, thus providing a built-in coping mechanism against depression. The rise in body temperature that results from a vigorous workout also has a tranquilizing effect on the body, not unlike soaking in a hot bath. Finally, the hour at the gym or pounding the streets might provide a break in your day's hectic schedule that provides a time-out from worries and unpleasant emotions.

Then there's the notorious "runner's high," that feeling of euphoria following any intense physical activity. This natural high has been attributed to an exercise-induced release of endorphins, the body's natural morphinelike chemicals that help boost pain tolerance and generate feelings of euphoria and satisfaction. However, the research on endorphins and exercise remains equivocal. "Exercise raises blood levels of endorphins up to ten-fold," says Ed Pierce, Ph.D., associate professor in the department of health and sport science at the University of Richmond. "But the key is whether or not brain levels of endorphins are increased and, while a correlation between blood and brain chemistry has been found in animals, we as yet have no research to show the same in humans."

Endorphins or no endorphins, one thing seems clear: Exercise is a great antide-pressant. "People want to categorize the mood-elevating effects of exercise, saying it's biochemical or psychological, but in reality it's probably a synergistic effect of these and, as yet, unidentified factors," says Pierce. "What we do know is that exercise relieves depression better than psychotherapeutic medications, counseling, or a combination of the two." For example, in a study on 357 adults at Stanford University, researchers compared the effects of no exercise versus various intensities of exercise on psychological outcomes. After twelve months, the exercisers reported significantly reduced stress, anxiety, and depression compared to their sedentary counterparts, regardless of whether or not they experienced any changes in fitness or body weight. The level of intensity and even the type of exercise doesn't seem to matter; intense and moderate activities, as well as both aerobic activities—such as walking, running, or swimming—and anaerobic sports—such as bodybuilding—alleviate depression and improve mood. But exercise is only effective at boosting mood if you stick with it: Depression can return within forty-eight hours of your last exercise session.

Natural Mood Boosters

The consensus among physicians and scientists is that a multitude of causes, ranging from purely medical ones through those that are diet and lifestyle-induced, or purely psychological, are recognized as contributors to depression. Stressful life events, such as the loss of a family member or friend, a difficult change in job or finances, or problems at home or at work, can contribute to depression. Medical conditions underlying depression might be detected in a routine medical checkup and include changes in blood sugar and any irregularities in blood or urine samples. Fatigue, memory loss, and depression frequently precede as well as result from an underactive thyroid, which is common in women and also can be detected in a physical exam. Even food sensitivities, such as a history of food allergies, physical reactions related to foods including skin or respiratory problems, or a family history of allergies, might contribute to the blues. Contrary to popular belief, depression is not a natural consequence of aging, nor is it a condition with which a person must just learn to live. There are numerous medications as well as natural dietary and lifestyle factors within your control that can help curb the symptoms of both dysthymia and depression. (See "Herbs and Supplements for Depression: What Works, What Doesn't, and Why," on pages 167–168.)

What you eat and how much you exercise is only part of the blues battle. Effective coping skills, a strong social support system, and limiting or avoiding cigarettes and medications that compound an emotional problem are additional important considerations. You also won't solve your mood problems by drinking. Alcohol lowers tryptophan levels in the brain, which impairs serotonin production and makes depression worse. There are ways you can get a natural high (possibly from endorphins): by laughing, listening to soothing music, and meditating. An added benefit is that people who soothe their mood with these strategies also reduce their risk for heart disease, high blood pressure, and cancer, as well as increase their alertness, self-esteem, and energy level.

You might find it interesting and helpful to keep a journal of your feelings.

Herbs and Supplements to Fight Depression: What Works, What Doesn't, and Why

Carnitine: Carnitine supplements might help improve mood and reduce cortisol levels in people with clinical depression. Doses used in these studies are 500 milligrams, given four times daily.

DHEA: Dehydroepiandrosterone (DHEA) is a steroid hormone produced in the adrenal glands and a building block for the sex hormones—estrogen and testosterone. Levels of the hormone drop at a rate of about 3 percent a year; by the time people reach seventy years of age, they have only about 10 to 20 percent of the DHEA they had in their twenties. Supplements of approximately 50 milligrams daily are supposed to improve mood, mental function, and sleep patterns; increase energy and libido; and counteract stress. However, DHEA has risks, including an increased likelihood for acne, prostate cancer, aggressiveness, and liver damage. Long-term consequences are unknown, and purity and strength of supplements are not regulated. Supplements made from wild Mexican yams claim to contain the building blocks for DHEA, but there is little or no evidence that the body converts these compounds into DHEA. "Unless people are advised by their physicians to take DHEA, supplementing with this hormone is a buyer-beware decision," says Huber Warner, Ph.D., acting associate director of the Biology of Aging Program at the National Institute of Aging in Bethesda. You can naturally boost DHEA levels by meditating.

Flax: Flaxseed is a rich source of the omega-3 fatty acids, which are low in people suffering from depression. No optimal dose has been established. To get the full benefits of flaxseed, choose the seeds or meal rather than the oil.

Saint-John's-wort: The herb Saint-John's-wort (also called hypericum) curbs the symptoms of depression in about half of all people who use it, possibly in a similar way, but to a lesser degree, as some serotonin-raising medications like Prozac. In a study from the University of Salzburg in Austria, 67 percent of people battling SAD felt better after taking Saint-John's-wort compared to only 28 percent taking placebos. This herb appears to be safe and relatively free from side effects. On the down side, an optimal dose of this herb in treating depression has yet to be identified, there is no assurance of product quality since herbs in the United States are largely unregulated, and the possible interactions with other medications are unknown. For those people interested in trying Saint-John's-wort, suggested doses range from 300 to 900 milligrams daily. Always discuss taking the herb with your physician, especially if you are already taking a mood-elevating medication.

Vitamin E: Back in the 1980s, a researcher at the Division of Reproductive Medicine at North Charles General Hospital in Baltimore reported that up to 300 IU of vitamin E daily reduced some symptoms of premenstrual syndrome (PMS), including depression, irritability, and tension. Subsequent research has not supported these early claims.

With each entry, note the time, place, and situation you are in so you can see over time what triggers depression. Using this information, you can develop a plan for countering those situations. Helping others by volunteering your time to improve the environment, raising money for a needy cause, delivering food to housebound people, or participating in any other volunteer effort of your choice can help take your mind off your own troubles and reconnect you with others. Even spending time in the outdoors, walking in the woods or on the beach, might help you boost serotonin levels and curb the blues. Depression can be a symptom of other problems, so always consult a physician if emotional problems persist or interfere long-term with your quality of life and health. In the meantime, keep in mind that what you choose to soothe your hunger also will be fueling your mood.

CHAPTER SEVEN

Stress and Diet

Have you ever:

- Caught a cold right after a big event?
- Craved candy bars when pressured to meet a deadline at work?
- Found yourself unable to think of a name, find the right word, or remember where you put your car keys when you're under stress?
- Lost your appetite when troubled or anxious?
- Gained or lost weight when a relationship ended?

If so, you've experienced firsthand what science is just beginning to understand: Stress, diet, mood, and immunity are interconnected.

For centuries scientists believed the mind ruled, yet remained separate, from the body. Recently research on stress has changed the way we look at the human experience. What was first called the mind-body connection by questionable philosophers in the 1970s is now a respected science called psychoneuroimmunology, or the study of how the mind, hormones, and immune system communicate. In recent years more and more proof points to the fact that the brain is not separate but is intricately intertwined with the body. What you eat, how well you cope with stress, how clearly you think today and in the future, your moods, and your risk for most major degenerative diseases are all interconnected. Let's first look at how stress affects the body, then investigate how diet can prevent the ravages of too much of the wrong kinds of stress.

Prehistoric Stress

To be alive is to be under stress. Everything from the ring of a doorbell to the loss of a loved one can trigger the stress response. Some things are stressful in a positive way. A new job, falling in love, or taking an art class are potentially stressful events that prompt us to reach our goals, become better people, or stretch our creative limits. Some stress is even fun, such as the thrill of a hot air balloon ride or watching a suspenseful movie. Stress also comes cloaked as worries, anger, jealousies, and fears, and these stressors—called distress—are the villains of health, although too much of any stress can be harmful.

Stress is your body's knee-jerk reaction to a threat. It is one of those survival-of-the-species basic instincts dating back to the beginning of life. Stress to the cave dweller meant physical danger. In those days a proper response to anything unusual or threatening was literally a matter of life and death. In Darwinian terms, those who responded quickly survived, while those who kicked back and ignored the threat didn't. The sight of a saber-toothed tiger triggered early people's nerves and glands to secrete numerous stress hormones such as cortisol. As a result the cave dweller's pupils dilated, nostrils flared, and vision improved, all in an effort to better identify the nature of the attacking beast. Muscles tensed and prepared the body to run, jump, or face the enemy. Breathing, pulse rate, and blood pressure increased, while blood vessels constricted, speeding oxygen and blood to the muscles and away from the internal organs. The liver released large amounts of glucose (sugar) into the bloodstream, and fat fragments (called free fatty acids) were released from fat cells to provide the fuel to "fight or flee." Within a split second the body was transformed from a peaceful state to war mode.

Today we are essentially cave dweller bodies dressed in designer clothes. We have traded the threat of a saber-toothed tiger for rush-hour traffic, intense time schedules, overextended lifestyles, and overcrowding. Stress comes from within as anger, unrealistic expectations, fears, and self-doubts. Our hearts still race, our blood pressures climb, our blood vessels constrict, and the stress hormones flood our systems in response to these modern-day tigers. But instead of expending our rallied defenses, as our ancestors did by running for cover or standing up to fight, we stew in our own juices. Stress hormones linger in the bloodstream, blood cholesterol and sugar levels rise, and nerve chemicals release in record numbers. It is this stressful stew pot that is linked to the loss of brain power and suppressed ability to fend off infection and numerous diseases—from peptic ulcers, asthma, and colds to cardiovascular disease and possibly cancer. How well do you cut back on your modern-day stress load? To find out, take Quiz 7.1, "Tally Your Stress Points," below.

Quiz 7.1   Tally Your Stress Points

Is your life balanced with some peace and an occasional bout of frenzy; always calm; or usually nuts? Rate each of the following statements depending on whether it is always true (1), never true (5), or somewhere in between.

1. I eat at least three nutritious meals or snacks a day.   _____
2. I drink less than three cups of coffee, cola, or other caffeinated
    beverages daily.   _____
3. I eat a minimal amount of sugary foods.   _____
4. I get at least seven hours of sleep.   _____
5. I give and receive affection and attention regularly.   _____
6. I have a circle of close friends and relatives who live close by on whom I
    can rely. I feel comfortable disclosing my feelings and beliefs to them.   _____
7. I believe most things will turn out all right and I am optimistic about the
    future.   _____
8. I set aside at least thirty minutes a day for quiet time.   _____
9. I do something fun at least three times a week.   _____
10. I exercise at an intensity that causes me to perspire at least five times
    a week.   _____
11. I avoid tobacco smoke.   _____
12. I drink less than five alcoholic drinks a week.   _____
13. I am able to pay my bills.   _____
14. I only worry about things that really matter and I usually handle daily
    stresses successfully and quickly.   _____
15. I am in good health.   _____
16. I usually feel secure and relaxed and seldom feel nervous, jittery, or high
    strung.   _____
17. I am happy with my home life.   _____
18. I am happy with my work and/or community involvement.   _____
19. I am able to quickly resolve conflicts at home and/or at work.   _____
20. I am a good time manager.   _____
21. I do not take street drugs, and I use prescription medications only when
    necessary and only with physician approval and monitoring.   _____

22. I laugh or chuckle daily and belly laugh regularly. (The average person laughs 540,000 times in his or her life. That equates to a minimum of twenty-one laugh episodes each day!)   _____

Scoring:

Under 36: Your stress level is relatively low.

37 to 46: You are moderately stressed and should take an inventory of your life to see what could be done to reduce your stress level.

47 to 57: Your life is very stressed and cannot support optimal health. Take action to reduce your stress load and increase your commitment to healthy habits and activities.

More than 57: Your life is extremely stressed. Don't waste another minute before making several changes to reduce the pressure. Choose a stress plan that will give you the greatest relaxation payoff for the least amount of effort.

The Mind-Body Connection

"The effects of stress on health and aging may be greater than we think," warns Robert Russell, M.D., professor of medicine and nutrition at Tufts University. In fact, stress is a major player in mood, food cravings, thinking, insomnia, and all aspects of emotional and physical health. The interactions between how you handle stress and your moods are far too complex to discuss in their entirety in this book. So here is a taste of how one stress hormone affects your mental and emotional well-being.

Within a split second of experiencing something stressful, a center in the brain called the hypothalamus secretes a hormone called corticotropin-releasing factor (CRF). This stimulates another brain center called the pituitary to release adrenocorticotropic hormone (ACTH), which, in turn, triggers the adrenal glands to release stress hormones into the system, including cortisol. When cortisol reaches peak levels, this tells the hypothalamus to shut off CRF release. Long-term or repeated bouts of stress, however, clog this feedback loop. As a result, cortisol levels remain high for extended periods of time.

Short bursts of cortisol are helpful to the stress response, but long-term or chronic exposure to this hormone is toxic to the brain and body. Cortisol reduces the brain's ability to use glucose, especially the hippocampus, which is a relay station for short-term memory. Cortisol affects the functioning of many nerve chemicals, including serotonin, dopamine, and neuropeptide Y, thus affecting eating habits, mood, and brain function (more on this on pages 176–177, 179–180). Excessive exposure to cortisol also is toxic to brain cells, increasing free-radical damage and ultimately killing them. This results in loss of memory, inability to retain new information, and reduced capacity to learn. Elevated cortisol levels also amplify the stress response, increasing anxiety, irritability, insomnia, eating disorders, and interfering with our ability to relax. The harmful effects of stress are magnified when people feel overwhelmed or "out of control." In contrast, people who handle stress effectively, eat well, exercise regularly to burn off those stress hormones, and who keep their cortisol levels low are healthier, live longer, and are most likely to maintain the brain power of a twenty-year-old!

Obviously, finding ways to both reduce unnecessary stress and effectively cope with the stress you can't avoid is critical to your health today and in the future. Dietary strategies for coping with stress are geared to:

1. Repairing any damage already done, and helping prevent future damage from cortisol and poor circulation that results from constricted blood vessels during stress.
2. Supplying the nutritional building blocks needed for optimal functioning of the brain, body, and immune system so these tissues can protect themselves against any harmful effects of the stress response.

How Stress Affects Your Nutrition

Stress and nutrition are closely intertwined. A nutritional deficiency is a stress in itself, since suboptimal amounts of one or more nutrients place a strain on all of the body's metabolic processes dependent on that nutrient. For example, even a slight iron deficiency reduces the oxygen supply to the tissues and brain; oxygen-starved tissues leave a person feeling tired, irritable, and unable to concentrate. Likewise, an inadequate intake of the B vitamins places stress on the cells' ability to convert carbohydrates and fats into energy. Suboptimal amounts of antioxidants like vitamin C weaken the body's antioxidant defenses, exposing the tissues to damage and disease. In addition, how well your body is nourished prior to and during a stressful event will affect how well you handle the stress. In short, a well-nourished person will cope better than a poorly nourished person.

On the other hand, stress affects nutrient needs by reducing absorption, increasing excretion, altering how the body uses the nutrients, or even increasing the daily requirements for certain nutrients. Yet people's eating habits often are at their nutritional worst during high stress. People who frequently diet tend to overeat all the wrong foods when stressed, and even people who eat well during the best of times can lose their appetites during high-stress times. Consequently, a person is more vulnerable to nutritional deficiencies when stressed than during almost any other time in life, and these nutrient deficiencies amplify the stress.

Any type of stress—from the physical stress of disease or surgery to the emotional stress of losing a loved one or the mental stresses at work—upsets nutritional balance, which in turn makes the stress just that much worse. If the stress is short-lived, such as a temporary increase in workload or anticipation of an upcoming event, and you are already well-nourished, you will handle the situation with less anxiety and the stress is not likely to significantly affect nutritional status. However, if you are marginally nourished prior to a stressful situation and/or the situation lasts for some time, such as a high-pressured job or years of juggling work and family responsibilities, you overtax your body's ability to handle this high-stress period, with nutritional status and overall health paying the price unless immediate action is taken to improve diet and coping skills.

Worry and the Common Cold

Emotional and mental stress suppresses the immune system, thus reducing your ability to fight off colds, infections, and disease. Let's first take a brief look at what makes the immune system tick, then discuss how stress and nutrition affect it.

The War Zone

Your body is like a fortress under siege. Everything in the environment, from the food you eat to the people you greet, exposes you to viruses, bacteria, and other microorganisms (or "germs") that can cause infection and disease. Whether or not you succumb to the daily attacks depends greatly on the strength of your immune system.

The immune system is your body's main defense against both foreign invaders and abnormal cell growth such as cancer. The armed forces of this system include organs, tissues, millions of cells, and numerous chemicals. For example, specialized white blood cells, called B-cells, circulate in the blood and other body fluids, where they neutralize the toxins produced by bacteria. B-cells secrete chemicals called antibodies, which act like Patriot Missiles specifically tailored to destroy foreign invaders. T-cells are the cornerstone of immunity within the cells. Among other things, T-cells produce chemicals called lymphokines, such as interferon, a protein that defends cells from viruses and is suspected to be a natural defense against cancer. Other specialized cells in the immune system include natural killer cells (free agents that act independently of other immune forces to locate and destroy germs), macrophages and monocytes, which surround and "neutralize" hostile substances, and other white blood cells.

This complex defense system provides constant feedback on the "state of the union." The result is a sensitive and intricate system of checks and balances that, in the presence of optimal nutrient intake and moderate to low stress, helps your body guarantee an armed defense against "germ warfare" and abnormal cell growth that is efficient, quick, and specific. On the other hand, a weakened immune system might fail to recognize an invader or fail to mount a strong attack. The results can be chronic or repeated infections, or more serious illnesses such as cancer.

Immunity, however, is not a black-and-white issue. "Whether the attacking organism or the immune system prevails depends on many factors, including a person's nutritional status, general health, stress level, and sleep patterns, as well as the force of the onslaught," says Darshan Kelley, Ph.D., research chemist at the Western Human Nutrition Research Center in Davis, California. It is the total picture that determines a person's resistance to disease.

The Stress Factor

As your heart starts racing and the perspiration appears on your brow, the stress response also is suppressing your immune system. As a result, antibody production decreases, T-lymphocytes retreat, and B-lymphocyte numbers decline. Even minor nuisances, such as loud noise and bright lights, can affect your body's natural defenses. Depression, loss of a loved one, and other major stresses suppress the immune system by as much as 50 percent in some people. Consequently, the more a person is stressed, the greater the need to support the defense system by:

- Eating breakfast.
- Eating a nutrient-packed and low-fat diet.
- Avoiding tobacco.
- Limiting alcohol consumption.
- Sleeping at least seven hours a night.

- Working less than ten hours a day.
- Exercising daily.
- Using effective stress-management skills such as time management, deep breathing, meditation, progressive relaxation, yoga, music therapy, or aromatherapy.
- Nurturing positive beliefs, attitudes, and expectations, including hope, trust, love, faith, and laughter, which enhance the immune system.

Stress-Fighting Nutrition Factors

Diet, immunity, and stress are so intertwined that it is difficult to know where one stops and the next begins. One thing is clear: You can help lower cortisol levels, boost your natural defenses, help calm yourself, and curb the negative effects of stress on your body and mind by fueling your body with the nutrients it needs to stay healthy. But it will take some focus and willpower to give your body what it needs rather than what it might be craving.

Why Do We Crave Sweets When We're Stressed?

The stress hormone cortisol scrambles our appetite-control chemicals, which affects food intake and mood. Cortisol turns on the production of neuropeptide Y (NPY), alters dopamine levels, and lowers serotonin. It's no wonder we make poor food choices when we're stressed, turning to sweets, salty snacks, and processed grains. (See chapters 1 and 2 for more on NPY and dopamine.) Consequently, weight gain during stressful times might be a result of this altered chemistry, which prompts overeating, especially of sugary foods. (See From Mood to Food and Back, on page 177.)

At a time when you need your mental, physical, and emotional reserves, sugar can leave you at wits' end with plummeting blood-sugar levels and a host of brain chemicals in disarray. Sugar is an accomplice to many health problems, since it either replaces nutritious foods or adds unwanted calories. When sugar intake increases above 9 percent of total calories, your vitamin and mineral intake progressively decreases, which compromises your immune system and adds further stress to a body already under pressure. A high-sugar diet also increases urinary losses of calming minerals, including magnesium and chromium.

From Mood to Food and Back to Mood:

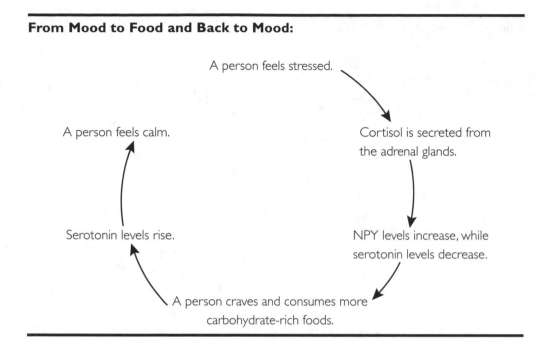

A person feels stressed.

Cortisol is secreted from the adrenal glands.

A person feels calm.

Serotonin levels rise.

NPY levels increase, while serotonin levels decrease.

A person craves and consumes more carbohydrate-rich foods.

Larry Christensen, Ph.D., at the University of South Alabama reports that people suffering from emotional stress feel better if they eliminate sugar and coffee from their diets. In his studies, people were less stressed and showed improved emotional stability within two weeks of initiating low-sugar, low-caffeine diets. Dr. Christensen admits the relationship between specific dietary factors and psychological problems is poorly understood and might vary dramatically from one person to another. However, you have nothing to lose and everything to gain by adopting a nutrient-packed, low-sugar, and low-caffeine diet. See Table 7.1, "Quick Fix Snacks," on page 178, for nutritious alternatives to high-sugar snacks.

Stress and Fat Don't Mix

As if there wasn't enough wrong with high-fat diets, a study from the University of Maryland at College Park reports that high-fat diets, especially vegetable oils, raise stress hormone levels and interfere with the body's ability to calm itself even after the stress is over. Cutting back on fat and adopting a low-fat vegetarian diet lowers cortisol levels.

Table 7.1   Quick-Fix Snacks

- 1 mango
- 4 cups of air-popped popcorn
- Drizzle 1 tablespoon of fat-free chocolate syrup over 2 cups of fresh strawberries.
- 1 large pear
- Strawberry-kiwi pudding: Mix $1/2$ cup fresh strawberries, two peeled and sliced kiwi, and one 6-ounce low-fat strawberry-kiwi yogurt. Place in a bowl and top with a sprig of fresh mint or one strawberry. Serve with two vanilla wafers.
- $1/2$ cup fresh pineapple chunks with $1/2$ cup 1 percent low-fat cottage cheese
- Candied-ginger fruit salad: In a bowl, mix one peeled and sectioned orange, $1/2$ peeled and sliced banana, $1/2$ peeled and diced mango or papaya, and one sliced plum. Toss fruit with 1 tablespoon orange juice concentrate, 1 teaspoon lemon peel, and 1 tablespoon crumbled candied ginger. Place in a parfait glass and serve with one ladyfinger cookie.
- Cranberry spritzer: Mix 8 ounces of cranberry juice with 8 ounces of sparkling water, ice cubes, and a twist of lemon.
- A large baked apple: Core an apple; fill its hollow with sugar-free cranberry soda pop and a dash of cinnamon and nutmeg. Bake at 350 degrees Fahrenheit for forty-five minutes.
- OJ ice cubes (a great alternative to munching on ice cubes!): Pour orange juice into ice cube trays and freeze.
- Large prawns, steamed and dipped in tomato-based cocktail sauce
- Low-fat tortilla chips with salsa
- Steamed pea pods with fat-free sour cream dip: Season with chili sauce, crushed garlic, lemon, grated orange peel, or curry.
- Orange slices dipped in fat-free chocolate syrup
- Glacéed grapes: Rinse grapes in water, then roll lightly in granulated sugar.
- Cherry tomatoes, cucumber slices, and hummus
- Cooked large white beans (fava) marinated in lemon juice, garlic, fresh sage, and wine
- Three fig bars and 1 cup of warmed nonfat milk flavored with almond extract and sprinkled with nutmeg
- $1/2$ cantaloupe filled with 6 ounces of low-fat lemon yogurt and topped with 1 tablespoon of lemon zest
- Two slices of extra-lean ham lunch meat, twelve fat-free whole wheat crackers, and water
- Fruit parfait: In a parfait glass, mix the following with 1 tablespoon orange juice concentrate, layer, and top with 1 tablespoon light whipped cream: one orange, peeled and sectioned; $1/2$ cup fresh strawberries; $1/2$ banana, sliced.

A low-fat diet also stimulates the immune system, while dietary fat—especially polyunsaturated fats found in vegetable oils, trans fatty acids (TFAs) in margarine and shortening, and saturated fats in meats and whole milk products—suppress the immune system. "Partially hydrogenated vegetable oils are a real problem," warns Mary Enig, Ph.D., former research associate at the University of Maryland and one of the first researchers to investigate TFAs in our food. What Dr. Enig began uncovering in the early 1980s has been confirmed by numerous studies since: TFAs, in amounts typically consumed by Americans, alter basic metabolic pathways, tamper with cell membranes, and generate free radicals that further suppress the immune response. The potential health risks of TFAs wouldn't be an issue except that we're eating a lot more than we think. Up until the turn of the century, the naturally occurring TFAs in meat and dairy products comprised a small portion of the diet (approximately 3 percent of total fat intake). But that changed dramatically when the food industry introduced hydrogenation into commercial food production, frying French fries and potato chips in hydrogenated vegetable oils. "People typically consume 10 to 15 grams of TFAs every day," warns Dr. Enig. Eliminating foods that contain these oils, including processed snack foods, fried fast foods, and margarine, would help maintain a strong immune system during times of stress.

Some fats boost immunity and reduce your risk for developing stress-related diseases, such as the oils in fish. Including two or three servings of fish in your weekly diet helps improve immune responses and reduce the risk for developing stress-induced colds, infections, and disease, including cancer. For example, in a study at the University of Marburg in Germany, fish oils lowered heart rates and blood pressure in a group of mentally stressed animals. Olive oil, on the other hand, appears neutral, neither raising nor suppressing immunity. Studies on animals support these findings and show that limiting total fat—by reducing saturated fats, corn and vegetable oils, and hydrogenated vegetable oils and holding constant or slightly increasing the intake of fish and olive oils—helps improve wound healing and immunity in stressed animals.

Fats, in the guise of sweet-and-creamy tastes like chocolate, desserts, ice cream, and even whole-milk yogurt, trigger the release of endorphins, the brain chemicals that calm and soothe. If these nerve chemicals are charting your course, then it is best to work with your chemicals, rather than against them. Plan nutrient-packed carbo snacks, such as raisin toast with all-fruit jam, or Cheerios and dried apricots, for your crave-prone times of the day. In addition, keep moving. Exercise helps use up the extra carbohydrates so they are not converted to fat. Until more is known about how fat affects the stress response and immunity, following a low-fat diet as outlined in the Feeling Good Diet in chapter 12 is the best bet.

Caffeine Jitters, High Anxiety

Caffeine gives coffee and cola their punch. Virtually all of the caffeine in these beverages is absorbed and quickly distributed throughout the body. Within half an hour, caffeine's stimulating effects can be felt. Caffeine has a direct effect on the brain and central nervous system. Thought processes and regulatory processes, such as heart rate, respiration, and muscle coordination, are affected after drinking even one cup of coffee. Three or more cups can give you the "coffee jitters." In addition, coffee consumed with food can reduce mineral absorption, especially iron, by as much as 90 percent and can rob the body of other minerals, such as calcium and magnesium, needed during times of stress.

Caffeine lingers in the body for hours, escalating the stress response. In fact, caffeine alone can cause anxiety symptoms. As a consequence, coffee can add to the stress equation by aggravating the stress chemicals and interfering with sleep (coffee drinkers take longer to fall asleep, sleep less soundly, and wake up more often than nonusers). Substituting a cup of tea or a diet cola for an evening cup of coffee is not the solution, since both the tea and the cola contain the same amount of caffeine as a cup of instant coffee.

The Minerals

Researchers at the U.S. Department of Agriculture studied the effects of work-related stress on mineral status and found that despite adequate dietary intake, blood levels of several minerals dropped as much as 33 percent, and tissue stores for certain nutrients were depleted, during a five-day "Hell Week" at work where employees were given extra work and asked to meet difficult deadlines.

This loss of minerals jeopardizes the immune system and aggravates the stress response. For example, stress triggers the release of the stress hormones, which drains magnesium from the body and increases dietary requirements for the mineral. The stress-induced magnesium deficiency raises stress hormone levels, escalates the stress response, and causes stress-related depression and irritability. Studies on laboratory animals show that a magnesium deficiency increases sensitivity to noise and crowding and escalates stress-induced diseases such as ulcers, while animals whose diets are high in magnesium cope better and are at lower risk for disease.

The link between magnesium and stress is so strong that researchers at the American College of Nutrition recommend people supplement with magnesium during times of stress. According to Mildred Seelig, M.D., M.P.H., at the University of North Carolina, taking calcium supplements without also increasing magnesium intake upsets the ratio of these two minerals and intensifies a magnesium deficiency, which could further escalate the stress response. So it's prudent to also supplement with magnesium along with calcium. Your needs for chromium, copper, iron, selenium, and zinc also increase during stress.

The Antioxidants

Vitamins C and E and other antioxidant nutrients help regulate the immune system and are affected by stress as well. (See chapter 8 for more on the antioxidants.) Both emotional and physical stress increase the amount of dietary vitamin C the body needs. The stress glands, including the adrenals and the pituitary, are major storage sites for vitamin C in the body. During times of stress, these stores are depleted, which could intensify the body's stress response by elevating stress hormone levels. This creates a catch-22 situation where stress-induced loss of vitamin C undermines the immune system's ability to defend against disease and escalates the stress response, which further depletes vitamin C levels and increases the likelihood of further stress. All it takes is an increase in vitamin C from fruits and vegetables or supplements to break this cycle. Vitamin E also is a key player in immunity; just supplementing with this vitamin can boost dwindling immune responses.

Typical American diets are low in vitamins C and E, and possibly other antioxidants, such as beta carotene. In addition, diet alone might not be enough during times of stress. "In our studies on seniors using 60 IU, 200 IU, and 800 IUs of vitamin E, we found that the 200 IU daily dose was most effective in boosting immune function," says Simin Nikbin Meydani, DVM, Ph.D., professor of nutrition and immunology at Tufts University in Boston. It would take two and one-half cups of safflower oil or forty-six cups of spinach to reach this level of vitamin E. Consequently, supplements are necessary.

According to the latest national nutrition survey from the U.S. Food and Drug Administration, 99 percent of Americans are not eating antioxidant-rich diets that include at least five, and preferably nine, daily servings of fresh fruits and vegetables.

Table 7.2   Calming Foods

The following snacks are low-fat, low-calorie, and packed with vitamins and minerals that help soothe a stressed body. Keep in mind that the total diet is what is important. No one food can transform an otherwise poor diet into a great eating plan.

SNACK	AMOUNT	GOOD SOURCE OF
SWEET:		
Apricots, fresh	3 medium	Beta carotene, potassium, iron
Bananas	1 medium	Potassium, vitamin B_6, magnesium
Raspberries, fresh	2/3 cup	Beta carotene, vitamin C, potassium, iron, magnesium, manganese
Orange slices	1 cup	Vitamin C, folic acid, beta carotene, calcium, potassium
Papaya	1 medium	Beta carotene, vitamin C, potassium, calcium
Mango	1 medium	Beta carotene, niacin, vitamin B_6, folic acid, calcium, vitamin E, potassium
Strawberries, fresh	2 cups	Vitamin C, folic acid, potassium, iron, manganese
Frozen blueberries	1 1/4 cups	Beta carotene, potassium, manganese
Peaches, canned in own juice, and	1 small	Beta carotene, potassium
nonfat yogurt	1/2 cup	Calcium, magnesium, vitamin B_2
Dried cranberries	2/3 cup	Vitamin B_6, potassium, calcium, iron, copper, manganese
Dried figs	2	Calcium, iron, magnesium, potassium, selenium
Baked Apple*	1 medium	Beta carotene, potassium, iron
Raisin bread dipped	1 slice	B vitamins, iron, calcium, magnesium,
in nonfat apple-spice yogurt	1/4 cup	vitamin B_2
Pumpkin Mousse Pie*	1 slice	Beta carotene, iron, calcium, vitamin D
CRUNCHY:		
Fat-free refried	1/4 cup,	B vitamins, iron, folic acid, vitamin C,
beans, chips, and salsa	1 ounce, 1/4 cup	magnesium, potassium, zinc

* See "Recipes for Feeling Your Best" at the back of this book.

Celery sticks filled with nonfat	4 stalks	B vitamins, calcium, magnesium,
ricotta cheese and unsweetened	1/3 cup	potassium, zinc
crushed pineapple	1/3 cup	
Shredded carrots and	1 cup	Beta carotene, B vitamins, calcium,
raisins, with	1 tablespoon	iron, potassium, selenium, zinc
nonfat poppy seed dressing	1 tablespoon	
on whole wheat toast	1 slice	
Red bell peppers with	2	Vitamin B_6, folic acid, vitamin C,
curried nonfat yogurt dip	1/4 cup	vitamin E, potassium
Baked tortilla chips	1 ounce	Iron, magnesium, zinc
Broccoli, raw, with	1 cup	B vitamins, folic acid, vitamin C,
nonfat sour cream dip	1/4 cup	vitamin E, calcium, iron, magnesium,
		potassium, selenium, zinc
Carrots with	1 1/3 cups	Beta carotene, calcium, iron, potassium
nonfat cream cheese and	1/4 cup	
garlic dip	1 clove	
Cantaloupe	1/2	Beta carotene, folic acid, vitamin C,
		calcium, magnesium, potassium

TASTY:

Veggie Flat Bread Pizza*	1	Beta carotene, potassium, vitamin C
Warm microwave	1	Iron, zinc
whole-grain pretzel with mustard		
Thai Wrap*	1	Vitamin C, folic acid, potassium, iron
Grilled Chicken Salsa Wrap*	1	Protein, B vitamins, vitamin C, potassium,
		iron, selenium, zinc
Open-Faced Black Bean	1	B vitamins, folic acid, calcium
Burrito*		iron, potassium, selenium, zinc
Vegetable Lentil Soup*	3/4 cup	Folic acid, calcium, iron, magnesium,
		potassium, selenium, zinc
Nonfat milk with almond extract	1 cup	Calcium, vitamin B_2, vitamin D
Wheat germ	1/4 cup	B vitamins, vitamin E, calcium, iron,
(sprinkled on anything)		magnesium, potassium, selenium, zinc

* See "Recipes for Feeling Your Best" at the back of this book.

If you're stressed and not consuming at least two fruits and vegetables at meals and snacks, then consider taking a supplement that contains at least 250 milligrams of vitamin C. (See Table 7.2, "Calming Foods," on pages 182–183, for more information.)

The B Vitamins

Our bodies' B vitamin requirements increase slightly during times of stress. Most of the B vitamins help develop or maintain the nervous system, which is in overdrive during stressful events. Your need for vitamins B_1, B_2, and other B vitamins increases as calorie intake increases, since these vitamins are essential in converting calories from food into energy in the body. Therefore, a deficiency results either from a vitamin-poor diet or from excessive intake of high-calorie, nutrient-poor foods, such as sweets and refined/highly processed foods. Even slight vitamin deficiencies further upset the nervous system and contribute to stress-related symptoms, such as irritability, lethargy, depression, and suppressed immunity.

Studies conducted at Loma Linda University and Oregon State University report that increasing vitamin B_6 intake raises blood levels of the vitamin and enhances the immune response. But large supplemental doses (250 milligrams or more) of vitamin B_6 can be toxic, so stick with a moderate-dose multiple that includes vitamin B_6 along with vitamin B_6–rich foods, such as bananas, avocados, chicken (without the skin), fish, baked potatoes, and dark green leafy vegetables.

Cholesterol and Hostility: Is There a Connection?

For years people were told to lower their blood cholesterol levels and to take it easy, because aggressive and competitive personalities, called Type A's, are more prone to developing heart disease. Then researchers switched gears, reporting that people with very low blood cholesterol levels or who consumed low-fat diets might avoid heart disease, but were more depressed and aggressive and likely to commit suicide or die a violent death.

The obvious, but erroneous, assumption is to draw a direct link between low cholesterol levels and hostility. Some people even came to the conclusion that low-fat diets make people angry enough to kill themselves. Wrong. It is more likely that some other variable is linked to low cholesterol and hostility, or that the link is nonexistent and only a fluke find in a few studies. For example, a study from the University of Edinburgh in the United Kingdom found no association between low cholesterol levels and anger. Some studies even reported that people's moods improved, showing less depression and aggressive hostility, when their blood cholesterol levels dropped. Even if low-fat diets did make people grumpy, a daily exercise program more than compensated by boosting mood, relieving depression and stress, and further lowering risk factors for heart disease such as elevated blood fats.

More recently, studies show that low intake of certain fats might aggravate an already stressed or angry disposition. Special fats found in fish oil, called the omega-3 fatty acids, help regulate mood by increasing serotonin levels, the nerve chemical that relieves depression. Low intake of fish oils lowers brain levels of serotonin in animals and increases aggressive and hostile behaviors. Similar effects have been noted in humans with lower fish oil consumption and serotonin levels, including increased rates of impulsive suicide attempts, according to researchers at the National Institute of Alcohol Abuse and Alcoholism in Bethesda, Maryland. (See chapters 6 and 8 for more on fish oils, mind, and memory.)

The lesson to be learned from this confusion is that one study does not a conclusion make. One study is like a thread in a tapestry of research that must be replicated over and over by other well-designed research studies before the results can be taken seriously enough to make general dietary and lifestyle recommendations. In the meantime, just make sure you add a few weekly servings of fish to the Feeling Good Diet!

Calm Down with Exercise

Our ancient ancestors knew what to do about stress: They ran away from it, or stood up and fought it. Exercise is still the best way to relieve stress, burn off those health-damaging stress hormones, boost your body's natural defenses against the ravages of stress, and prevent the wear and tear of the body that results in infection today and disease later in life. Exercise increases blood flow, encourages the growth of new cells in the brain and body, lowers cortisol levels, improves mood, and helps you see the bright side during stressful times. It acts as a natural tranquilizer and reduces fatigue, anger, and tension associated with stress. People who exercise regularly report less stress, are calmer, and handle stress better than sedentary folks.

Researchers disagree on whether strenuous or moderate exercise is the best, but they do agree that the more exercise you do, the better.

Stress-Proof Basics

Obviously, too much stress isn't good for you, but sometimes it is unavoidable. So, when you can't beat stress, join it, but go into battle nutritionally well armed. When stressed, every bite counts. The Feeling Good Diet is the foundation of your defense strategies, with some modifications.

1. Cut back on colas. Granted, most people don't drink enough fluids when under stress and would benefit by hydrating their high anxiety; however, soda pop is not the best choice. Americans consume more than 450 servings per person per year of soft drinks; at five to nine teaspoons of sugar per serving, that equals 2,250 to 4,050 teaspoons of sugar from soft drinks alone, not counting the caffeine load. Limit your intake to no more than one 12-ounce serving of soda a day, preferably a decaffeinated, diet variety.

2. Savor a cup of coffee, but don't go back for seconds. Too much caffeine only increases anxiety. Switch to decaffeinated, grain-based beverages such as Postum, or mix regular coffee or tea with decaffeinated to cut back. For every cup of coffee or tea you have, drink two glasses of water.

3. Cut out sweets until the stress subsides. You don't have nutritional room for high-fat, high-sugar, or low-nutrient foods. Plus, sweets fuel the stress response. Instead, turn to naturally sweet fruits, whole grains, and other nutritious foods recommended in the Feeling Good Diet. (See Table 7.2, "Calming Foods," on pages 182–183.)

4. Keep fiber in mind. Often the digestive tract is hit hard by stress. To ensure normal bowel function, include at least five fiber-rich fresh fruits and vegetables, six servings of whole-grain breads and cereals, and one serving of cooked dried beans and peas in the daily diet. A variety of fibers is important, so don't depend on processed "bran" cereal for your daily fiber needs.

5. If you lose your appetite when you're under pressure, try to eat six to eight mini-meals throughout the day rather than force yourself to

Table 7.3   Breakfast Quick Fixes

Are you burning the candle at both ends, with no time left for breakfast? The following meals can be prepared in five to ten minutes, so there is no excuse for not eating breakfast. Remember to allow yourself a few minutes to sit down, relax, and enjoy the meal!

BREAKFAST #1

1 cup oatmeal and 2 tablespoons toasted wheat germ, cooked in 1 cup nonfat milk, topped with 2 tablespoons raisins, 2 tablespoons chopped walnuts, and 1 tablespoon brown sugar. Serve with one sliced banana sprinkled with cinnamon powder. (Can be made in microwave to save even more time.)

BREAKFAST #2

One toasted whole wheat English muffin, topped with 2 tablespoons peanut butter. Serve with 1 1/4 cup fresh blueberries sprinkled with lemon zest and 1 cup nonfat milk flavored with vanilla, nutmeg, and/or NutraSweet.

BREAKFAST #3

1 cup shredded wheat minibiscuits, topped with 1 cup nonfat milk, 1 tablespoon chopped almonds, 2 tablespoons dried cranberries, and 1 tablespoon brown sugar. Serve with 1 cup fresh strawberries.

BREAKFAST #4

Two small or 1 large bran muffin with 2 tablespoons cashew butter. Serve with 3/4 cup hot cocoa made with nonfat milk and sugar-free mix and 1/2 cantaloupe or honeydew melon, drizzled with lime juice.

BREAKFAST #5

Two slices low-fat French toast (made with nonfat milk), sprinkled with powdered sugar. Serve with 1/2 cup stewed prunes and 1 cup fresh-squeezed orange juice.

BREAKFAST #6

Two pancakes, made with low-fat Bisquick, nonfat milk, eggs, and 1 tablespoon wheat germ per pancake, topped with 2 tablespoons nonfat sour cream, 1/4 cup apricots canned in their own juice, and one banana, peeled and sliced. Serve with 1 cup nonfat milk or vanilla-flavored soy milk.

BREAKFAST #7

Veggie omelette: Whip one whole egg and two egg whites and pour into nonstick, 10-inch frying pan coated with vegetable spray. Cover and cook over medium heat until cooked through and firm. Remove in one piece, place on plate, fill with steamed vegetables (onions, garlic, zucchini, mushrooms, red peppers, etc.) and fresh herbs. Fold egg mixture over vegetables-herbs to form an omelette. Serve with one slice whole wheat bread, toasted, topped with 1 tablespoon apricot preserves, and 6 ounces grapefruit juice.

BREAKFAST #8

Breakfast burrito: Sauté chopped onion, garlic, and green pepper in 1 tablespoon water until tender. Add $1/2$ cup egg substitute, salt and pepper to taste, and scramble. Heat a 10-inch flour tortilla and fill with egg mixture, $1/2$ ounce grated sharp cheddar cheese, and 1 tablespoon fresh salsa. Serve with 1 cup fresh orange juice and a decaffeinated latte made with skim milk.

BREAKFAST #9

Two whole-grain frozen waffles, toasted and topped with 2 tablespoons fat-free sour cream and 1 cup fresh blueberries. Serve with 1 cup orange juice.

---

eat a few big meals. Listen to your body and eat foods that sound good, as long as they are wholesome choices. If you overeat when stressed, snack on low-fat goodies and eliminate high-fat temptations until your willpower returns. Stash nutritious foods in your glove compartment, desk drawer, briefcase or purse, or in the employee kitchen so you won't be caught off guard by a craving. Increase your exercise to compensate for the extra calories. (See Table 7.3, "Breakfast Quick Fixes," on pages 187–188.)

6. Eliminate alcohol or limit intake to five drinks a week or less. Alcohol adds further stress to the body and contains empty calories you can't afford to waste right now.

7. Take a moderate-dose multiple vitamin and mineral supplement that supplies a wide variety of vitamins and minerals, including the B vitamins, calcium, magnesium, chromium, copper, iron, manganese, molybdenum, selenium, and zinc. Follow the guidelines in chapter 14 for choosing the best supplement. Vitamin E is safe in adult doses up to 400 IU, and vitamin C is safe up to 1,000 milligrams for most adults.

Avoid supplements labeled as "stress" or "therapeutic" formulations. At best, these products are a waste of money. At worst, their imbalanced formulations could aggravate a preexisting nutrient deficiency, which would further compromise your immune defenses and ability to cope with stress. "Balance is the key with the minerals," says Dr. Adria Sherman, Ph.D., professor of nutritional sciences at Rutgers University. "These nutrients interact and it is their unified effect on immunity that is important." Dr. Sherman also emphasizes that this balance is best found in nutritious foods, not supplements. (See Table 7.4, "Herbs and Supplements to Fight Stress: What Works, What Doesn't, and Why," below.)

Table 7.4   Herbs and Supplements to Fight Stress: What Works, What Doesn't, and Why

Chicken soup: Chicken soup contains cysteine, a compound that thins the mucus in the lungs, making it easier to expel.

Echinacea: This herb appears to naturally stimulate your immune system by turning on blood chemicals that regulate the duration and intensity of the immune response. Thus, either the capsules or the drops taken several times during the day might curb cold and flu symptoms. Make sure the product states on the label that it is standardized, or you're likely to see little or no results. Don't take echinacea for more than two to three weeks at a time, however, since its protective effects might wear off with prolonged use.

Garlic: Garlic contains potent antibacterial and antiviral compounds that might help fend off stress-induced colds and infections.

Ginseng: This root might enhance immunity and act as a tonic in animals; there are no well-designed scientific studies to show a similar effect in humans. Many products on the market contain little or none of the active ingredients in ginseng, the ginsenosides. So look for products that contain the root or a standardized ginsenoside content.

Herbs and spices: Licorice soothes an irritated throat, fenugreek lubricates and soothes coughs, and capsaicin in red and cayenne peppers relieves nasal stuffiness. The herb horehound is an effective expectorant, and hyssop helps treat upper respiratory infections. Teas made from chamomile also might soothe a stressed body.

Kava: This South Pacific plant has antianxiety effects, might reduce pain, and improves mental clarity. Kavalactones in kava act on the part of the brain where emotions and moods are processed. Optimal doses are unknown, although 100 milligrams of kava extract taken three times daily has proven effective in some studies. Look for products standardized to contain at least 70 percent kavalactones (60 to 75 milligrams/capsule). Do not take with prescription drugs, when driving or operating heavy equipment, with alcohol, if you are under eighteen, or if you're pregnant or nursing.

Valerian: This root might act as a mild tranquilizer, depressing the central nervous system and relieving muscle spasms. The herb is typically taken an hour before bedtime in a dose of 50 to 100 drops of the tincture or tea prepared from 1 teaspoon of dried root. Might cause stomach upsets.

Zinc lozenges: This form of zinc might not prevent the common cold, but a handful of studies show that it might shorten the duration and severity of some symptoms, such as coughing, headaches, hoarseness, congestion, and sore throat. Taking one or two of these daily is worth a try, but watch out for overdoses. More than 35 to 50 milligrams of zinc taken daily over time actually suppresses the immune system and could interfere with your body's efforts to get well.

CHAPTER EIGHT

Smart Foods

- Are you frequently stumped midsentence, with the right word on the tip of your tongue?
- Can't remember what's-his-name's name, let alone where you put the keys?
- Do you punch in a number on the telephone and, as it's ringing, realize you've forgotten whom you called?
- Do you walk into a room and can't remember why you went in there?
- Do you forget whether you did something, like lock a door or turn off the coffeepot?

About the time you start appreciating how vital your memory is, you're losing it. In fact, by the time people reach their fifties, their scores on memory tests are reduced to about half of what they scored in their twenties. Reaction times also slow, affecting how fast we hit the brakes when a car pulls in front of us and how quickly we learn new skills on the job or remember what's-his-name's name. Mental slumps, poor concentration, slowed reaction times, forgetfulness, and loss of creative thinking aren't limited to the middle years; they can hit us at any age. Don't worry—it's unlikely you're suffering from anything more serious than being tired, stressed, depressed, lonely, or just plain not taking good care of your health. There is much you can do to stop the progressive mental funk; you even might restore your thinking to peak performance.

The History of Smart Foods

What you eat could have profound effects on how you think, on your intelligence level, and on your memory. For example, what you eat affects the following:

1. The level of nerve chemicals in the brain that regulate all mental processes.
2. The development and maintenance of brain cell function and structure.
3. The insulating sheath surrounding nerve cells that speeds the transport of messages from one neuron to the next.
4. The level of enzymes and their activity, which enhances brain functions.
5. The amount of oxygen that reaches the brain.
6. The rate of accumulation and removal of cellular waste products.
7. The ability of brain cells to transmit electrical messages.
8. The efficiency of brain cell membranes to transport nutrients into, and debris out of, the cell.

When we don't consume the right mix of brain-boosting nutrients, our brain cells (all 100 billion of them!) don't function optimally and can even die. The results show up as memory loss, reduced ability to think clearly and quickly, poor concentration, acceleration of the age-related changes in brain tissue, reduced ability to learn and reason, leading to a lowered IQ, and a dwindling desire to learn.

On the other hand, choosing the right mix of foods and nutrients could keep you thinking quickly and remembering well throughout life. Take, for example, a study from the University of New Mexico School of Medicine in Albuquerque, where researchers investigated nutritional status and brain power in a group of people aged sixty-six to ninety years old. Their performances on a battery of mental tests were directly related to how well nourished they were in the present and in the past. As nutritional status went up, so did cognitive performance. Optimal vitamin intake enhanced abstract thought and boosted test scores. And that's just the start of what nutrition can do! How's your mental health? To find out, take the quiz on page 193.

Quiz 8.1   How's Your Mental Health?

Answer yes or no to the following statements:

1. Lately, I've had trouble naming things that are familiar to me.
2. My memory isn't as good as it used to be.
3. I often forget important meetings, appointments, or other planned responsibilities.
4. I find it more difficult to concentrate than in the past.
5. I sometimes get confused about what time it is or where I am.
6. I rely on coffee to stay alert.
7. I sometimes repeat the same story to the same people within a short amount of time.
8. I'm not as interested in learning and trying new things as I used to be.
9. My attention span isn't what it used to be.
10. I often walk into a room and can't remember what I came in to get.
11. I have trouble listening to people because my mind wanders.
12. I frequently find myself blankly staring out the window.
13. My verbal skills and vocabulary are not as good as they used to be.
14. I have trouble keeping up with conversations and often bluff my way through a conversation.
15. My work performance has dropped recently.
16. I put things away and then can't remember where I put them.

Few people can answer no to all of the above statements. However, the more times you answered yes to these statements, the more likely it is that you are suffering from mental fatigue. In most cases, memory loss, confusion, or other mental problems are only minor irritants that are easily corrected by changes in your diet or lifestyle. More serious problems always should be discussed with your physician.

It Starts Earlier Than You Think

What your mother, and possibly even your grandmother, consumed during pregnancy could be affecting how smart you are today. Recent research shows that the developing baby is much more sensitive to the mother's nutritional status than previously thought, with the consequences not always appearing until much later in life. The phenomenon is called "programming," which means that poor intake of one or more essential nutrients during critical periods in an organ's growth can permanently alter or program the structure, size, or function of that organ. "There are very good data that indicate fetal growth affects adult disease risks," says Irvin Emanuel, M.D., professor of epidemiology and pediatrics at the University of Washington in Seattle. Researchers suspect that inadequate nutrition during fetal development compromises intellectual development and increases the child's risk later in life for disease and even obesity. According to Dr. Emanuel, even the nutritional status of our grandmothers affects our health by influencing how well our mothers developed in the womb. "The changes are subtle, but accumulate over generations," he says.

Skimping on specific vitamins and minerals before, during, and following pregnancy also can backfire. For example, an inadequate supply of iodine in a mother results in severe mental retardation of her child; too little folic acid results in neural tube defects; and not enough protein and calories results in a small head and brain size and reduced desire to learn, IQ, and intellect. A shortage of iron in a pregnant woman's diet results in apathy and lowered IQ scores later in the life of her developing child. Not enough vitamin B_6 results in seizures and irritability in newborns, while too little calcium results in low calcium levels in a nursing mother's breast milk, jeopardizing the health of the nursing baby.

We also know that babies who are breast-fed are smarter than formula-fed babies, probably because breast milk contains special fats called the omega-3 fatty acids, which are essential to normal brain development but are not found in commercial formulas. (See below for more on the omega-3 fatty acids.)

Since the cause-and-effect link between diet and the brain is clear during this critical fetal growth period, it is likely that poor nutrition at other stages of life also affects how we think, remember, learn, and concentrate. Current research shows that poor lifelong dietary habits and failure to supplement with the necessary nutrients probably speeds the progression of age-related memory loss and other cognitive functions. Chronic stress bathes the brain in cortisol (a stress hormone), which also speeds age-related memory loss. On a more positive note, many of these effects are reversible if unhealthy habits are permanently changed. At most stages in your life you can boost brain power by making a few simple changes in what, when, and how much you eat, as well as in how you handle stress and how frequently you exercise.

A Word of Caution

Don't take feeling well as a sign of thinking well. Nutrient requirements are based on physical symptoms of vitamin, mineral, and protein deficiencies. Yet the brain shows changes in thinking, memory, personality, and intelligence long before symptoms appear in the body. You might have trouble remembering things or you may feel "under the weather," but don't feel ill enough to seek medical attention. Even if you did, it's unlikely a physician would detect subtle dietary problems that are undermining your thinking. Consequently, vague, yet profound, changes in mental ability can progress undetected because you otherwise feel fine. In fact, impaired mental function always precedes physical problems, so look to your diet first before blaming your age or heredity factors for lapses in memory, thinking, or concentration.

As You Eat, So Shall You Think

Even if you're the most absentminded person, thinking clearly is within your grasp and can be as simple as taking five minutes to eat breakfast; keeping lunch light; approaching weight loss with a little common sense; or including a few more fruits and vegetables in your daily menu.

Take the Morning Train to Forgetville

People who eat breakfast think better and faster, remember more, react quicker, and are mentally sharper than breakfast skippers. They also miss fewer days of school and work. Just about every measure of thinking ability improves after eating a good breakfast—from math scores and creative thinking to speed and efficiency in solving problems, concentration, recall, and accuracy in work performance. Compared to breakfast skippers, people who eat breakfast communicate more effectively, make fewer mistakes, get the job done more quickly, and are more creative throughout the day.

The link between breakfast and the brain starts with energy. The brain is a very metabolically hungry tissue. The 100 billion nerve cells and an equal amount of supporting cells in the brain account for only 2 percent of body weight but use between 20 and 30 percent of the calories you eat in a day. The brain also is fuel fussy, demanding that all its energy come from glucose (the fuel found in sweets and starchy foods).

The trick to thinking clearly and avoiding mental fatigue is to eat a breakfast but to stick with carbohydrate-rich cereal or pancakes, since eating a high-fat breakfast will leave you feeling "less vigorous, [less] imaginative," and less alert, and "more feeble and fatigued," according to researchers at the University of Sheffield in the United Kingdom. That is as simple as having a bowl of whole-grain cereal or a whole-grain waffle with milk, a piece of fruit, and a glass of orange juice. (See Table 7.3, on pages 187–188, for more breakfast ideas.)

The Midday Doldrums

Carbohydrate-rich pancakes, toast, waffles, and cereal at breakfast help fuel your thinking during the morning hours, but they make you sleepy and less able to concentrate at lunch. Bonnie Spring, Ph.D., professor of psychology at Harvard University, reports that seniors are particularly susceptible to the effects of carbohydrates. Her studies show that mental alertness and the ability to concentrate decrease after a midday meal of carbohydrate-rich foods. This effect is compounded if the carbohydrates come primarily from sugar-laden foods, because these foods also supply few vitamins, minerals, and other brain-enhancing nutrients.

As mentioned in chapter 4, high-fat or calorie-packed meals (more than 1,000 calories) make you drowsy, not alert. So keep lunch light and combine a little protein with lots of minimally processed carbohydrate-rich foods, such as a turkey sandwich on whole-grain bread with mustard, a piece of fruit, and a glass of tomato juice or a salad (with oil-free dressing).

Sweet Delusions

When it comes to brain power, Paul Gold, Ph.D., commonwealth professor of psychology at the University of Virginia in Charlottesville, says that a spoonful of sugar might sharpen your mind. In Dr. Gold's studies, giving healthy seniors, Alzheimer's patients, or college students lemonade laced with 50 grams of glucose enhanced learning and memory.

The trick is knowing how much is enough. "There's an optimal zone of [sugar] ingestion," says Dr. Gold. "Consume too little and there's no response, while too much actually produces memory impairment and amnesia, at least in animals." According to Dr. Gold, sugar consumed while the brain is actively learning might stimulate the release of acetylcholine, a neurotransmitter that enhances nerve cell communication and memory (see chapter 1).

Other studies report sugar has no effect on thinking, and there also is evidence that an all-carbohydrate snack, whether it's crackers or candy, makes some people sleepy. In a study from Kansas State University, college women were less alert within an hour of drinking a sugar-sweetened beverage compared to women who drank water or an aspartame-sweetened beverage. The sugar probably raised brain levels of serotonin, a neurotransmitter that has a calming effect and promotes sleep.

Larry Christensen, Ph.D., chair of the department of psychology at the University of South Alabama in Mobile, believes any benefit from sugar on memory is short-lived, and that in the long run a high-sugar diet probably undermines cognition in some individuals. Dr. Christensen's research on clinically depressed individuals, who also suffer from pessimistic thinking and a negative view of the future and self, found that depression often vanishes when sugar is removed from the diet. "Although we don't understand the exact mechanisms," says Dr. Christensen, "the long-term effects of chronic sugar consumption might contribute to the fatigue associated with depression and the depressive thinking pattern."

So what should you do? Since sugar is not an essential nutrient, it's safe to abstain for a few weeks and see if you notice a boost in mood, thinking, or energy level. Or try having an all-sugar snack just before a board meeting or other task that requires brain power. If it works, great. If it doesn't, then your best bet is to include sweets in moderation, keeping portions small and adding them as a dessert to the end of a meal rather than as a solo snack.

Dieting Makes You Dumb

Most of us know that crash diets don't work, but did you know they also make you dumb? Michael Green, Ph.D., former senior research psychologist at the Institute of Food Research in the United Kingdom, studied the effects of diet on mental performance. In one study, fifty-five women between the ages of eighteen and forty—some of whom were on weight-loss diets while others were not—were seated in front of computer terminals where a continuous flow of single numbers was displayed. The women were asked to press a response button whenever they noticed a sequence of three odd or three even numbers.

"The women on very-low-calorie diets displayed poorer reaction speeds, immediate memory, and ability to sustain attention," concludes Dr. Green. In short, compared to the nondieting women, they processed information slowly, took longer to react, and had more trouble remembering sequences. This mental funk was even noted in dieters who hadn't lost weight and in nondieting women who had severely restricted their food intake. Although poorly understood, Dr. Green suspects that the preoccupation with body shape, food, and the dieting experience might overload the dieter's mental capacity. Or, the inability to concentrate or pay attention might result from lowered iron status, which is common in people who are following quick-weight-loss diets. While dieting might make you dumb, losing weight the good old-fashioned way—that is, a gradual weight loss of no more than two pounds a week—allows you to lose the right kind of weight (fat weight), keep it off, and stay clearheaded in the process.

Fish Really Is Brain Food

The human race evolved on diets rich in fish and low in saturated fats. "For millions of years, in fact for more than 99 percent of the time the human species has been on earth, our ancestors ate and evolved on diets of plants and very lean wild game," says S. Boyd Eaton, M.D., adjunct associate professor of anthropology at Emory University. Although plants were the mainstay of our evolutionary diets, our ancestors also ate their fair share of meat. But unlike today's meat, which comes from domesticated animals and is high in saturated fat, the meat on ancient plates was fish and wild game, which is low in fat (4 percent fat versus 25 to 30 percent in today's domesticated meat), very low in saturated fat, and very high in omega-3 fatty acids.

These diets served us well, according to Dr. Eaton, who adds that when our Paleolithic ancestors survived childbirth, infection, and violent deaths, they lived relatively disease-free to an old age. Since evolution takes millions of years, today we remain basically cave dwellers dressed in designer jeans, genetically programmed to thrive on diets of nuts, seeds, leaves, honey, and fish, but gorging on fatty beef, French fries, doughnuts, and cheese puffs, which might contribute to memory loss and dulled thinking.

About 50 percent of the brain is fat, especially highly unsaturated fats like the omega-3 fatty acids and arachidonic acid. One omega-3 in particular, called docosahexaenoic acid (DHA), is an important component in nerve cell membranes. DHA gives brain cells their ability to readily transport nutrients into the cell and quickly remove debris and waste products. DHA also helps regulate hormonelike compounds called prostaglandins, leukotrienes, and cytokines, which further influence brain function and the release of brain chemicals, such as serotonin.

The hitch is that DHA is obtained only from the diet, and our diets are sorely lacking in this fat compared to the amounts to which our bodies grew accustomed during evolution. Today we drown salads in corn oil, fry food in hydrogenated fats, and eat meats loaded with saturated fats, but we consume little or no fish. To add insult to injury, we drink alcoholic beverages and smoke, which further deplete levels of omega-3 fatty acids in the brain.

The research in this area is new and reflects mostly the impact that fish oils have on preventing and treating depression by boosting serotonin levels (see chapter 6). Research on infants shows that DHA is essential for normal brain development, thinking, and concentration in infants. While breast-fed infants are smarter than formula-fed infants, a study from the University of Dundee, United Kingdom, found that term infants fed DHA-fortified formulas for the first four months of life scored higher on problem-solving tests at ten months of age. The researchers conclude ". . . [these fats] may be important for the development of childhood intelligence."

Low DHA levels in children also affect behavior and learning. In a study from Purdue University in Indiana, behavior, learning, and health problems were assessed in boys ages six to twelve and compared to blood levels of omega-3 fatty acids. Low omega-3 fatty acid levels were associated with more temper tantrums, sleep problems, and behavioral problems. In addition, boys with low omega-3 levels were more likely to develop learning problems.

What's good for children is also essential to adults. Researchers at the National Institute of Public Health and the Environment in The Netherlands found that people who eat fish regularly show less cognitive decline as they age compared to people who consume more vegetable oils. The diets of men between the ages of sixty-nine and eighty-nine were compared with cognitive ability during a four-year period. The results showed that high intakes of vegetable oils impaired thinking, while people who regularly ate fish maintained more youthful thinking and memory.

Limited evidence also links low DHA levels in brain tissue to serious mental disorders, such as bipolar disorders and schizophrenia. Supplementing diets with DHA or other omega-3 fatty acids (as an adjunct to regular therapy) improves symptoms in up to 64 percent of patients. In some cases the benefits are so dramatic, the researchers stopped the studies early so that all the patients could benefit from the supplements rather than continue with placebos.

The bottom line? More research is needed before specific recommendations can be made regarding the omega-3 fatty acids and brain function. In the meantime your best bet is to limit red meat consumption to no more than three extra-lean servings a week and to eat more fish, especially omega-3–rich fish, such as salmon. (See Table 8.1, "Clean Fish," below.)

Table 8.1   Clean Fish

Although a few fish should be avoided or eaten in small amounts because of pesticide contamination, many more fish are safe and tasty to eat.

1. Select lean fish (most chemical contaminants concentrate in fatty tissues). Cod, flounder, haddock, Pacific halibut, ocean perch, pollack, and sole are relatively safe from chemical contamination.
2. Select Pacific- and offshore-caught fish (limit or avoid near-shore saltwater or inland-caught freshwater fish). Salmon (caught in the Pacific, or farmed in Chili or Norway) also is safe.
3. Choose small, young fish. It's the older, fattier fish that have had time to bioaccumulate pesticides and PCBs.
4. Cook shellfish and select clams and oysters harvested on the Pacific Coast, if possible.
5. Limit tuna, swordfish, and shark to one serving a week; women who might become or are pregnant should limit these fish to once a month. Canned tuna contains less mercury than fresh tuna steaks, but limit intake to no more than two medium-sized cans a week (about six sandwiches).

Crank Up Cognition with Coffee

Within half an hour of drinking a cup of coffee, you'll notice a mental boost. That's because the caffeine in coffee (or tea, cola, and chocolate) halts the depressant effects of adenosine, a neurotransmitter that calms the brain; thus, the nervous system stays revved and you think more clearly, are more alert, have a faster reaction time, and can concentrate better.

Just because some caffeine boosts thought processes, that does not mean drinking more of it makes you smarter. The stimulating effects of caffeine linger in the system for up to fifteen hours. A cup of coffee or a cola midafternoon could disrupt sleep at ten P.M., resulting in mental fatigue and poor judgment the next day. Caffeine also is effective only up to your "jitter threshold"; add more coffee after this and you're too buzzed to think clearly. You also might experience caffeine withdrawal within hours of your last cup, which leaves you grumpy and mentally slug-gish. Finally, coffee and tea contain compounds called tannins that reduce other brain-boosting nutrients, such as iron, by up to 75 percent. So gradually cut back on coffee to no more than two cups a day, have two cups of water for each cup of cof-fee, and drink your coffee or tea between meals.

Antioxidants and the Brain Drain

One reason why our memory fades with age is that we don't protect this precious tissue with enough antioxidants. The brain is only 2 percent of your total body weight but consumes 20 percent of your daily oxygen, which exposes it to a huge daily dose of oxygen fragments called free radicals. These molecules enter the body in cigarette smoke, fried foods, smoggy air, or as a natural consequence of normal metabolic processes. Cortisol, one of the stress hormones, floods brain cells in a free-radical bath.

Free radicals are troublemakers, attacking, damaging, and destroying every brain cell in sight. They damage cell membranes and the genetic code within the cells, generate toxic by-products that further damage cells, and contribute to the underlying causes of aging itself. To make matters worse, the brain also is rich in polyunsaturated fats, which are highly susceptible to free-radical attacks. The wear and tear that decades of free-radical attacks have on the brain contributes to the gradual loss of memory and thinking associated with aging.

Fortunately, the body has an anti–free-radical army comprised of the antioxidant nutrients, including vitamins C and E and beta carotene. Other nonvitamins also boost brain defenses, including lipoic acid, coenzyme Q10, and the phytochemicals in many fruits, vegetables, and green tea. This dietary militia deactivates free radi-cals, but only if their forces match or exceed those of the attacking free radicals. The body's antioxidant system can be overwhelmed when exposed to excessive amounts of free radicals. Even if 99.9 percent of all free radicals were erased by an active anti-oxidant system, the damage done by the remaining 0.1 percent accumulates over time. A rate of ten thousand free-radical "tears" in each cell's genetic code, proteins, and membranes each day results in millions of wounds over the course of a lifetime. It is this backlog of cellular debris that contributes to the aging process.

Maintain antioxidant levels in brain tissue throughout life and you might keep more youthful brain power. You also will offset the damage from stress that other-wise leads to age-related memory loss. A study from Erasmus University Medical

School in The Netherlands found that thinking ability remained high throughout life when people consumed lots of beta-carotene–rich foods. Studies from all over the world have found similar benefits. Healthy centenarians with little memory loss and great concentration also have the highest antioxidant levels and consume the most antioxidant-rich fruits and vegetables. Even animals fed diets fortified with vitamins C and E retain brain tissue that resembles that of young animals, and they learn faster and remember more than fellow animals without antioxidants. In a study from the University of Sydney in Australia, men and women who consume ample vitamin C performed the best on tests for attention, recall and memory, and calculation. (See Table 8.2, "Antioxidant-Rich Foods," below.)

Table 8.2   Antioxidant-Rich Foods

FOOD	SERVING	AMOUNT (MILLIGRAMS)
VITAMIN C		
Green pepper	1 large	128
Orange juice	6 ounces	90
Grapefruit	1 medium	76
Brussels sprouts	1/2 cup	68
Strawberries	1/2 cup	66
Broccoli	1/2 cup	52
Collard greens	1/2 cup	44

FOOD	SERVING	AMOUNT (IU)
BETA CAROTENE		
Carrot juice	1 cup	11,520
Carrot	1 raw	11,000
Sweet potato	1 small	8,100
Spinach	1/2 cup cooked	7,300
Apricots, dried	8 halves	5,500
Collard greens	1/2 cup cooked	5,400
Beet greens	1/2 cup cooked	5,100
Cantaloupe	1/4 melon	3,400
Peach	1 medium	2,170

VITAMIN E		AMOUNT (IU)
Wheat germ oil	1/4 cup	63.6
Wheat germ	1/2 cup	27.0
Almonds	1/4 cup	25.0
Safflower oil (preferably cold-pressed)	1/4 cup	19.5

SELENIUM		AMOUNT (MICROGRAMS)
Organ meats	4 ounces	149.6
Seafood	4 ounces	37.9
Lean meat or chicken without skin	4 ounces	22.7
Whole grains	1 slice or 1/2 cup cooked	12.0
Nonfat milk	1 cup	3.6
Vegetables*	1 serving	Average = 1.6
Fruits*	1 serving	Average = 0.9

* Amounts vary depending on the selenium content of the soil in which the food was grown.

The antioxidants, especially vitamin E, also might help slow the progression of Alzheimer's disease, the major cause of dementia in older persons. The brains of Alzheimer's patients have all the signs of massive free-radical damage. A study from Columbia University College of Physicians and Surgeons in New York City found that people with Alzheimer's disease who took vitamin E supplements were able to slow the progression of the disease. Other antioxidants that might help curb the symptoms of Alzheimer's include ginkgo biloba, lipoic acid, and compounds called flavonoids in fruits and vegetables.

To keep your antioxidant defenses strong, consume daily at least six to eight servings of fresh fruits and vegetables, such as orange juice, strawberries, carrots, sweet potatoes, spinach, broccoli, kiwi, and cantaloupe. Prunes are especially good sources of antioxidants. A recent study from Tufts University found that prunes ranked the highest in antioxidant activity of any fruit or vegetable tested. Also take daily supplements of vitamin E (400 IU) and vitamin C (250 to 1,000 milligrams).

Table 8.3   Effects of the B Vitamins on Thought, Memory, and Mood

VITAMIN B$_1$

Effects of Deficiency: Aggressiveness, anxiety, apathy, confusion, depression, fatigue, irritability, memory loss, nerve damage, poor concentration and attention span, psychosis.
Dietary Sources: Wheat germ, brewer's yeast, green peas, collard greens, oranges, cooked dried beans and peas, asparagus.

VITAMIN B$_2$

Effects of Deficiency: EEG abnormalities, irritability.
Dietary Sources: Low-fat milk, yogurt, oysters, avocados, spinach, broccoli, brussels sprouts.

NIACIN

Effects of Deficiency: Nerve damage, apathy, depression, anxiety, irritability, mania, memory loss, delirium, dementia, mood swings.
Dietary Sources: Chicken, salmon, extra-lean beef, peanut butter, green peas, potatoes, brewer's yeast, low-fat milk, wheat germ.

VITAMIN B$_6$

Effects of Deficiency: Acute sensitivity to noise, EEG changes, fatigue, depression, irritability, reduced learning ability, seizures.
Dietary Sources: Bananas, avocados, extra-lean beef, chicken, fish, potatoes, collard greens.

PANTOTHENIC ACID

Effects of Deficiency: Depression, fatigue, irritability, restlessness.
Dietary Sources: Oranges, collard greens, potatoes, broccoli, brown rice, cantaloupe, wheat germ.

BIOTIN

Effects of Deficiency: Depression, fatigue and lethargy, sleepiness.
Dietary Sources: Oatmeal, soybeans, peanut butter, salmon, low-fat milk, brown rice, chicken.

VITAMIN B₁₂

Effects of Deficiency: Abnormal EEG, confusion, delusions, depression, irritability, hallucinations, memory loss, paranoia.
Dietary Sources: Oysters, tuna, yogurt, low-fat milk, fish, chicken, cheese, extra-lean beef.

FOLIC ACID

Effects of Deficiency: Apathy, dementia, depression, delirium, forgetfulness, insomnia, irritability, psychosis, mental retardation in infants.
Dietary Sources: Brewer's yeast, spinach, orange juice, romaine lettuce, avocados, broccoli, wheat germ, cooked dried beans and peas, bananas.

VITAMIN C

Effects of Deficiency: Lethargy; personality changes, including depression and hysteria.
Dietary Sources: Oranges, brussels sprouts, strawberries.

B's on the Report Card

Inadequate intakes of several B vitamins also could be at the root of any brain drain you are experiencing. In some cases, such as in the case of psychiatric patients, the deficiency is secondary to the mental illness. In other cases, poor dietary intake of one or more nutrients initiates a vicious cycle of mild depression, apathy, or lowered mental function that further reduces food and nutrient intake. (See Table 8.3, "Effects of the B Vitamins on Thought, Memory, and Mood," on pages 204–205.) Poor intake of other nutrients, including zinc, iodine, and vitamin D, also clogs thinking, shortens attention span, sidetracks motivation, and slows learning capacities.

When a mental funk is caused by a poor diet, boosting the intake of vitamins (and minerals, such as boron, iron, and zinc) revs brain power. For example, in a study from the University of Reading in England, school-aged children took either multivitamin and mineral supplements or placebos, after which they were retested on a variety of cognitive tests. The supplementers fared far better the second time around on nonverbal IQ compared to the nonsupplementers: They processed information faster, allowing them to complete the test on time and resulting in more correct answers. In most cases it doesn't require megadoses of vitamins, only an emphasis on healthful eating, to supply your brain with the nutrients it needs to function in high gear.

Vitamin B₁

It is difficult to believe anyone could consume inadequate amounts of vitamin B_1, since this B vitamin is even added to highly refined white breads and cereals. However, marginal deficiencies are not uncommon, especially in adolescents, seniors, and people who abuse alcohol. The deficiency affects the nervous system, probably because vitamin B_1 is essential for extracting energy from the brain's number one fuel source: glucose. Fatigue, loss of appetite, weakness, mental confusion, memory loss, emotional instability, reduced attention span and concentration, aggressive behavior, personality changes, and irritability are a few of the symptoms characteristic of poor vitamin B_1 intake.

In a study from the University of Swansea in Wales, 120 young women took daily either a placebo or vitamin B_1 supplements. After two months, the supplementers reported they were more clearheaded, composed, and energetic. Those who took the supplements found their reaction times improved. Other studies, such as one from the University of New Mexico School of Medicine in Albuquerque, also report that people who consume diets rich in B vitamins score higher on tests measuring memory than do people who eat poorly. Even children show improvements in reaction times, memory, and intelligence scores when their intakes of vitamin B_1 are increased. If poor diets are the cause of these mental problems, then consuming more vitamin B_1–rich foods, including wheat germ, brewer's yeast, green peas, collard greens, oranges, and cooked dried beans and peas, should alleviate the symptoms.

Niacin

The link between niacin and mental health swings between the ridiculous and the sublime. This B vitamin was once advertised as the cure-of-the-century for schizophrenia, yet later proved at best only moderately effective as a therapy. Later research showed that niacin can cause liver damage when consumed in large doses, so no one should self-medicate without physician monitoring.

On the other hand, more than fifty body processes are dependent on niacin, including the release of energy from carbohydrates and the manufacture of many nerve chemicals and hormones that regulate thinking and memory. Consequently, it is no surprise that even a mild deficiency produces symptoms that include depression, confusion and disorientation, anxiety, irritability, and short-term memory loss. A severe deficiency results in dementia and psychosis. In contrast, consuming several servings daily of niacin-rich foods, such as chicken, salmon, peanut butter, green peas, and wheat germ, will correct these problems if they are caused by a deficiency.

Vitamin B$_6$, Folic Acid, and Vitamin B$_{12}$

Even marginal deficiencies of vitamin B$_6$, folic acid, or vitamin B$_{12}$ contribute to a variety of mental problems, including dementia, depression, poor concentration, moodiness, confusion, reduced learning ability, and even convulsions. Vitamin B$_6$ also might help soothe the mental distress experienced during times of grief.

These B vitamins perform a variety of functions in the brain:

- All three contribute to the manufacture and release of nerve chemicals, such as serotonin, dopamine, and GABA, while the incomplete by-products of these nerve chemicals accumulate and irritate the surrounding nerves.
- Vitamins B$_6$ and B$_{12}$ aid in the manufacture and maintenance of the insulating sheath, called myelin, that surrounds nerve cells and speeds the transfer of messages through the brain. Deficiencies of either vitamin damage this sheath and result in reduced memory, slower reaction time, and impaired thinking.
- Vitamin B$_{12}$ and folic acid are essential for normal cell reproduction, including the manufacture of red blood cells. Inadequate intake or absorption of this B vitamin and/or folic acid results in poorly formed red blood cells that cannot carry oxygen to the brain. Fatigue, impaired mental function, decreased attention span, listlessness, and anemia result.
- Folic acid helps maintain our bodies' genetic code within each cell, and helps manufacture new cells. Too little folic acid means cells do not replicate or new cells are made imperfectly. Tissue function is hampered because of the reduced number of cells and the possible increase in abnormal cell growth. The symptoms are widespread since every cell in the body is affected by a folic acid deficiency. Anemia, irritability, behavior problems, and loss of appetite are only a few of the symptoms.

- All three B vitamins are needed to maintain normal blood levels of a compound called homocysteine (HC). When intake of these B vitamins is low, blood levels of HC rise (a condition called hyperhomocysteinemia), which damages blood vessels, reduces blood (and oxygen) flow to the brain, and compromises mental function. High HC levels also might kill nerve cells critical to thinking, and is common in Alzheimer's patients and in seniors; up to 30 percent of this population has elevated HC levels that contribute to age-related memory loss.

The need for these B vitamins increases with age. Vitamin B_{12} deficiency is prevalent in up to 42 percent of seniors, partially because secretion of stomach acid and a compound called intrinsic factor, both necessary for vitamin B_{12} absorption, decrease with age. Consequently, the diet can be adequate in vitamin B_{12}, but little is absorbed. The deficiency goes undetected, since up to 40 percent of these people don't develop other symptoms of deficiency, such as anemia. The standard test for vitamin B_{12} malabsorption, called the Schilling test, recently was found ineffective in identifying many cases of deficiency. Unless more sensitive tests for B_{12} status are undertaken, a deficiency can progress undetected, resulting in impaired mental status, memory loss, reduced attention span, dementia, paranoia, and depression. In the past, neurological dysfunction resulting from B_{12} deficiency was considered irreversible. However, recent studies on seniors show that supplementing with B vitamins, including vitamin B_{12}, often improves, and even reverses, mental impairment in at least 50 percent of patients. In severe cases where the body no longer makes any intrinsic factor, physician-supervised injections of vitamin B_{12} might be necessary.

Folic acid deficiency also is linked to several serious psychiatric disorders, including clinical depression, organic brain syndromes, and schizophrenia. Some patients who supplement with extra folic acid show greater improvements and have shorter hospital stays than do patients who don't supplement. In one study, eight out of nine folic acid–deficient patients who took supplements for six months had excellent recovery successes compared to patients who did not supplement. Supplementing with vitamin B_6 also improves symptoms of autism in some people. Granted, not all serious psychological disorders are so easily treated; however, increasing your intake of folic acid to 400 to 800 micrograms in conjunction with optimal intake of vitamins B_6 (2 to 25 milligrams daily) and B_{12} (2.4 to 10 micrograms daily), is safe and potentially helpful in the prevention and treatment of some mental disorders. (See Table 8.4, "Smart Foods and Snacks," on page 209.)

Table 8.4   Smart Foods and Snacks

The following foods and snacks are packed with the nutrients that stimulate brain function. (For each recipe, see "Recipes for Feeling Your Best," at the back of this book.)

The Zinger Smoothie	Vegetable Lentil Soup
Brain Teaser	Curried Squash Soup
Gazpacho Smoothie Over Ice	Vegetable Beef Soup
	Curried Turkey Vegetable Soup
Open-Faced Black Bean Burritos	Pumpkin Mousse Pie
Black Bean and Cheese Roll-Ups	
Spicy Grilled Salmon with Ginger	
Sautéed Shrimp and Vegetables	
Crunchy Pea and Shrimp Salad	
Vegetable Tabbouleh	
Wild Greens Topped with Pears, Blue Cheese, and Walnuts	
Fresh Green Bean Bundles with Dill	
Apricot-Glazed Carrots	

What Do Eggs, Wheat Germ, and Your Brain Have in Common?

Choline is a building block for a special category of fats called phospholipids (fats containing the mineral phosphorus) found in cell membranes and the nerve chemical acetylcholine, which regulates memory. Although the body manufactures choline, boosting brain levels with supplements of choline might improve memory or slow age-related memory loss.

Brain cells need choline to function properly. In fact, Alzheimer's disease is characterized by an underproduction of acetylcholine. Although the body can manufacture some choline with the help of folic acid and vitamin B_{12}, sometimes it doesn't produce enough to maintain normal brain function; consequently, blood choline levels drop when people consume choline-poor diets, which could have far-reaching effects on their thinking processes, interfering with the storage and retrieval of information. For example, people flunk memory tests when they are given a drug that blocks acetylcholine function, but pass with flying colors when they are given a drug that raises acetylcholine levels. Choline supplementation during pre- and postnatal development in animals produces marked improvements in memory that last into adulthood, while people suffering from memory loss who are given choline supplements sometimes show improvements in short-term memory and abstract thinking.

The best dietary sources of choline are wheat germ, egg yolks, liver, peanuts and peanut butter, and brewer's yeast. Small amounts of choline are found in potatoes, tomatoes, whole wheat bread, milk, oranges, cauliflower, and cucumbers. The suggested average daily intake of choline is between 700 and 1,000 milligrams. Deficiency symptoms develop when intake falls below this amount, which might be common as people decrease their intakes of cholesterol-rich foods, such as eggs, that also are primary sources of choline. Richard Wurtman, Ph.D., professor of neuroscience and the director of the clinical research center at the Massachusetts Institute of Technology (MIT), believes that choline intake is probably low enough in some diets to cause memory problems.

Whether choline reduces a person's risk for developing dementia, such as Alzheimer's disease, is controversial. While one study showed slight improvements in long-term memory when patients took 1,000 milligrams of choline daily for one month, most studies found that supplements of either choline or lecithin only sometimes raised blood levels of choline, yet had no effect on memory. Even if choline supplements raised brain levels of acetylcholine, there is no evidence that damaged brain cells use the extra nerve chemical. If choline supplementation is effective at all, it probably is most useful in the early stages of memory loss before pronounced structural changes in the brain produce irreversible damage.

Choline supplementation always should be discussed with a physician. In addition, it can produce side effects, such as diarrhea, and is not advised in certain psychological conditions. For example, manic depressives should not supplement with choline, since the nutrient can aggravate the depressive phase of the illness.

Phosphatidyl What?

Choline has a cousin that might boost brain power, especially as we age. It's called phosphatidylserine (PS), another phospholipid consumed in soy-based foods and lecithin, manufactured in the body, and found in especially high concentrations in the brain. PS acts as a revolving door for brain cells, allowing nutrients easy access to the cell and providing a quick escape for toxic cellular debris. PS helps brain cells conduct nerve impulses, enhancing communication within the brain. Finally, the body uses PS to make acetylcholine, the memory-enhancing nerve chemical. These are some reasons why researchers believe increasing intake of PS might boost brain power.

Our memories peak in our twenties, then slowly wane, so that by our fifties, we're making lists, forgetting names, and losing our keys. PS supplements might be effective in limiting, and possibly even reversing, a portion of this decreased mental ability. PS supplements restock brain cell membranes, boosting nerve chemical activity such as dopamine and serotonin, stimulating nerve cell growth, lowering levels of the stress hormones, possibly generating new connections between cells, and stirring activity in all brain centers, especially higher brain centers such as the cortex, hypothalamus, and pituitary gland.

The few studies that there are on PS supplements show that they improve memory and learning in animals, depressed or Alzheimer's patients, healthy people, and seniors, and with no side effects. Parris Kidd, Ph.D., of PMK Biomedical-Nutritional Counseling, in El Cerrito, California, presented this information at the American College of Nutrition Conference in October 1998. He speculates that PS can turn back the mental clock by up to fourteen years. Unfortunately, no specific effective dose for PS has been identified, although some researchers speculate that 300 milligrams taken for the first few weeks followed by a 100-milligram maintenance dose is safe. No benefits are noted for daily doses of less than 100 milligrams. If you're considering taking PS supplements, be sure to purchase only standardized products from reputable manufacturers, since these products are not regulated by the U.S. Food and Drug Administration (FDA). You also might naturally boost PS levels by including more fish in your diet, since the omega-3 fatty acid DHA (see pages 198–200) appears to boost the body's ability to make PS.

Iron Intelligence

Iron deficiency is the most common nutrient deficiency in the United States, and could be a major contributor to shortened attention spans, lowered IQ and intelligence, lack of motivation, poor hand-eye coordination, lowered scores on vocabulary tests, inability to concentrate, limited educational achievement, and suboptimal work performance in children and adults. While adult men and post-menopausal women have relatively low iron needs compared to their calorie intakes, infants, children, teenagers, women during their childbearing years, pregnant and breast-feeding women, and seniors are at particularly high risk for developing iron deficiency.

Iron is essential for transporting oxygen to the brain and within each brain cell. Your brain literally suffocates without sufficient oxygen, and the cells cannot convert glucose and other calorie-containing fuels into energy quickly enough to meet cellular needs, so many of the cells' functions slow down or stop. By-products of cellular activity accumulate, and nerve chemicals, such as dopamine, are impaired. When you don't have enough iron, you are tired, cannot think clearly, and are more irritable.

Increasing iron intake in deficient people stimulates brain activity, especially in the left hemisphere of the brain, the region of the brain responsible for analytic thought and abstract thinking. Optimal iron intake also is linked to greater verbal skills and overall improved mental functioning. Even infants who are optimally nourished in iron are more likely than iron-deficient infants to be happy, calm, relaxed, trusting, outgoing, and show more interest in exploring their environments. They also grow up to be smarter than iron-deficient babies. The good news is that iron-deficient adults show reversal of these and other symptoms when iron intake is increased. To prevent or correct iron deficiency, follow the guidelines in Table 4.3, "Ironclad Rules," on page 116, and have a blood test done to make sure your serum ferritin levels are above 20 micrograms/liter. (See chapter 4 for more information on how to increase iron intake.)

Exercise and De-Stress Your Brain

Want to win at Jeopardy? Then stay in shape. Exercise stimulates blood flow to the brain, supplying it with a hefty dose of oxygen and nutrients. It also minimizes plaque buildup inside blood vessels, so blood flows unhindered. Exercise is a stressbuster that lifts the spirits and builds self-esteem. Preliminary studies show exercise also supplies the brain with natural substances called neurotropins that enhance cell growth and help process all kinds of information. Neurotransmitter levels—in particular, norepinephrine, which helps in memory storage and retrieval—also increase as much as 29 percent with exercise. Convert couch potatoes into exercisers and they show dramatic improvements in thinking ability, reaction times, memory, and concentration. In fact, they regain the quick-wittedness of youth.

If you take steps to de-stress your life, you will notice an improvement in your thinking. The stress hormone cortisol interferes with the brain's ability to use glucose. The resulting energy shortage inhibits the brain's ability to store memories and slows mental function. Cortisol also blocks nerve chemical activity, which interferes with the brain's ability to relay information, and affects reaction times, memory, creative thinking, and concentration. Finally, cortisol kills brain cells by disrupting brain cell activity, slowing removal of waste products from brain cells, and generating excessive amounts of free radicals. Whatever it takes to reduce the stress in your life, do it. Build a supportive network of family and friends, cut back on your responsibilities, meditate, take a yoga class, and/or exercise daily.

Attitude is another factor that either boosts brain power or undermines it. People who expect to lose mental abilities as they age inevitably do so at much higher rates than people who expect to think clearly. Living an active life that is mentally stimulating, being married to a smart partner, and being well educated also hedge your bets against memory loss.

Reprogramming your body's aging process and revving your brain's motor takes time. If you think you can pop a pill, walk a mile, meditate for ten minutes, or order a "Smart Drink" at a local juice stand and be smarter overnight, think again. Ideally, providing the body and mind with optimal levels of all the essential brain-building nutrients, exercising daily, and learning to cope effectively with stress should begin in childhood and be maintained throughout life for a healthy, active, and long life of clear thinking and feeling good. The good news is, it is never too late to halt the damage and start building a better brain. Optimal nutrition, daily exercise, and healthful living help rebuild and regenerate these tissues gradually so that within three months to one year you should notice an improvement in memory, concentration, alertness, and thinking. (See Table 8.5, "Herbs and Supplement for Brain Power: What Works, What Doesn't, and Why," on pages 214–215.)

Table 8.5   Herbs and Supplements for Brain Power: What Works, What Doesn't, and Why

Aspirin: Regular use of nonsteroidal antiinflammatory drugs, such as aspirin and ibuprofen, might delay the onset of Alzheimer's disease. Side effects include stomach upset and bleeding.

Carnitine: Carnitine might help slow the progression of Alzheimer's disease when given in 2-gram daily doses.

Coenzyme Q10 (CoQ10): This antioxidant aids in energy production in brain cells, improves blood circulation to the brain, and boosts energy. No recommended dose has been established, but 100 to 200 milligrams appears safe.

DHEA: Dehydroepiandrosterone (DHEA) is a hormone that decreases with age. Animals given DHEA supplements learn faster and remember more than their unsupplemented friends. It's unclear whether similar effects can be expected in people. Side effects of DHEA supplementation include acne and an increased risk for prostate cancer, aggressiveness, and liver damage. DHEA is not regulated by the U.S. Food and Drug Administration (FDA), so there are no guarantees of product safety or efficacy. One study found that only seven out of sixteen DHEA products tested contained the amount of DHEA listed on their labels; the rest contained little or no DHEA or contained dosages exceeding safety levels.

Ginkgo biloba: Ginkgo biloba might help increase oxygen flow to the brain and protect brain tissue from free-radical damage. This herb also might help relieve mild dementia, and a 120-milligrams daily dose might slow the progression of Alzheimer's disease. Look for products standardized to 24 percent flavone glycosides and 6 percent terpene lactones.

Guarana: This Brazilian plant is believed to stimulate brain function; however, studies have found it ineffective.

Lipoic acid: This antioxidant protects brain tissue from free-radical damage and enhances the action of other antioxidants, such as vitamins C and E. Dietary sources include spinach, broccoli, and organ meats. Researchers at the University of California, Berkeley, report that lipoic acid raises intracellular glutathione levels, making it an ideal defense against oxidative damage of nerve and brain cells. Preliminary evidence shows lipoic acid exerts a protective effect in brain injury, mitochondrial dysfunction, diabetes and diabetic neuropathy, and other acute or chronic damage to brain or nerve tissue. A recommended dose has not been established.

Pycnogenol, or pine bark extract: This plant-derived compound contains flavonoids, which are antioxidants that might protect cells from free-radical damage. However, the research is limited, and not enough evidence exists yet to support claims that pycnogenol is any more effective than other antioxidants in protecting brain cells from age-related disease.

Tyrosine: This amino acid is the building block for the nerve chemicals dopamine, epinephrine (adrenalin), and norepinephrine (noradrenaline). These three help regulate levels of arousal and anxiety. Stress depletes tyrosine from the blood, which limits the amount available for manufacturing nerve chemicals. Supplements of tyrosine might boost memory, but only when there is a deficit caused by stress or aging. Whether supplements improve thinking ability in other people is unknown.

CHAPTER NINE

Can't Sleep?

- Do you stare at the clock in the middle of the night, wishing you could go to sleep?
- Do you fall asleep, but can't stay that way?
- Do you sleep fitfully at night, then feel tired and tense all day because you're not well rested?
- Do you have trouble concentrating and doze off during the day?
- Do you sleep right through the alarm and then can hardly rouse yourself from bed?

A good night's sleep should be a simple matter of plumping up the pillow, closing your eyes, and counting a few sheep before you nod off. Instead, you are tossing and turning, watching the clock, or waking up at four A.M. If it is any consolation, you are a restless bedfellow with some very famous people, including Napoléon Bonaparte, Winston Churchill, Charles Dickens, Cary Grant, and Marilyn Monroe, who spent many a sleepless night. The good news is that with a few diet and lifestyle changes, most people can improve their sleep habits.

You're Not Alone

The statistics on insomnia are eye-opening. A recent Gallup poll found that nearly half of all Americans say they frequently have problems getting to sleep—that's

33 percent more sleepless people than just five years ago. Researchers estimate that 95 percent of adults experience some form of insomnia during their lives. Approximately 40 million people suffer from chronic sleep disorders or sleep apnea, which is repetitive episodes of impaired breathing that interfere with sleep. Seventeen percent of adults consider the problem serious enough to seek medical attention.

Even those who aren't insomniacs often get too little sleep. While insomniacs lie in bed wishing they could fall asleep, sleep-deprived individuals would gladly fall asleep if they could just get to bed. Since the late 1800s, people gradually have spent less time sleeping. Today, many people get less than seven hours of sleep each night, while our grandparents snoozed about nine hours a night. Missing a night's sleep won't seriously affect your health, but it might reduce your attention to detail, slow your reaction time on the freeway, and clog your creative thinking. Researchers at the University of California report that losing even a few hours of sleep also impairs the functioning of your immune system the next day, leaving you more vulnerable to colds and infections. Just one sleepless night can reduce the activity of natural killer (NK) cells—infection-fighting immune cells that help prevent colds, flu, and other viruses.

People who have chronic insomnia suffer from all of these ailments and more. Insomniacs are more likely to be depressed, be short on tolerance, be more irritable and less attentive, and suffer temporary memory loss. Repeatedly missing a good night's sleep can affect relationships at home and at work, job satisfaction, sanity, and general happiness. Insomniacs often give up hobbies, recreational activities, or socializing because they are too exhausted, while the quality of their lives deteriorates. They also are accident-prone; one out of every five freeway traffic accidents is the result of a driver falling asleep at the wheel.

Sound sleep solves most, if not all, of these problems. It also comes with some added advantages, like weight loss. Researchers at Walter Reed Army Medical Center, in Washington, D.C., report that men effectively treated for sleep apnea also lost one-half pound a week, which over the course of the six-month study produced a ten-pound drop per person in weight. It is unclear whether the men were more active as a result of a good night's sleep or whether adequate rest rebalanced hormone levels that resulted in weight loss. What is clear is that insomnia is much more than a sleep disorder, since the quality—and possibly the quantity—of life depends on the quality of sleep.

What Is Your Sleep Quotient?

A common misconception is that everyone needs eight hours of sleep nightly. While this is the average required rest, it is by no means typical. Some people need only four hours, while others require a minimum of ten hours to feel refreshed and rested. The "short" sleeper is not overactive, just as the "long" sleeper is not lazy. Sleep needs differ just like fingerprints, shoe size, and personalities.

How much sleep do you need? That depends on you. If you wake up refreshed and ready for the day, then you probably are sleeping enough. If you feel tired and have trouble functioning during the day, you probably aren't getting enough sleep. Are you sleep deprived? Take the quiz on page 219 to find out.

What Causes Insomnia?

We spend a third of our lives in bed, yet have a very sketchy idea of what causes sleep disturbances. A multitude of "sins" can tip the sleep scale in favor of insomnia. Stress is a major factor. Even worrying that you won't fall asleep is enough to keep you awake. Sometimes sleep disturbances result from depression, sporadic sleeping habits, disruption in normal sleeping patterns, such as being on vacation or sleeping in an unfamiliar bed, or taking afternoon naps. More than half of the time, insomnia is caused by psychological and emotional stress. People often report they can't sleep because they are "all wound up," have too much work to do, or have to juggle children, work, and home responsibilities, leaving little time for sleep. In these cases, following the dietary guidelines for relieving depression and stress outlined in chapters 6 and 7 could be all it takes to solve your sleeping problems.

The hot flashes during menopause, and chronic fatigue syndrome (CFS) also are associated with poor sleep habits. People who exercise are much less prone to insomnia than are sedentary people; however, exercising, or even meditating, within four hours of bedtime can invigorate the body and interfere with falling asleep for some people. Ironically, sleeping pills disrupt normal sleeping rhythms and can lead to insomnia if taken long-term. Even snoring or grinding your teeth can interfere with a good night's sleep.

Hormones also might influence sleep patterns. Some women report needing more sleep during the premenstrual phase of their cycle. A woman might sleep more during the first trimester of pregnancy and less during the last trimester. Sleep disorders also increase as a person ages and during other health problems, such as

Seasonal Affective Disorder, SAD (see chapter 5). Numerous factors upset your sleep patterns, including medical conditions such as allergies or heartburn, medications such as antidepressants and blood pressure–lowering drugs, smoking, and even your surroundings (noise, a restless bed partner, or a change in weather).

Quiz 9.1 Are You Sleep Deprived?

While occasionally not getting a full dose of shut-eye won't hurt, night after night of insufficient sleep can jeopardize your health. If you answer yes to more than three of the following questions, you might be a member of the sleep-deprived set.

1. I fall asleep five minutes after my head hits the pillow at night.
2. I drink caffeinated beverages, such as coffee, tea, or colas, during the day to stay alert.
3. I often have an alcoholic beverage at night to relax.
4. Getting up in the morning is a struggle. I need an alarm clock to get me up, and even then I sleep through my alarm or turn it off and go back to sleep.
5. I am easily irritated by minor upsets or am grumpy with family members or co-workers because I am tired.
6. I have trouble keeping my eyes open when I drive in the late afternoon or at night.
7. I have trouble concentrating and I even nod off occasionally during the late afternoon and evening.
8. I have powerful waves of drowsiness at work, at school, or even at a social function.
9. I would participate in more social activities or hobbies if I wasn't so tired.
10. I often wonder where my get-up-and-go has gone.
11. I've had two or more bouts with the common cold, flu, or other minor health nuisances in the past six months.
12. A single glass of beer or wine hits me harder than usual.

The Sleep Journal

Many people have trouble sorting out the reasons why they can't sleep. Keeping a sleep journal for two weeks is a proven method for identifying your sleep busters as well as your natural sleep-wake rhythms. Worksheet 9.1, "Your Sleep Journal," on pages 220–221, is such a diary. Keeping a journal will tell you when and how you sleep, your activity, eating habits, the amount of daily stress, and other factors that might be contributing to your poor sleeping habits. The journal can be used alone

Worksheet 9.1 Your Sleep Journal

Answer the following questions each day for at least one week. Then, look for patterns. On which days did you sleep the best? The worst? What happened during the day or at night that might have contributed to these sleep patterns? You also may note daily occurrences or habits that do not affect your sleep. Use this worksheet as a master to make additional copies.

DATE

DAYTIME HABITS:

	Mon.	Tues.	Wed.	Thurs.	Fri.	Sat.	Sun.
1. How much caffeine?							
2. How much alcohol?							
3. Any medications?							
4. How big/spicy was dinner?							
5. What was the evening snack?							
6. How would you rate your overall food intake?*							
7. What type and how much exercise did you have?							
8. What was your stress level?**							
9. What was the source of your stress?							
10. Were you around tobacco smoke?							
11. Were you energetic or tired?							
12. What was your worry level?**							
13. What was funny or gave you pleasure?							
14. How happy and satisfied are you?***							

	Mon.	Tues.	Wed.	Thurs.	Fri.	Sat.	Sun.
15. Did you take anything to help you sleep?							
16. Did you nap during the day?							
SLEEP HABITS:							
17. When did you go to bed?							
18. When did you fall asleep?							
19. How often did you wake up during the night?							
20. What did you think about when you were in bed?							
21. How many minutes were you awake last night?							
22. What did you do when you woke up?							
23. When did you get up for the day?							
24. Compared to your typical sleep, how would you rate last night's sleep?*							
25. How refreshed and alert were you when you got up this morning?*							

* Scale: 5 = excellent; 1 = poor
** Scale: 5 = low; 1 = high
*** Scale: 5 = very happy and satisfied; 1 = very unhappy and dissatisfied

or in conjunction with other treatments, such as biofeedback, hypnosis, or relaxation therapies. People with chronic insomnia might require the help of trained personnel at a sleep clinic. A list of accredited sleep disorders clinics in your area can be obtained from the American Sleep Disorders Association (see the "Resources" section at the back of this book).

Some Sleep-Stealing Foods

Your problem might not be in the bedroom but at the table, since many dietary habits can interfere with getting to sleep, staying asleep, or how peacefully you doze. For example, people are sleepiest, have difficulty concentrating, lack ambition, and are more fatigued within one and a half to three hours after a big or high-fat meal. Several dietary habits—including consumption of coffee and alcohol, the size and spiciness of the evening meal, quick-weight-loss dieting, and even some food additives—could keep you tossing and turning.

I Dream of Caffeine

Coffee keeps you awake, which is usually why people drink it. This drug revs the nervous system and lowers melatonin levels, the hormonelike chemical that puts us to sleep. A cup of coffee or tea in the morning or even a glass of cola or a chocolate doughnut in the early afternoon is a quick-pick-me-up and usually won't affect most people's sleep that night. However, even one caffeinated cola, cup of coffee or hot cocoa, or even a caffeine-containing medication taken in the early afternoon can leave some caffeine-sensitive people wide-eyed at night. Even if you are not particularly sensitive, too much caffeine can cause shakiness, nervousness, irritability, and insomnia. Often people either are unaware of how sensitive they are to caffeine or underestimate how many cups of caffeinated beverages they consume. They might not experience coffee jitters, but they are listening to the radio at two A.M. Coffee also is a diuretic, and the increased need to urinate can cause night awakenings.

If you suffer from insomnia and drink more than two cups of coffee during the day or drink coffee after one P.M., try eliminating caffeine from your diet. If you feel and sleep better after two weeks of being caffeine-free, then avoid caffeine permanently. Some people experience withdrawal symptoms, including depression, irritability, headaches, fatigue, or even tearfulness, within a few hours of giving up coffee. These symptoms might last up to four days, after which energy level and mood should improve, leaving you feeling better than ever.

For some people, "just saying no" to coffee is harder than it sounds. If you're convinced you really need a cup of coffee to keep you going, then gradually add back a cup here and there after the two-week trial and monitor how each cup affects your mood, energy level, and sleep patterns. You are consuming too much when coffee addiction and insomnia reappear.

To cut back on caffeine:

- Drink decaffeinated or grain-based beverages, such as Postum, as alternatives.
- Substitute carob for chocolate.
- Throw away the first cup of tea made from a tea bag, since it has the most caffeine, and drink the second cup.
- Replace caffeinated colas with sparkling water.

Children, pregnant women, and caffeine don't mix. Insomnia in children can result from excess cola or chocolate consumption. Keep in mind that a twelve-ounce cola for a small body has the caffeine equivalent of a cup of coffee to an adult! Pregnant women should avoid all caffeinated beverages, since caffeine crosses the placenta, disturbs sleep patterns in the growing baby, and might increase the risk for birth defects, spontaneous abortion, and delayed growth.

Don't Drink and Doze

A nightcap might make you sleepy at first, but you'll sleep less soundly and wake up more tired as a result. Alcohol and other depressants suppress a phase of sleep called rapid eye movement (REM) sleep, during which most of your dreaming occurs. Less REM is associated with more night awakenings and more restless sleep.

People who abuse alcohol have abnormal sleep patterns, with hundreds of mini-awakenings throughout the night. Their REM sleep is low, and they spend little or no time in deep sleep, called delta sleep. They might spend more time in bed, but they sleep poorly and are groggy throughout the day. Even during recovery, an alcoholic's sleep problems can linger for months or years. Babies born to women who drank alcohol during pregnancy also are irritable and show disturbed sleep patterns.

A glass of wine with dinner probably won't affect your sleep; however, it's best to limit the amount to two glasses and avoid drinking any alcohol within two hours of bedtime. You should start sleeping better within two weeks of being alcohol-free, if alcohol is a contributing factor to your sleep problems. You should *never* mix alcohol with sleeping pills!

The Evening Meal May Be Doing You In

What and how much you ate for dinner could be at the root of your insomnia. Large, fat-laden dinners make you drowsy but they won't help you sleep through the night. Heavy meals stimulate prolonged digestive action, which can keep you awake. Instead, try eating your biggest meals at breakfast and/or lunch and eating a light evening meal of approximately 500 calories and a small, low-fat snack before bedtime. Include some chicken, extra-lean meat, or fish at dinner to help curb middle-of-the-night snack attacks.

Spicy or gas-forming foods also can contribute to sleeping problems. Dishes seasoned with garlic, chilies, cayenne, or other hot spices can cause nagging heartburn or indigestion. Foods seasoned with monosodium glutamate (MSG), a taste-enhancer often added to Chinese food, can cause sleep disturbances, vivid dreaming, and restless sleep in some people. The higher the dose, the greater the likelihood of a reaction. Eating gas-forming foods or eating too fast and swallowing air also can leave you bloated and uncomfortable, which in turn interferes with sound sleep. Try avoiding spicy foods at dinnertime, limit your intake of gas-forming foods to the morning hours, and eat slowly to thoroughly chew the food and avoid gulping air. (See Table 9.1, "Gas Control," on page 225.)

Are You Allergic to Sleep?

Several other food-related habits can interfere with sleep. Food allergies (corn, wheat, and chocolate are some of the more common causes of food allergies) do not directly cause insomnia but can trigger allergic reactions, while lactose intolerance can cause bloating and cramping that can disturb sleep patterns. Termed food-allergy insomnia, these conditions cause intestinal discomfort, which can interfere with getting to sleep and staying asleep. They are most common in infants who are intolerant to milk products and are rare in adults. Usually the disorder spontaneously subsides between ages two and four. Many adults mistakenly blame food allergies for their insomnia, when in reality this is seldom a cause of poor sleep habits.

Table 9.1   Gas Control

The following foods are possible gas-formers. Since people differ on which foods they can tolerate, try eliminating one of these foods at a time and observe the results. Avoid eating any foods that cause discomfort after noon.

Apples, raw	Kohlrabi
Avocados	Leeks, onions, and shallots
Broccoli	Legumes, including beans, lentils, and split peas
Brussels sprouts	Peppers, green
Cabbage and sauerkraut	Pimentos
Cantaloupe	Radishes
Cauliflower	Rutabagas
Corn	Turnips
Cucumbers	Watermelon
Honeydew melon	

Rare cases of medically diagnosed hypoglycemia (low blood sugar) can trigger discomfort and hunger, even in the middle of the night, and can lead to night awakenings. Hypoglycemics should not snack on cookies, ice cream, or other high-sugar foods before bedtime, since these foods only aggravate low blood sugar and sleep problems.

Night Awakenings

Some people's sleep problems are night awakenings, when they wake up and can't get back to sleep without first having a snack. Although most common in small children, anyone can develop this sleep problem at any stage in life. These midnight snack attacks might be triggered by hunger, a medical condition such as an ulcer that requires food to soothe the pain, or they might just be habit. "Often these nighttime eaters have eaten too few calories during the day," says Gary Zammit, Ph.D., director of the Sleep Disorders Institute at St. Luke's Hospital in New York City. "Night eating is reduced by 50 percent or more in some people when they increase their daytime food intake," he says.

In most cases, your best bet is to break the cycle. First, include some protein-rich foods with dinner, such as chicken or fish, or eat a light snack just before bedtime to curb hunger pangs. Also make sure you eat enough throughout the day to adequately fuel your body. Sleep problems escalate when we drastically cut calories. The most severe examples of this are people suffering from serious eating disorders, such as anorexia and bulimia, who also are prone to sleep disturbances. They wake up more frequently, awaken too early, and dream less than normal eaters. All of these symptoms resolve with weight gain and resumption of normal eating habits. Your best bet for long-term weight management and sound sleep is to make dietary changes gradually and eat at least 2,000 calories a day of nutrient-packed, low-fat foods.

Second, stop rewarding your stomach by feeding it every time it wakes you up. Instead, read a book, drink a glass of water, or ignore the craving. Or, according to Dr. Zammit, some people can wean themselves off midnight snack attacks by gradually eating less food, less frequently, in the middle of the night. It takes about one to two weeks to break a midnight snack habit.

Boosting Serotonin: From Supplements to Popcorn

Tryptophan is nature's sleeping pill. As discussed in chapter 1, this amino acid is a building block for the neurotransmitter serotonin, which regulates sleep. Taking tryptophan supplements increases serotonin levels, reduces the time necessary to fall asleep by as much as 50 percent, and enhances the quality, depth, and length of sleep. Tryptophan supplements must be taken at night to be effective sleep-inducers. During the day, one of the body's enzymes counteracts the effects of serotonin on sleep; blood levels of this enzyme fall at night, which frees serotonin to influence sleep centers in the brain. Tryptophan supplements are not currently available in the United States. In the late 1980s, the Food and Drug Administration (FDA) banned all tryptophan products because of a contaminated supply from Japan.

A supplement called 5-hydroxy-L-tryptophan or 5-HPT is promoted as the building block for serotonin, as well as a mood-elevator, brain stimulant, and sleep-enhancer. The research on this chemical is limited but hopeful. Unfortunately these products also might contain contaminants similar to those found in tryptophan. Safety is questionable, and no known optimal dose has been established.

The next best thing to tryptophan and 5-HPT supplements is to self-regulate natural tryptophan levels by eating a high-carbohydrate, low-protein snack.

"According to our preliminary studies," comments Dr. Zammit, "a light carbohydrate-rich snack [before bedtime] may not influence how fast you fall asleep, but it may help some people sleep longer and more soundly." So have an evening snack one to two hours before bedtime, and make it high-carbohydrate and light, such as air-popped popcorn or half of a bagel topped with jam. See Table 9.2, "Late-Night Munchies," on page 228.

In contrast, a high-protein bedtime snack, such as a slice of turkey or a glass of milk, is a great source of tryptophan but also provides large quantities of other amino acids that compete with tryptophan for absorption and entry into the brain. Consequently, these snacks do not produce the serotonin rise and might even produce a drop in brain levels of serotonin, which could aggravate insomnia. (The advice to drink a cup of warm milk before bedtime won't raise serotonin levels, but the liquid is soothing and provides a feeling of satiety.)

B Vitamins, Minerals, and Your Snooze Control

Ignore your vitamin and mineral needs and you'll pay for it at night. Common symptoms of poor nutrition include fatigue, sleep disorders, irritability, tension, depression, and other mood and energy problems. Regardless of worries, tensions, and other factors, the bottom line is: Well-nourished, healthy people sleep better than unhealthy people.

To be more specific, marginal intake or elevated requirements for several of the B vitamins have been linked directly to sleepless nights. In a study conducted at the National Center of Neurology and Psychiatry in Tokyo, researchers gave vitamin B_{12} supplements to chronic insomniacs who, within days, began sleeping better. Sleep problems returned when the vitamin B_{12} supplements were discontinued. Researchers suspect this vitamin exerts an influence on melatonin, a hormonelike compound that helps regulate sleep. A study from the National Institute of Mental Health in Bethesda, Maryland, replicated these findings and found that people who respond favorably to vitamin B_{12} supplements required higher than usual amounts of the vitamin to maintain normal sleep patterns. However, the dosages used in these studies were very high, up to 3,000 micrograms per day (the typical requirement is 2 micrograms), and any experimentation with megadose vitamin therapy always should be done with physician supervision.

Table 9.2   Late-Night Munchies

Keep your evening snack light and carbohydrate-rich with any of the following:

- A piece of fruit and graham crackers
- Whole-grain toast, and jam
- A baked potato seasoned with chives and nonfat sour cream
- Savory Cilantro Dip with Baked Tortilla Chips*
- A Baked Apple*
- Air-popped popcorn
- Oven-roasted potato chips
- A small dish of sherbet or sorbet
- A small serving of a commercial fat-free dessert
- A low-fat oatmeal-raisin cookie
- Lemon Chiffon Pie*
- $1/2$ cinnamon-raisin bagel with a drizzle of honey
- Cheerios and raisins
- A fruit parfait with vanilla wafers

* See "Recipes for Feeling Your Best" at the back of this book.

Vitamin B_6 also is a suspect in insomnia. This B vitamin is essential for normal production of serotonin. A diet low in vitamin B_6 increases the risk for developing insomnia, while optimal intake of this vitamin improves sleep. Increased intake of other B vitamins, including folic acid and vitamin B_1, also improves sleep in some people. Vitamin B_1 supplementation, for example, reduced the need for daytime naps, improved sleep patterns, and increased activity levels in eighty healthy seniors studied at the University of California, Davis. In some cases, the vitamin corrects a marginal deficiency and is only effective for people who are consuming vitamin-poor diets, while in other cases the vitamin appears to work at larger doses despite apparent adequate dietary intake. In all cases you should discuss with a physician and dietitian the appropriateness of using pharmacological doses of vitamins before self-medicating with supplements.

Other nutrients are indirectly linked to sleep and wake patterns. Calcium and magnesium work as a team to relax and contract muscles and stimulate and subdue the nerves. Deficiencies of either mineral can cause muscle cramping, abnormal nerve function, and changes in deep-sleep eye movements that, theoretically, might affect sleep patterns. Insomnia drains magnesium from the body, and low magnesium is associated with a reduced ability to cope with stress. To be on the safe side during times of poor sleep habits, consume extra servings of magnesium-rich foods, such as whole grains, cooked dried beans and peas, nuts, and green vegetables, or take a supplement that contains 250 milligrams of magnesium.

Sleep patterns also might be affected by low copper or iron intake. One study showed that low copper intake (a trace mineral found in avocados, potatoes, soybeans, bananas, fish, chicken, and green vegetables) increased the risk for earlier bedtimes, longer latency to sleep, longer total sleep time, and feeling less rested upon awakening. Low iron intake also has been linked to an earlier bedtime, more nighttime awakenings, longer total sleep time, and restless legs syndrome (a crawling, aching, or fidgety feeling deep inside your legs). Increasing your daily intake of copper- and iron-rich foods certainly won't hurt and it might help reduce your restless nights. (See Table 9.3, "Eat to Sleep: The Twelve Diet Rules for Insomnia," on page 230.)

Stacking the Deck in Favor of Sleep

"The lamb and the lion shall lie down together, but the lamb will not be very sleepy."

—Woody Allen

Stress is the most common cause of insomnia. Often, controlling the source of stress will improve or completely eliminate sleep problems. Ironically, sleep deprivation increases the stress load and interferes with the ability to problem solve, thus producing a downward spiral unless you intercede to stop the cycle.

Besides practicing effective coping skills during the day, don't allow stress into the bedroom. Set aside a different time during the day to deal with worries, then turn to more relaxing thoughts in the evening. To help condition your body to relax, take a soothing hot bath or shower, read a nonsuspenseful book, or concentrate on a television comedy before bedtime. Save the bed for relaxation and sleep only. Don't pay bills, argue with your spouse, or watch television in bed. Also, set a bedtime ritual that helps program your body to expect sleep. Have a high-carbohydrate snack or a warm glass of milk, then brush your teeth, close the curtains, get clothes ready for the next day, set the alarm, and tuck yourself in. Follow the same ritual every night.

Table 9.3   Eat to Sleep: The Twelve Diet Rules for Insomnia

The following dietary guidelines—when combined with effective stress management skills, avoiding tobacco, and other sleep-enhancing habits—will help you make it through the night, asleep that is.

1. Avoid all caffeinated beverages, foods, and medications.
2. Limit alcohol to two drinks or less each day, and do not drink alcoholic beverages within two hours of bedtime.
3. Eat your biggest meal at breakfast or lunch and a light meal at dinner. Include some protein at the evening meal.
4. Avoid spicy foods at dinnertime.
5. Limit your intake of gas-forming foods to before noon.
6. Avoid MSG-containing foods, such as Chinese restaurant food.
7. Eat slowly and chew the food thoroughly.
8. Avoid strict dieting or dramatic changes in dietary habits.
9. Consume a carbohydrate-rich, low-protein snack one to two hours before bedtime.
10. If a carbohydrate-rich snack doesn't help you sleep, try drinking a cup of warm milk at bedtime.
11. Make sure your dietary intake of the B vitamins, calcium, magnesium, copper, and iron is optimal. If not, take a moderate-dose supplement that contains 100 percent of the Daily Value for these nutrients.
12. Break the middle-of-the-night snack attack cycle by not rewarding your stomach with food.

Don't program your body to toss and turn. If you are tired but can't fall asleep within thirty minutes, get up. Do something monotonous, such as read a boring book, knit, mend clothes, or listen to soft, repetitious music. Don't watch television. Stay up until you are sleepy, and then go to bed. Repeat this process until you fall asleep. If you can't fall asleep and are wide awake, use the "extra" time to do something fun. Work on a hobby, write letters, or make something. (See "Natural Sleep Aids," on page 231.)

Natural Sleep Aids

5-HPT: 5-hydroxytryptophan (5-HPT) supplements are advertised as natural sleep aids. However, the limited research on this substance shows that 5-HPT might not do the trick. Although a building block for serotonin, 5-HPT inconsistently induces and maintains sleep, and triggers vivid dreaming in some people.

Acupressure: Acupressure relies on the same principles as acupuncture. Try steady finger pressure directly below the inside of the anklebone and on the first indentation directly below the outer anklebone.

Herbs: Chamomile, catnip, hops, lemon balm, passionflower, Saint-John's-wort, and valerian. In one study, Swiss researchers found that valerian extract helped insomniacs drop off to sleep faster and stay asleep longer. Valerian has an unpleasant taste, so try it in capsule form or as a tincture. Measure one to two teaspoons per cup of hot water, and steep for ten minutes. Overdoses of valerian can cause blurred vision, changes in heartbeat, and excitability. The other herbs can be made into a tea an hour before bedtime, or you can soak in a warm tub that has been infused with one or more of them.

Kava: Try kava if sleep disturbances are related to anxiety. Try an extract standardized to 60 to 75 milligrams of kavalactones per capsule and take two or three capsules one hour before bedtime. Do not take long-term, since kava can be addicting.

Melatonin: Melatonin—a hormone secreted by the pineal gland in the brain—regulates the ebb and flow of wakefulness and sleepiness. Levels drop with age, so that by age sixty-five, a person has one-third to one-quarter the melatonin levels of a twenty-five-year-old. Melatonin supplements might improve sleep, especially if insomnia results from jet lag, but the sleep is a light sleep almost devoid of the deep sleep that gives the most rest. Common doses range from 1 to 3 milligrams daily, although recommendations have not been established. Side effects include drowsiness, confusion, and headaches. Melatonin also might aggravate preexisting depression. Long-term effects are unknown. You can get a natural melatonin boost from daily exercise and a low-fat diet.

You've Got to Move to Sleep

A major difference between good sleepers and poor sleepers is not what they do at bedtime but what they did all day. Good sleepers are more likely to be physically active. They exercise daily, walk or bicycle to work rather than drive, park far away from their destination and walk, take the stairs rather than the elevator, and use every opportunity to move. The physical activity helps a person cope with daily stress, produces a surge in sleep hormones, and tires the body so it is ready to sleep at night. Exercise also counteracts daytime grogginess that results from not sleeping well by raising calcium levels in the brain, which turns on brain dopamine production and improves mood and energy level. In a study from the University of Washington in Seattle, people who exercised vigorously for forty-five minutes at least three times a week got 33 percent more deep sleep than did people who were relatively inactive. In another study from Stanford University in Palo Alto, California, healthy adults with mild sleep problems who exercised for at least forty minutes a day, twice a week, fell asleep faster and slept about forty-five minutes longer than people who didn't exercise.

Working with Your Body Clock

Irregular sleeping habits also can cause insomnia. A person who slept poorly last night is likely to take a nap during the day or go to bed earlier the next night. The nap or early bedtime, however, makes it harder to fall asleep at the normal time the following evening. If you slept little or poorly, do not take a nap the next day (or, if you must, limit the nap to less than thirty minutes), try to go to bed at your normal time the next night, and do not take sleeping pills. Going to bed and getting up at the same time each day will help your body reset its internal sleep-and-awake clock.

Some people unconsciously reset their sleep clocks to a later hour. They can't fall asleep before midnight, but must get up at six A.M. They are tired all day, but seem to catch a second wind as the evening progresses. If you are one of these people, you can slowly reset your body's sleep clock by going to bed fifteen minutes earlier each night but still getting up at the same time. Develop an evening ritual that helps the body learn to expect sleep at a given time. Avoid coffee, eat a light evening meal and a carbohydrate-rich snack in the evening, and avoid overstimulating activities for the hour or two prior to bedtime. It might take two weeks or more to retrain your body's sleep clock.

Are you a lark or an owl? Do you awake at sunrise or snooze until noon? Are you more productive in the morning or at night? Larks go to sleep early and rise early, while owls excel when they go to bed late and get up late. These differences in body rhythms might be biological or inherited, but they can't be ignored. Once you know your natural rhythms, you can work with this ebb and flow. You will achieve your best results with the least amount of effort if you coordinate the demands of your life with your most productive times of the day and sleep when your energy level is at its lowest point.

II.

REINING IN OUT-OF-CONTROL APPETITES

CHAPTER TEN

Why Do You Overeat?

- Why do you crave doughnuts, but your friend can't keep her hands off the sugar cookies?
- Why is it that the more you diet to manage your weight, the more weight you gain?
- Why do we become hungry at the smell of cinnamon rolls baking?
- Why do you taste the off flavors in cabbage and coffee, while these are a friend's favorite foods?
- Why does a harmless plate of chocolates beckon? You try to ignore them—even leave the room—but it's no use: The cravings can be as strong as an addiction. Your willpower usually drains away, and there you are eating one, then another and another. You couldn't stop. No matter how many pieces you eat, you don't get full. You probably will realize later that you weren't even hungry. So you're left wondering why you gorge on chocolate but can't find room for those vegetables.

Those aren't easy questions to answer. There are almost as many theories about what governs appetite and triggers out-of-control eating as there are enticing foods on a grocery store's shelves. "We have a lot to learn about appetite and satiety and it's likely we'll find in the long run that the underlying reasons why people overeat are a combination of factors," says Barbara Rolls, Ph.D., a professor of nutrition at Pennsylvania State University.

Are You Overeating?

Women often think they are overeating, when in fact they're not eating enough. The Food and Nutrition Board (the same group that developed the Recommended Dietary Allowances) recommends that a moderately active woman who is five feet five inches tall and weighs 128 to 138 pounds should consume about 2,200 calories daily; yet women average about 1,500 calories daily, according to national nutrition surveys.

If you're eating less than 1,600 to 2,000 calories daily, then you're undereating, not overeating. But how do you know if you're eating too much or not enough? What does a real meal look like?

The basic day's menu should include at least six whole grains, five (preferably nine) fruits and vegetables, three calcium-rich selections such as nonfat milk or yogurt, and three iron-rich selections such as extra-lean meat, chicken, fish, or legumes. You should eat regularly throughout the day, or at least five times, so every mini-meal or snack should include one or more grain and one to two fruits or vegetables. At three of those meals/snacks, you also should include a calcium-rich and an iron-rich selection. (See Table 10.3, "Size Matters," on page 249 to learn about serving sizes.) All in all, about three-fourths of your plate will be grains, produce, and legumes; the other one-fourth will be meat and/or milk products. Here's what a sample plate should look like:

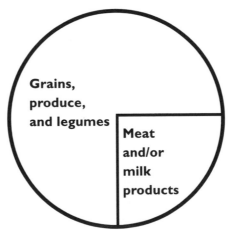

Even the definition is tricky. Hunger, or the inborn instinct to eat, is a facet of appetite. But if hunger was all there was, then eating would be a process of feeling physiological hunger, seeking food, eating in response to that need, and pushing back from the table at the first signal of fullness.

That certainly doesn't explain an addiction to chocolate . . . or potato chips, cheesecake, meat loaf, steak, or any other food eaten in excess. Obviously many of us sometimes eat more than we need, whether we're hungry or not, and often all the wrong stuff. In fact, overeating has become a national pastime. So while hunger is a physiological response orchestrated by a flood of neurotransmitters, hormones, and chemicals in the brain and body, appetite also encompasses a psychological or learned response to food that includes sensory qualities of food, social and emotional influences, individual preferences, cravings, and aversions. Not to mention the final stage of appetite: satiety, or the sensation of fullness that should follow eating and that also has both physical and psychological origins.

If all these sensations worked in harmony, none of us would have a problem with overeating. We would feel hunger and appetite simultaneously when our bodies needed food, and we would be satisfied after eating just enough to meet our needs. Unfortunately, this is not always the case. Sometimes the chemicals and hormones regulating appetite run amok or the sensory overload of a tantalizing snack drowns out our appetite clocks. Other times, we ignore hunger and override satiety signals; eat to fill emotional, not physical, hungers; or eat too much in an effort to satisfy a need for flavor. In still other cases, a lack of knowledge about what, when, why, and how much to eat contributes to our out-of-control appetites. Before you grab the bag of chocolate chip cookies, read on. Scientists know a lot about why our appetites sometimes rage out of control, as well as how to rein them in. (See "Are You Overeating?," on page 236.)

Born to Be Hungry

A discussion of appetite and overeating is peculiar to the twentieth century. For millions of years there was little more to eat than roots, nuts, leaves, and an occasional bison. "The human body evolved an elaborate and powerful appetite system to ensure we eat—and eat well—when food is around, with fat being the most efficient way to obtain energy," says Adam Drewnowski, Ph.D., director of the Nutritional Sciences Program at the University of Washington. This drive works best when the food supply is scarce and unpredictable, but as aptly said by B. G. Galef,

Ph.D., at McMaster University in Hamilton, Ontario, ". . . there is no reason to expect the wisdom of the body to lead humans to make wise food choices when faced with the superabundance of the modern supermarket." In short, our chemistry hasn't kept up with the food supply.

If we were faced with only an abundance of broccoli (or even chocolate, for that matter), overeating still might be a moot point. It's the variety of tasty foods that gets us. Dr. Rolls coined the term "sensory-specific satiety" to explain why we are more likely to overeat when offered different foods than if we're offered one food at a time. The first two or three bites are the most satisfying, while a food's pleasurability drops off dramatically after that. But alternate a host of high-fat, tasty items, such as a hot dog and French fries, with popcorn, soda pop, and an ice-cream cone at a baseball game, and we're likely to eat beyond fullness, and much more than if we'd snacked only on popcorn.

Dr. Rolls recently discovered another reason we overeat. It's a weight thing. No, not body weight—food weight. According to Dr. Rolls's studies, people stop eating when they have consumed a given weight or volume of food, regardless of its calories. "When we gave people either 300-, 450-, or 600-milliliter drinks that contained the same calories, the people who drank the greatest volume ate less a half hour later," says Dr. Rolls. In short, if you fill up on a pound of food, you would be overeating if you chose chocolate at 2,000 calories, but munching for health if you chose a pound of carrots at 195 calories.

Foods weigh the most when they're packed with water and fiber, which could be the reason why low-calorie, fiber-rich foods fill us up quicker, while calorie-dense, fatty, or sugary foods spur us to eat more. A Satiety Index was created by researchers from the University of Sydney in Australia who fed people thirty-eight common foods and measured their hunger and food intakes for the two hours following their meals. They found that people consumed fewer calories yet felt more satisfied after eating fiber-rich potatoes, oatmeal, oranges, pasta, and beans than when they ate high-fat yet fiber-poor croissants, cake, doughnuts, or candy.

When Chemicals Run Amok

At the basis of our highly evolved appetites is a symphony of neural and chemical cues. The conductor is housed in the brain's appetite-control center, called the hypothalamus, but the music is played from all parts of your body—from the nervous system to your liver, blood, and fat cells.

Take, for example, the neurotransmitters serotonin and neuropeptide Y (NPY). As discussed in chapters 1, 2, and 3, when serotonin levels are low or when NPY levels are high, we unknowingly turn to oatmeal, cookies, jelly beans, waffles, or any other carbohydrate-rich food, which in turn boosts serotonin and drops NPY levels, shutting off the cravings. These neurotransmitters work with an orchestra of nerve chemicals, including noradrenaline and gamma aminobutyric acid (GABA). Our preference for fat is fueled by another set of chemicals, including the endorphins and galanin. These and other hypothalamic messengers communicate with other brain centers and receive input about digestion and the body's fuel needs via chemicals such as cholecystokinin (CCK) from the digestive tract, enterostatin from the pancreas, fluctuating blood sugar and insulin levels, and the female reproductive hormone estrogen. This array of chemistry is set off by even the sight or smell of food. In short, our appetites, hungers, and cravings are essentially the result of riding internal chemical swells. Any imbalance in one or more of these chemicals could undermine the best of intentions to eat sensibly.

Eating disorders are possibly fueled by the same nerve chemicals, just at more extreme levels. More than two out of every three persons with bulimia (an eating disorder characterized by excessive food intake in a short amount of time—also called binge eating—followed often by self-induced vomiting or the use of laxatives) report that a binge is triggered by cravings for specific foods—in particular, sweets. Since NPY and serotonin, the neurotransmitters that trigger cravings for carbohydrates, are disturbed in anorexia and bulimia, some researchers speculate that eating disorders might be fueled by imbalances in neurotransmitters. When animals are injected with NPY, they gorge on carbohydrate-rich foods until they become obese. NPY levels are elevated in anorexics who vacillate between starvation and bingeing, and are very high in bulimics, which might override normal signals of satiety and contribute to their compulsion to overeat sweet and starchy foods. In addition, altered serotonin levels cause depression, which contributes to the eating disorder and loss of self-esteem.

Whatever begins the dieting spiral, it is likely that resulting imbalances in this chemical stew pot are major reasons why eating disorders progress. A person might start out with a normal balance of nerve chemicals, but the starvation or binge-and-purge cycle upsets the appetite control chemicals in his or her system. (This is the most common explanation, since most appetite-control chemicals normalize when normal eating habits are resumed in both anorexics and bulimics.) (See Table 10.1, "Are You a Food Addict?," on page 241.)

Even erratic eating habits or dieting in an otherwise healthy person can interact with an already touchy neurotransmitter balance, swinging the pendulum from balance to binge. "Appetite-regulating chemicals are upset when a woman goes on a quick-weight-loss diet," says Dr. Sarah Leibowitz at Rockefeller University. Skip meals and levels of NPY, endorphins, galanin, or other neurotransmitters rise, making it harder to have willpower when a craving occurs. Even our fat tissues get into the act, releasing 3-hydroxybutyrate, a fat fragment that heralds our need to eat when more than about four hours have passed since the last meal. Consequently, stressed-out dieters are more likely to overeat than are stressed-out nondieters. "Many people skip meals in an effort to save calories," says C. Wayne Callaway, M.D., at George Washington University in Washington, D.C. "This plan backfires and inevitably increases cravings, lowers resistance [to sweet, salty, or high-fat foods] later in the day, and leads to overeating." (See the nine components of the Feeling Good Diet in chapter 12, on pages 272–274, for suggestions on taming your neurotransmitters.)

Savor the Taste

Has an uncontrollable urge to eat ever driven you to the kitchen without a clue what you're hungry for? You take a bite of leftover lasagna. Crunch on a carrot. Drink some cranberry juice. Dish up a bowl of ice cream. Dive into the bag of potato chips. You graze on hundreds of calories, yet never feel satisfied. Or do you binge on pizza because you're in a diet rut, bored with the same foods day in and day out? This could be a sign that you are overeating because you need a flavor fix.

A desire for something savory outweighs even our basic hunger signals, yet many of us ignore the finer flavors, opting for the same old familiar foods. "In our effort to eat healthful, low-fat fare, sometimes we forget food's greatest qualities—it's supposed to taste scrumptious, look appetizing, and smell like heaven," says Evelyn Tribole, M.S., R.D., author of *Intuitive Eating* (St. Martin's Press, 1995). Granted, some people overeat for emotional reasons or because they're stressed, bored, or lonely (see chapter 11). But could it be that some of us overeat or choose all the wrong foods not because we're hungry or that our appetite chemicals are out of balance but because we haven't had a truly satisfying meal all day?

"Many people are craving taste and don't stop eating until that need for flavor is satisfied," says Rozanne Gold, award-winning chef and author of *Little Meals* (Little, Brown and Company, 1999). We often live on sensory-deficient diets, and even when we binge, it's on the same old salty, sugary, or fatty stuff. "We tend to eat

---

Table 10.1   Are You a Food Addict?

Eating disorders often progress from normal to moderately abnormal to binge eating to more serious or overlapping problems, such as bulimia, bulimia-anorexia, and anorexia. The sooner you detect the early warning signs, the more likely you can stop a bad habit from progressing to a serious problem. A yes to any one of the following questions is a red flag that you're putting too much emphasis on food.

1. Are you preoccupied with food or are you constantly dieting?
2. Do you sneak food, eat in secret, or hide food wrappers?
3. Are you uncomfortable in situations where there is no food available, or do you avoid situations where there will be food?
4. Are you constantly concerned about your weight or weigh yourself more than twice a week?
5. Do you lose control over how much food you intended to eat?
6. Has eating become increasingly more unmanageable?
7. Do you hide food in drawers, closets, the laundry hamper, the sewing machine, or other unusual places?
8. Do you nibble at a party and gorge when you get home?
9. Do you arrange to be home alone so you can eat?
10. Do you make excuses for overeating or not eating at all?
11. Has food or eating interfered with any part of your life?
12. Do you stay up late at night when everyone is in bed so you can eat?
13. Do you feel panicky about food?
14. Is food a primary source of security? Do you use it to feel better, calmer, less shy or anxious?
15. Has anyone ever said you have an eating problem or that you are too thin?
16. Do you think you have a problem with food and eating?
17. Do you eat large amounts of food in a short amount of time—i.e., less than two hours?
18. Have you ever used vomiting, laxatives, diuretics, enemas, fasting, excessive exercise, or amphetamines as methods to lose weight or to control your weight?
19. Have you ever felt ashamed of how much you eat?
20. Do you overeat more than twice a week or skip more than five meals in a week?
21. Are you more than ten pounds below the recommended weight for your height?

To learn more about eating disorders, contact any of the organizations that specialize in eating disorders listed in the "Resources" section at the back of this book, or see your physician.

---

one-dimensional diets these days, but if we chose foods that excited all the senses, we would feel more satisfied with smaller meals," says Gold.

What Is This Thing Called Taste?

Taste is the number one reason why we choose the foods we do, but most of us don't have a clue what it is. Taste is divided into four "primary taste qualities": salty (sodium chloride), sweet (sugar), sour (lemon juice), and bitter (quinine). A fifth taste, called *"umami,"* is a Japanese word that describes a proteinlike taste or savoriness but also denotes the total flavor gestalt of a dish. Scientists once thought that these taste receptors were housed in specific spots on the tongue (sour and salty were on the sides, bitter along the back, and sweet was on the tip), but now realize they are interspersed over the surfaces of the tongue, the epiglottis, the larynx, and the upper one-third of the esophagus, and work in tandem with bundles of nerve fibers that also react to stimuli.

The mouthwatering experience of eating a leg of lamb with apricot stuffing, or curried butternut squash soup, or a dark chocolate and raspberry layer cake is more than just taste. "Usually what we mean by taste is really the *flavor* of food, and we can't perceive flavor without our sense of smell," says Richard Mattes, Ph.D., R.D., professor of foods and nutrition at Purdue University in West Lafayette, Indiana. To appreciate how important smell is to flavor, try holding your nose while taking a bite of an apple and then an onion. You might taste some vague sweet or bitter qualities, but you won't be able to distinguish the fruit from the onion from a bite of cardboard.

Aromatic chemicals released in the mouth drift up the back of the throat to stimulate receptors in the nose, which relay the information to the olfactory nerve and then into the brain. The nose can detect hundreds of variations in smell and taste compared to the measly four or five taste sensations. "Up to 90 percent of the ability to detect food flavors can be attributed to the sense of smell," says Dr. Mattes. These same olfactory receptors also send messages to the limbic system in the brain, which processes information associated with emotion. This might explain why odors conjure up some of our most emotionally charged memories, why learning is enhanced when paired with the presence of a novel aroma, or even why some women have a love-hate relationship with chocolate. When researchers at the University of Pennsylvania gave chocoholics a chocolate bar, a calorie-equivalent in white chocolate, or a capsule filled with cocoa powder, only the chocolate bar satisfied the cravings. The researchers concluded that it was the aroma, not the sweetness, texture, or calories, that soothed the cravings.

But flavor is more than taste and smell. Other sensations, such as texture (is the food crunchy, creamy, or chewy?), temperature (we like our chef's salad cold and our winter soups warm), and pungency (such as ginger, black pepper, and horseradish), rely on the "common chemical sense," which relays information from the mouth via cranial nerve V to the brain. We also eat with our eyes, so it's not surprising that the very sight of a scrumptious meal also stimulates the brain's appetite center and gets the digestive juices churning before we've even unfolded our napkins.

The Snap, Crackle, and Fizz of Taste

The satisfying burn of salsa and the tingly fizz of a cola are classified as irritants. "Chemosensory irritation is separate from taste and smell and is mediated by a different set of nerves located on the palate, tongue, and the back of the throat; it's a skin sense more than a taste sense," says Mark Friedman, Ph.D., associate director of the Monell Chemical Senses Center in Philadelphia. Chili peppers, red peppers, and horseradish cause tingling, burning, and even itching sensations. There is even a novel compound in a Nepalese plant that produces a sensation much like a mild electrical current. "We don't understand why people are turning more and more to these spicy foods," says Dr. Friedman. "It could be an increasing willingness to accept other cultural cuisines; there is even a theory that thrill-seeking behaviors are somehow linked to a liking for foods flavored with these chemosensory irritants."

In short, our entire nervous system perks up to the savoriness of food in a sort of holographic way within the brain. Full-blown satisfaction comes from engaging the whole sensory system with a flavorful, aromatic meal.

Tastefully Yours

What you serve at a candlelight dinner will depend on the company. Granted, our basic tastes are hardwired into our taste buds and into our brains starting at birth. But taste also is a very individual matter, with our preferences as unique as our fingerprints. While one person might love scalloped potatoes with ham, that same meal might make another person nauseous.

That's because taste is genetically programmed, to a certain degree. During taste-test studies, identical twins like and dislike similar foods, while fraternal twins show few similarities in food choices. The reason could be differences in sensitivity to specific bitter compounds in foods, such as phenylthiocarbamide (PTC) or 6-n-propylthiouracil (PROP) in cabbage. To about 25 percent of the population, these compounds are extremely bitter (the supertasters), to another 50 percent they're only mildly bitter, and the rest of us can't taste them at all. For supertasters with their overabundance of taste buds, the world is like a rock concert of flavors—too many, too loud, and too crowded. Consequently, they like mild or subtle flavors and are most apt to shun salt substitutes like potassium chloride, the nonnutritive sweetener saccharine, pepper, coffee, and cabbage because all these items are too bitter. Supertasters also are more likely to avoid chili peppers because they're too hot, whipped cream because it's too creamy, and alcohol because of the "off" flavors. Nontasters eat much more of these foods.

Food preferences also vary between the sexes. Women have a more acute sense of smell, and that translates into a more vivid sense of taste and a greater likelihood of being supertasters. They are most likely to turn to the sweet-and-creamy combinations found in ice cream, cookies, cakes, pies, and doughnuts, while men define a meal by what meat is served. These preferences mirror the rise in galanin, a neurotransmitter that starts whispering fat cravings in our ears from midday until bedtime. Why the gender difference exists is anyone's guess. The theory proposed by Dr. Leibowitz that our fuel choices go hand in hand with reproduction and survival of the species could explain why men instinctively choose the protein-fat mixture in meat for muscle building, while women prefer the sugar-fat mixture to add pounds that will ensure healthy pregnancies. The female hormones also enhance women's perception of taste and smell during the childbearing years as a natural protection against eating anything toxic that could harm a fetus.

Of course we can't ignore the overall euphoria of eating chocolate. It could be that some foods, usually the ones we eat too much of, are so pleasurable that they override our complex system of satiation. Some of us also are more hedonistic than others, reveling in the pleasurability of the taste, aroma, and feel of food. These gourmet prodigies are born to enjoy the experience of eating and must learn to temper that appreciation by tasting, not gorging.

Genetics and euphoria aside, Dr. Mattes believes the number one cause of our food preferences is availability. "The driving force behind our flavor preferences is frequency of exposure; deprive people of salt and they learn to like unsalted foods more, cut back on fat intake and people learn to like lower-fat diets," says Mattes. But we live in a glut of high-fat, salty foods, so it is these that we learn to love. While fat in food carries many of the aromas and makes chocolate creamy, potato chips crunchy, and meat juicy, it doesn't leave us satisfied. So we end up overeating fatty foods in an effort to feel full.

The good news is we *can* reprogram our food preferences. According to researchers at the Fred Hutchinson Cancer Prevention Research Center in Seattle, people lose their love for fatty foods the longer they stick with low-fat diets. The secret is to make the adjustment gradually and avoid feeling deprived. "You also can trick your instincts to eat high-fat foods by dining on stews, soups, and other water-based foods that taste calorie-dense when they're not," says Dr. Drewnowski. You also can wean yourself off fat but still include creamy, rich textures in your diet by including more custard-style low-fat yogurts, chocolate syrup (which is fat-free), mangoes and papaya, and nonfat sour cream and cream cheese. Moderate use of aspartame can sweeten the diet without adding calories.

Lip-Smacking Rules

"Flavor has a major effect on whether or not we feel satisfied after a meal," says Zoe Warwick, Ph.D., professor of psychology at the University of Maryland. In her studies and in studies from the University of Pittsburgh, increasing the flavor of foods reduced hunger; successful dieting and weight loss were most likely when savory, carbohydrate-rich meals were consumed. Other studies show that people are most likely to lose weight when they eat small, frequent meals rather than three big square meals. A recent study found that people who ate soup for lunch consumed fewer calories at that meal and ate less for dinner that night; thus, a well-seasoned, low-fat soup might be just what you need to drop those extra pounds while curbing an out-of-control appetite. The trick is to make these mini-meals and filling foods satisfying by following these guidelines:

1. *Know which flavors turn you on.* "Think about the tastes, smells, and textures of food that are most satisfying to you," recommends Dr. Warwick. Are they hard and crunchy foods like peanuts, creamy foods like chocolate, sweet or salty foods like watermelon or feta cheese, or spicy foods like mango salsa? Then incorporate low-fat alternatives to these foods into your diet. "I used to crave Doritos and potato chips; now I'm happy with pretzels," confesses Dr. War- wick. (See Table 10.2, "How to Make Foods Tasty," on pages 247–248.)

2. *Think quality, not quantity.* Adding flavor and savoriness to your meals tantalizes the taste buds and accents the sensuous side to food— its colors, textures, and aromas. The more you combine flavors, the

more interesting is the meal. Experiment with sweet, spicy, and sour tastes by adding fruit, red pepper flakes, and arugula to a salad; combining lemon and mint in a marinade; or blending roasted red peppers and cayenne and drizzling it over a creamed vegetable soup. Then serve yourself small portions of the best flavors.

3. *Eat mindfully.* You still will overeat if you gobble your food. "For thousands of years, our spiritual ancestors regarded food as our connection to the mystery of life; yet today we reduce it to a functional fuel," says Deborah Kesten, M.P.H., author of *Feeding the Body, Nourishing the Soul* (Conari Press, 1997). Kesten reminds us that food sustains not only our body but also our mind and soul. To connect with this life force, she suggests eating with awareness, "listening" to each bite, "hearing" the subtle flavors, "tasting" the colors, and experiencing the aromas. Bring your attention inward as you chew food by sensing the changes in texture, temperature, and taste. Listen to your hunger signals; stop periodically during a meal and sit back, then return to eating only if you are truly enjoying the food and are still hungry. "So many times people take a bite of something that doesn't really taste all that good, yet they eat it anyway; if they would stop and ask themselves, 'Is this worthy of my tastebuds?,' they might stop the overeating before it begins," says Tribole.

4. *Pay attention* to the ambiance of the meal and its preparation. Set the table in style. Arrange the plate attractively. Dim the lights. Put on calming music. Relax before eating—say a prayer or just be silent. "We must take time to lovingly prepare and mindfully enjoy flavorful meals; it is then that our food will truly nourish us, since it will be spiced with spirit, stirred with soul, and served from the heart," says Kesten.

Know How, No Way

The more you know about nutrition, the better you eat. People well versed in accurate nutrition information consume fewer calories, less fat, and more fruits and vegetables. The catch is that many of us know less than we think. According to a Gallup poll conducted by Weight Watchers International and the American Dietetic Association, 90 percent of women surveyed said their diets were healthy, yet only 1 percent of us really meet even minimum standards for a healthful diet.

Table 10.2   How to Make Foods Tasty

Do you need an inspirational boost when it comes to flavoring your meals? Stock your kitchen with flavor-enhancing ingredients and you can muster a tasty meal even in a pinch. Here are nineteen items that pack a taste punch for little or no calories:

1. *Canned chilies:* Add whole chilies to a grilled chicken sandwich or diced chilies to soups, scrambled eggs, pita sandwiches, or on tortillas.
2. *Canned roasted red/yellow peppers:* Add to a grilled cheese sandwich; blend them with some cayenne and drizzle over a creamed vegetable soup, egg dishes, pasta sauces (cold and hot), or add as a topping with cheese for crackers.
3. *Fresh cilantro:* Add to bottled salsa, a bean burrito, a summer soup, fruit or vegetable salads, vinaigrette dressings, black beans, or rice dishes.
4. *Sun-dried tomatoes:* Use in pasta salads, sandwich spreads, vegetable dips, or as an extra topping on pizza. Mix into sautéed zucchini or as an accompaniment to grilled eggplant. Blend with olives, garlic, and balsamic vinegar to make a spicy spread for grilled vegetable sandwiches.
5. *Fresh ginger:* Combine with curry to flavor chicken, add to hot or iced tea, season steamed vegetables such as pea pods or carrots. Use as a topping along with green onions on roasted fish. Add to stir-frys, tofu dishes, or salad dressings.
6. *Balsamic vinegar:* Mix with olive oil for a bread-dunking dip, drizzle over steamed broccoli, or use instead of other vinegars in salad dressing. Add to soups or cold rice or pasta salads.
7. *Horseradish:* Use in potato dishes, vegetable dips with dill, vegetable or chicken wraps with sour cream, spicy soup like gumbo, turkey burgers (ginger is good here, too), cold potato salad, or cold green beans.
8. *Lemon:* The grated rind (called lemon zest) can be added to sorbets, frozen yogurts, or fruit salads. The juice can put a tangy taste into couscous, gazpacho, and dressings, and can be used as marinade for fish.
9. *Fresh herbs:* Fresh always tastes better than dried, so either grow herbs yourself or purchase them fresh in the produce section. Add fresh basil to pasta, tomatoes or other vegetables, bread dough, or even mango slices (basil and lemon are a good match). Fresh rosemary accents any meat, as well as pasta dishes, roasted vegetables, lima beans, peas, or squash. Fresh dill is an excellent flavorant for fish, chicken, omelettes and other egg dishes, salads, beets, cabbage, potatoes, or cucumbers. Fresh oregano is excellent in Italian, Greek, or Mexican dishes.

10. *Crushed red pepper flakes or Tabasco:* Sprinkle on pizza, pasta dishes, salads, or soups. Add to olive oil or sour cream dips, rice dishes, or bean salads. Mix into corn bread batter or bread dough.

11. *Apricot preserves:* Roll into a crepe with sour cream; use with rice vinegar and soy sauce or oranges and garlic in marinades for chicken or lamb; mix into fruit salads or couscous; add to batters for scones, muffins, or tarts.

12. *Black peppercorns:* Add to pasta, salads, eggs, fish, and beef dishes. Grind some into brown bread batters, stewed fruits, hot chocolate, or spiced cider. White peppercorns are good on grilled meats, shish kebab, and creamed soups. Or mix black, white, and green peppercorns in a mill.

13. *Cloves:* Add whole cloves to a bouquet garni in stews or soups; add a pinch of ground cloves to chili or glazed carrots; mix into coffee cake batter; or flavor your sugar bowl by adding a few cloves.

14. *Nut oils:* Use walnut or hazelnut oils instead of olive oil in vinaigrettes. Drizzle over potato salad instead of using mayonnaise. Try on hot steamed vegetables, such as asparagus, broccoli, or green beans, or use almond oil and sherry vinegar on a wild rice salad.

15. *Fruit:* Add fruit to make an unusual dish: Cook chicken with mangoes or grapes, or add pears, fresh berries, or peaches to a tossed salad. Accent a marinade with mandarin oranges.

16. *Gourmet lettuce:* Throw out the iceberg and toss a great salad using radicchio, endive, escarole, baby lettuce, arugula, treviso, puntarelle, frisee (curly endive), purslane, watercress, young spinach, and large red oakleaf lettuce. Add pineapple, plums, or other fruit, or grilled vegetables or meats as a topping.

17. *Fresh mint:* Use it to flavor iced tea. Toss it with new potatoes, fresh peas, or steamed carrots. Mix mint and basil for pesto sauces. Use as an accompaniment to any fiery foods, such as Southwest Asian dishes. Add to fresh fruit or citrus salsas or chutneys.

18. *Salsa:* Make your own by experimenting with grilled corn, vine-ripened tomatoes, garlic, red onions, and chilies. Or try fruit salsas made from mango, jicama, and black beans. Try adding rice wine vinegar, fresh mint, lime juice, fresh herbs, avocados, or cilantro.

19. *Honey:* Drizzle over fruit salads. Use with fresh herbs in a glaze for roasted meats. Coat slices of sweet potato and roast. Blend with olive oil, vinegar, and mustard for a vinaigrette. Mix with soy sauce, ginger, orange juice concentrate, and rice wine for a marinade.

Table 10.3   Size Matters

Take a look at people's portions and you'll find that one person's snack could be another person's meal. The moderate servings on which the Feeling Good Diet is based are in stark contrast to what many people think is a serving. Here are a few guidelines to keep your portions in line with a fork rather than a forklift.

ONE SERVING OF:	IS THE SIZE OF:

MILK PRODUCTS

8-ounce glass of milk or a tub of yogurt	two filled wineglasses ($3^1/2$–4 ounces)
1 ounce of cheese	a large marble or a pair of dice

GRAINS

$^1/2$ cup of rice, noodles, or cooked cereal	a tennis ball
1 slice of bread or $^1/2$ small bagel, an English muffin, or a hamburger bun	a CD case
1 pancake	a CD

MEAT/BEANS

3 ounces of meat, chicken, fish	the palm of your hand, a deck of cards, or a cassette tape

VEGETABLES AND FRUIT

1 cup raw	a baseball
$^1/2$ cup cooked	a medium-sized fist
1 piece	
$^3/4$ cup juice	

FATS AND SUGARS

1 teaspoon of butter or margarine	1 pat or the size of a stamp the thickness of your finger
2 tablespoons salad dressing, or peanut butter	a standard ice cube or a Ping-Pong ball
2 tablespoons pancake syrup	a shot-glass full

Part of the problem is that we're painfully confused about basic nutrition facts. According to a U.S. Food and Drug Administration (FDA) survey of people's knowledge about fat, only one out of every five people knew that all fats—be it olive oil, butter, or lard—provide the same number of calories; seven out of ten had not heard of monounsaturated fats, and almost 40 percent were unsure or wrong about what foods supply saturated fats. We also downplay the fat in foods, underestimate portion sizes, and downright lie about how much we eat. Consequently, we've cut our fat percentages not because we've actually cut fat grams, but because we've increased our calories. (See Table 10.3, "Size Matters," on page 249.)

Knowledge also backfires. Tell us we're eating low-fat, and we eat more. In another study conducted by Dr. Rolls, women ate more for lunch when they thought they were snacking on low-fat yogurt than they did when they were told the yogurt was full-fat, regardless of the actual fat and calorie contents. This mind-over-calories phenomenon might explain why obesity rates continue to rise despite increasing use of fake sugars (it's too soon to tell if fake fats will help us cut back on calories). See Table 10.4, "Those Little Habits," on page 251, for guidelines on how to nurture your culinary literacy.

Overeating All the Right Foods

"The critical issue is that it is fat, sugar, and salt we overeat; you never hear anyone say, 'I just can't stop eating celery,'" says Dr. Drewnowski. So the whole issue of out-of-whack appetites might come down to focusing on natural foods and your health, not fake fats and waistlines. First fill your tummy with strawberries, baby carrots, whole wheat pasta, plain nonfat yogurt flavored with fresh-cut mangoes, and the like. If there is room left over, then turn to the cakes, cookies, snack foods, and French fries. You won't eat as much, will feel full longer, and will find that even when confronted with that plate of chocolates, you'll be more likely to have just one, not the whole platter! Of course, there is always exercise. "Daily physical activity shifts the body from energy excess to energy need, so what is considered overeating when you're sedentary is just fueling your body when you're fit," says Dr. Drewnowski.

Table 10.4   Those Little Habits

If lack of knowledge is the reason why you overeat, then the answer is easy: Start taking this nutrition thing seriously.

1. *Get fat-free savvy.* "What a fat-free cookie loses in fat, it gains in sugar; consequently most fat-free desserts have about the same calories as regular ones," warns Adam Drewnowski, Ph.D., director of the Nutritional Sciences Program at the University of Washington. Fat-free cream cheese might be lower in calories, but not if you slather three times as much on a bagel. Use sparingly both regular and fat-free versions of anything sweet or creamy.

2. *Read labels.* Look for foods that supply no more than 3 grams of fat for every 100 calories. Also note the serving size, which might be unrealistically small, giving the false impression of being low-calorie.

3. *Watch those portions.* We've become accustomed to gigantic servings. A 2-ounce bagel is now a 500-calorie, 4-to-7-ounce meal. The local deli heaps 6 ounces of turkey on your sandwich, not the 3 ounces considered a serving. Also, watch out for those high-fat items that are easy to nibble, such as that plate of chocolates, a bag of chips, or a half-gallon of ice cream. "You are better off deciding what you want to eat, then putting a serving on a plate," says Barbara Rolls, Ph.D., professor of nutrition at Pennsylvania State University. "That way you get the full range of information on how much you're eating and are less likely to overdo it."

4. *Never socialize on an empty stomach.* People eat more when they're with friends and family. So have a healthful snack before a party, split an entrée when dining out, and don't mix alcohol with socializing since even one drink breaks down the best of intentions, leaving you more likely to overeat.

5. *Do the grease slick test.* Some foods don't come with labels, such as that bran muffin at the coffee shop or the doughnuts after church. But you usually can tell if something is high-fat by the slick feel in your mouth. If your doughnut leaves a grease stain on your fingers or a napkin, you can bet several teaspoons of fat went into its making.

6. *Take conscious control.* "Unless people make a conscious decision to choose more fruits, vegetables, and whole grains, they will automatically and inevitably turn to high-fat, high-sugar items like cakes and cookies," says Dr. Drewnowski.

CHAPTER ELEVEN

Food Abuse: Eating for All the Wrong Reasons

- "My date the other night didn't go well. I came home sure that I would never find a life mate, stood at the kitchen counter, and finished off half a tub of ice cream."
- "My eating is pretty normal while I'm at the office. But when I'm home alone at night I seem to lose all willpower to resist the chips."
- "After an argument with my boss today, I reached for a candy bar."
- "While shopping at the mall, I saw a heavy person in a store window, then realized it was me. I headed straight to the bakery and ate two cinnamon rolls."

One of the main themes of this book is that many of our food cravings, desires, preferences, and compulsions are fueled by a mixture of nerve chemicals. These neurotransmitters are intrinsically linked to the body's basic drive to survive and are as instinctive as breathing. Most attempts to "will" them away only make them worse, so individuals must learn to work with—not against—their cravings. But while our appetite-control chemistry is the foundation of when and why we eat, it is strongly influenced by our moods, beliefs, and habits.

The Psychology of Eating Habits

Most people at one time or another turn to food to soothe their feelings. In fact, emotional eating is so common that many people consider it unavoidable and normal. The red flag for emotional eating is when you eat in response to a mood rather than in response to hunger. The former fuels the feelings; the latter fuels the body.

There is nothing wrong with an occasional snack to calm you down or make you feel better. Somehow life seems less depressing when we are satiated with cookies and ice cream, leftover turkey, corn chips and dip, or a dish of rich chocolate pudding. You have a problem, however, when emotional eating leads to compulsive eating, obesity, malnutrition, or other health issues. It also is a problem if it is used as a way to deal with emotions or to escape negative feelings, covering up underlying problems that should be addressed.

Anxiety, worries, tension, upset feelings, stress, and fear are common causes of emotional eating. Food becomes the tranquilizer that calms the nerves and soothes anxiety. The anxiety is caused by anticipation of an event, such as having to give a presentation, or a thought, such as, "I can't do this." In either case, the result is that you turn to food to soothe yourself. Or it might be that turning to food during times of stress is a learned response: Whenever you were anxious in the past, you reached for the symbol of caregiving—food—to help you through the tough times. If those associations date back to childhood, when you were given food whenever you were upset or cried, then your adult eating habits become an unconscious way to deal with your tension.

The bigger the assignment, the higher the demands, or the tighter the deadline, the more likely you are to eat. Women might be more vulnerable to this stress-eating scenario than are men. Researchers at the University of Michigan in Dearborn sat women and men at tables loaded with munchies, and had them watch either a bland film about travel or a high-anxiety film about gruesome accidents on the job. The women who watched the gory film ate twice as many cookies, candies, and crackers as the people who watched the travel film, while the men who viewed the gory film actually ate less food. As mentioned in chapter 7, this food-mood link might be reinforced because eating raises levels of endorphins and serotonin, which in turn calm us down.

In situations such as boredom and loneliness, eating becomes a way to fill the emotional void. It is the interesting activity to curb boredom or the satisfying relationship to cure loneliness. While preventing boredom and developing meaningful relationships take time and effort, eating is easy and relatively effortless. Unfortunately, it is a quick fix that only adds to the problem in the long run. Boredom, anxiety, anger, depression, jealousy, and other emotions are a normal part of life, but using food to treat them or to avoid resolving them is not a long-term solution for feeling better.

Confusing Food with Love

Food is the most common tangible symbol of love and nurturing. At birth a baby learns to rely on someone else for food, and finds that feeding time also is a time for nurturing from and bonding with the caregiver. Our strong emotional link between food and love continues throughout life. Our culture's major events revolve around food, from birthdays and weddings to secular holidays and major religious celebrations. Socializing and celebrating are synonymous with eating.

There also might be a physical link between our body chemistry and a need to be nurtured. A hormone called oxytocin links food with love. This hormone is released in new mothers after delivery and stimulates milk production while also strengthening the mother-child bond. Kerstin Uvnas-Moberg, M.D., a researcher at the Karolinska Institute in Sweden, theorizes that an adult with high levels of this hormone might experience physical hunger when feeling lonely or in need of love, which can lead to overeating and possibly weight gain.

We also learn to confuse our emotions, rewards, and consequences with food. A child is told to eat his spinach before he can have dessert. Another child is instructed that unless she eats her sandwich, she cannot go outside and play. Another child is told to "eat something; it will make you feel better." Chocolates are a gift on Valentine's Day that say "I love you." Overeating on Thanksgiving is expected; indeed, you might be suspected of not liking the dinner (and therefore the cook) if you don't overindulge. These and other messages during childhood help strengthen the links between food, reward, punishment, and love.

Food also is a source of self-nurturance, self-love, and self-protection for someone who silently deals with a past trauma. According to researchers at the University of California, San Diego, childhood abuse (including sexual and physical abuse), losing a parent to death or divorce during childhood, or experiencing a sad or violent childhood can cause an adult to be fearful and to unconsciously use food to gain weight. In their study, 40 percent of obese subjects reported having had one or more alcoholic parent compared to only 17 percent of the slender subjects. The obese subjects also were twice as likely to have grown up in families where beatings, verbal abuse, and other violence were common.

Weight gain creates a protective shell that allows such people to feel less vulnerable and to keep other people at a distance. For them, eating also is a way to cope with and numb the pain, and to nurture themselves. Or people might be so overcome with rage resulting from the trauma that they turn the anger inward. The self-hatred then leads to overeating, substance abuse, or other self-destructive behaviors. It is increasingly difficult to distinguish body needs from emotional needs when eating becomes a way to satisfy both physical hunger and emotional pain.

The irrational thoughts and beliefs that develop as a result of a trauma further confuse emotions with eating. For example, thoughts that you are unlovable, flawed, or unworthy fuel feelings of loneliness and erode self-confidence, self-esteem, and self-acceptance. Rather than identify a childhood trauma or the sources of a bad experience in a relationship, people internalize the trauma and label themselves as inadequate. In all cases, the origin of the emotion must be identified and dealt with in a supportive, trusting way, usually with counseling. Once that pain has been treated, the emotional eating can be addressed or might stop on its own.

Beyond Fad Diets

"So great is man's hunger for forbidden foods!"

—Ovid, *Metamorphoses*

Diets not only don't work, they probably are a main reason many Americans overeat and are seven pounds heavier today than they were ten years ago. That's because people don't take well to deprivation; the more food is off-limits, and the more we worry about what we're eating, count calories and fat grams, and lament our lack of willpower, the more we eat, says Carol Munter, coauthor with Jane Hirschmann of *Overcoming Overeating* and *When Women Stop Hating Their Bodies* (Fawcett Books, 1995), who warns, "The end result of dieting is compulsive overeating." The best that can happen from dieting is that we overeat once in a while. At worst, we develop severe eating disorders like binge eating or bulimia. "Foods that are forbidden on a diet start to glitter and it is those foods a person will turn to when he or she needs a reward or to feel better," says Munter. Combine this taboo with our cultural and social obsession with sugar, fat, and salt, then place those foods on every street corner across America, and *voilà*—overeating!

Comfort Foods, Holiday Style

There is more to holiday festivities than just the "groaning table" (an old phrase to express the table groaning under the full weight of the feast). Ritual, atmosphere, and togetherness are the true magic this time of year. So, light candles, decorate with fresh-cut holly, hang up a little mistletoe, put on some memorable holiday music, and set your most elegant table. At each setting, place a festive card with a short prayer for each person to read. (Include more than just Bible or Torah readings, such as Chinese or Muslim blessings, cowboy graces, and Indian songs.) Either before or after dinner, have each person share a special holiday memory, read a portion of a favorite holiday story, or describe what the holidays mean to them. After dinner, round up everyone for a group walk or an indoor game like Charades to work off a few of those ho-ho-ho calories!

HOLIDAY MENU #1 (You'll find all these recipes at the back of the book)

1/2 Cornish Game Hen with Caramelized Onion
1/2 cup Wild Rice with Mushrooms
1 cup Wild Greens Topped with Pears, Blue Cheese, and Walnuts
1/2 cup Apricot-Glazed Carrots
4 Fresh Green Bean Bundles with Dill
1 slice Apple-Cranberry Upside-down Pie

Nutritional information:
882 calories; 27 percent fat (26.4 grams);
53 percent carbohydrates; 20 percent protein; 18.4 grams fiber.

HOLIDAY MENU #2 (You'll find all these recipes at the back of the book)

4 ounces Roast Turkey with Herb Rub
1/2 cup Apple-Raisin Stuffing
1/2 cup Cranberry-Orange Relish
Fresh Green Bean Bundles with Dill
Wild Greens Topped with Pears, Blue Cheese, and Walnuts
Pumpkin Mousse Pie

Nutritional information:
925 calories; 25 percent fat (26 grams);
53 percent carbohydrates; 22 percent protein; 13.1 grams fiber.

The link between dieting and food obsession is nothing new. During World War II, Ancel Keys, past professor emeritus at the University of Minnesota, studied the effects of food restriction on a group of conscientious objectors who cut calories by 25 percent for six months. As the men lost weight, their interest in food intensified. They talked about food, they fantasized about food, they collected recipes, they developed bizarre eating rituals. Sound like someone you know on a diet? Today's dieters are under even more pressure; unlike the conscientious objectors, they are constantly exposed to food and dieting messages from the media, society, and friends. It's no wonder they eat more when told not to, or after a high-calorie meal, than their nondieting friends.

Dieting numbs the hunger response, so people lose the ability to know when they're hungry or full. When people go on fad diets, they unknowingly set up a chain of negative consequences that lead them away from normal hunger and eating. Their internal cues to eat are replaced by external signals from a diet or the environment, which is a setup for overeating. Hunger becomes an unacceptable reason to eat. In their attempt to substitute willpower for normal physical drives, dieters lose their ability to listen to their body's cues. Their faulty hunger awareness means they have trouble regulating their food intake once the diet is over. They might mistakenly associate feelings of anxiety, loneliness, or other physical or emotional sensations with being hungry.

Dieters also are more likely to interpret all troubling feelings as hunger. It's an understandable trade-off. Probably nothing else in life is as firmly rooted in security as is food. "As babies, the most powerful comforter when we are distressed is food, so it makes sense that we would continue to turn to that symbol of comfort as adults. Grabbing a cookie is like trying to return to that security, that home, that safe place," says Munter. Thus, food becomes a tranquilizer when we're anxious and a mood elevator when we're depressed. It fills us up when we're emotionally starved, comforts us when we're lonely, and entertains us when we're bored. Unfortunately, turning to food for something other than physical nourishment only temporarily trades one problem for another. (See "Comfort Foods, Holiday Style," on page 256.)

It's a slow road back to getting in touch with our bodies, hungers, and physical needs, but the rewards are worth it. Women who give up the diet mentality and relearn how to nurture themselves experience a new lease on life. So how do you stop eating for all the wrong reasons? Begin by following the guidelines in Table 11.1, "Starting Over," on pages 258–259.

Table 11.1   Starting Over

How do we stop the dieting madness and get back in touch with our bodies and real hungers? First and foremost: Stop dieting, and never diet again. Then:

1. *Listen to your body.* Tune in to your natural hunger signals, making a distinction between what author Carol Munter calls mouth hunger (psychological hunger) and stomach hunger (true hunger symptoms include an emptiness in your stomach and stomach rumblings). If you are truly hungry, don't deny yourself. Ask yourself, "What would satisfy this particular hunger?" Then eat what seems like a good match.

2. *Eat mindfully.* Pay attention to and enjoy every mouthful. Then stop halfway through a meal, sit back, and pay attention to your body. If you still feel physically hungry, then have another few bites, stop, and listen again. Stop when you are comfortably full.

3. *Graze, don't gorge.* "Start feeding yourself on demand, like you would feed a baby," recommends Munter. By reparenting ourselves, we learn to trust that food will always be there and we begin to feel more secure in general. Eat mini-meals every four hours or whenever you are physically hungry.

4. *Be patient with yourself.* Until you have reprogrammed your attitudes toward food and no longer feel deprived, there's always the chance you'll overeat. Your goal is to *gradually* lean in the direction of eating for physical hunger and away from emotional hunger.

5. *Focus on health, not weight.* "Women who have dieted all their lives are often afraid to give up the diet mentality and eat at will; they're afraid they'll gain an enormous amount of weight," says Munter. In reality, your weight will stabilize when you "legalize food," and even if you gain a few pounds in the beginning, over time you will return to what for you is a normal, healthy weight.

6. *Reformat your thoughts.* Throw out perfectionist thinking. Stop labeling foods "good" or "bad," diets as something you are "on" or "off," weight as something you lose "all of" or "none at all," or yourself as someone who is a success or failure based on your weight. In short, erase the diet mentality from your mind, your attitudes, and your life.

7. *Seek comfort elsewhere.* "Talk through, rather than eat through, those feelings," recommends Thomas Wadden, Ph.D., professor of psychology and the director of the Weight and Eating Disorders Program at the University of Pennsylvania. Learn to identify your feelings and fulfill your needs by means other than food, such as daily exercise, spending time in nature, developing close friendships, meditating, or even counseling.

8. *Start small.* Defat high-fat recipes, cut back on added fats at the table, substitute lower-fat

ingredients for fatty ones (splashes of citrus juice, wine, or vinegar for oils; yogurt for mayonnaise; evaporated fat-free milk for cream; or lean meats for fatty beef).

9. *Keep a journal.* Keeping track of what and when you eat is the single most important step in reprogramming your taste buds. Most people grossly underestimate their food intakes, sometimes by 600 calories or more! The more we eat, the more we forget what we've eaten. A journal will help you identify what and where unwanted calories and foods are creeping into your diet, as well as where you want to start making changes.

10. *Believe in yourself.* It takes great mental strength to make a dietary change. Have faith in yourself, tell yourself repeatedly you can do it, and reward yourself (with a nonfood) every step along the way.

11. *Exercise.* Daily exercise helps you get—and stay—in touch with your body, curbs unruly appetites, and balances brain chemistry. It also helps you manage your weight and allows you to eat a little more of what you want without feeling guilty.

From Dieting to Eating Disorder

As emphasized throughout this book, restrictive diets often send the appetite-control chemicals into a tailspin. The eating pendulum swings from restraint to binge, sometimes resulting in obsessive eating, fear of food, desperation, and anger. The more dieters fail at dieting, the more likely they are to struggle with emotional eating and to be fearful about weight management and eating in general. They might even become paralyzed by the fear that they will lose all restraint and eat compulsively—a fear not unlike that in eating disorders such as anorexia and bulimia. Consequently, these people might develop a diet-induced fear of food.

Binge eating is a less serious form of bulimia that is not usually accompanied by purging and is more common in overweight people. The binge is usually not triggered by hunger but rather by a negative emotion, such as anger, stress and tension, irritability, or depression. A third of dieters admit they binge eat at least twice a week and another 22 percent confess they binge at least once a week. (Although the word "binge" often is used subjectively, some people consider any quantity of a "forbidden" food, even three cookies, to be a binge.) Binge eaters might be less likely to lose weight and maintain weight loss compared to nonbingers and are more likely to battle food cravings, especially cravings for carbohydrate-rich snacks. In fact, low-calorie diets often trigger binge eating in these people.

Why Thinness Becomes an Obsession

Given the profound social pressure to maintain thinness, it is amazing that more women do not develop eating disorders. Almost 90 percent of women wish they were thinner. What causes some to resort to self-destructive eating behaviors while others just diet a little and complain a lot about their weight? No one knows exactly. Anorexics and bulimics might have emotional struggles or problems stemming from childhood that underlie their eating disorders. Others might be genetically programmed to anorexia or bulimia (i.e., if one identical twin has an eating disorder, the other twin has a fifty-fifty chance of also developing eating problems, while other siblings only have a 10 percent chance). Social and family values, psychological issues (personality disorders, poor reasoning skills, and poor coping skills are a few of the problems common to people with eating disorders), hormone imbalances, and a history of physical or psychological trauma also are possible factors that contribute to the onset of eating disorders.

As time passes, without exception, food disorders get worse. In many cases, what begins as seemingly harmless comments about a person's weight or the social pressure from other dieting friends can fuel a determination to lose weight and, once the person has jumped onto the dieting bandwagon, she cannot get off. In essence, if dieting wasn't a trend, these people would never have fallen into the eating disorder spiral. Often people with eating disorders report they start to diet, but then find they can't do without the food that helps soothe both hunger and emotional pangs. The next step is to binge and purge (in the case of the bulimics) or to control eating even further (in the case of the anorexics). Dieting spirals into an eating disorder as the fear of fat becomes an obsession that is fueled by diet-induced imbalances in the body's appetite-control chemicals. In essence, even if psychological issues (i.e., a desire to lose weight) initiate the condition, physiological factors help perpetuate it. Hormones and nerve chemicals from growth hormone, prolactin, cortisol, and estrogen to NPY, the endorphins, serotonin, vasopressin, and CCK are turned topsy-turvy as a result of eating disorders.

The ABCs of Food Abuse

The solution to serious eating disorders is to seek professional help by physicians, psychologists, and dietitians trained specifically in how to handle the complexities of anorexia, bulimia, or even binge eating. The solution for the more common, garden-variety emotional eating is simple enough: Grow up. Put more gently, people must relearn some basic skills from childhood, such as the ability to comfort themselves when they feel blue, stressed, or afraid, and to set limits on their actions. In short, people need to take emotional inventories of themselves and find ways to fulfill these needs by something other than food.

The first step in undoing the harm done by fad dieting is to just say no forever to any restrictive diet that reduces daily energy intake below 1,500 calories. The second step is to regain a sensitivity to body signals, especially hunger. Ask yourself:

- Do I try to ignore hunger? If so, why? What happens when I ignore my hunger?
- Is hunger an enemy or a friend? Why?

Whenever you have the desire to eat, ask yourself whether or not you are physically hungry and to what extent. If you are not hungry or are only moderately hungry, think about what other factors might be influencing your desire to eat. If you are hungry, identify exactly what food would satisfy your hunger. Pay attention to the taste, texture, and aroma of food when you are eating. Eat slowly and listen for your body's signal that it is full. For more advice, refer to Table 11.1, "Starting Over," on pages 258–259.)

Another place to start is by identifying why you overeat. People often believe that events just happen. They find themselves snacking from the refrigerator after work or eating while watching television in the evening—for no apparent reason. But behavior doesn't just happen. There always is a reason—something that preceded the eating—that caused the behavior to occur. More importantly, a person always has a choice; no one is ever a victim of food abuse.

Food abuse follows a pattern. The underlying cause of emotional eating is called the antecedent—something that precedes the eating. The antecedent can be an event, such as being criticized at work; a negative thought such as, "I can't do anything right"; or a feeling, such as depression, anger, or irritation. The antecedent is followed by behavior, such as eating a bag of chips. The behavior is always followed by consequences—the chips taste good and you momentarily forget about the scuffle at work, but you have eaten a food that does not fuel your best mood and you might feel guilty later. Thus consequences can have both positive and negative effects. These are the ABCs of food abuse.

Learning Your ABCs

The best way to tone down your emotional eating is to identify the ABCs of why you eat: what causes you to start eating and what happens as a result. To do this, you need to keep a journal, such as the Food & Mood Journal in chapter 12, for at least one week. Record everything you eat and drink, or only those items you think are related to emotional eating. Also record when you ate, how you felt before and how you felt afterward, and anything else that might be related to the experience (any other consequences or thoughts). Always record the information at the time of eating, since memory fades and is inaccurate even an hour afterward.

At first it might be difficult to target your feelings associated with eating, so at least write down any related thoughts. Try to recall what you were thinking just before you had the urge to eat. What brought on the thought? Keep in mind that these thoughts always are in response to something—an antecedent. For example, do you often feel sad or depressed just before a food craving? What triggered the depression? What negative or irrational thoughts contributed to the experience? Is the emotional column in your journal empty? This could be a sign that you are eating to avoid boredom. Do you eat chips when angry? Mushy foods when depressed? Caffeinated beverages or chocolate when sad? When you are feeling lonely, guilty, or in need of nurturing, do you crave comfort foods that your mother served when you were a child?

Negative thoughts, beliefs, and emotions fuel food-abusive behaviors, so identify them and nip them in the bud. Listen to your self-talk, that internal dialogue that precedes emotional eating. Write down these thoughts in your journal to help you see them objectively. Are they rational or irrational? Once you have identified the thoughts and beliefs, you can begin replacing irrational ones with positive thoughts using a technique called thought stopping. Thought stopping is a way to stop negative thoughts. You yell, "Stop!" in your head at the first recognition of a negative thought. (Some people even picture a stop sign in their minds.) For example, a negative thought such as, "This is too hard. I can't do it," can be stopped before it gains strength by silently saying, "Stop!" (see Table 11.2, "Some Irrational Beliefs," page 263). The technique works best when the negative thought is replaced with a positive one such as, "This is challenging, but I can do it." Once you identify the negative thoughts that precede emotional eating, you can develop a repertoire of positive thoughts to use when the need arises.

Note the time of day you are most likely to eat inappropriately. Do you crave foods in midafternoon? Is this a low-energy time of day, when you are likely to be

---

Table 11.2   Some Irrational Beliefs

Many times emotional eating stems from irrational beliefs. Here are a few:

1. *The "all-or-nothing" belief.* If you are a perfectionist, this might apply to you. It is the "if you are going to do it, do it right" motto. For example, a person mistakenly believes he must follow an eating plan exactly or not at all, everyone must like him, or he should be good at everything. In reality, many things worth doing are not necessarily worth doing perfectly, and even small changes might be better than no changes.

2. *The overgeneralization belief.* If you tend to take one event and generalize it to apply to everything, then this might apply to you. For example, one slip from following the Feeling Good Diet is viewed as proof you will never succeed rather than as just one small experience in an otherwise successful venture.

3. *The "too big/very insignificant" belief.* If you exaggerate your flaws and underestimate your strong points, this might apply to you. In this case, a minor slip—such as not exercising one day—overshadows all the days you did exercise.

4. *The "should/have to" belief.* If you often find yourself saying should/must/have to, then this might apply to you. Irrational beliefs about what a person "should" do can cause unrealistic standards for performance that often lead to guilt and resentment. Examples include: "Life should be fair," "I should follow my plan," or "I should be able to do this."

5. *The "I feel, therefore I know" belief.* If you justify your thoughts based on your feelings, this might apply to you. For example, the thought that "I feel guilty, therefore I must have done something wrong" is an irrational thought often used to justify a feeling. Feelings are not proof that a thought is correct, since feelings are created by thoughts and those thoughts might be irrational.

6. *The labeling belief.* If you categorize, label, or stereotype people or yourself, this might apply to you. Often using labels such as "loser" or "failure" results in redefining all your actions based on these stereotypes. For example, labeling yourself as "weak" might result in not making decisions or taking charge of your life.

7. *The entertainment committee belief.* If you feel responsible or blame yourself for everything that happens, this might apply to you. For example, a friend doesn't call when he said he would, so you mistakenly assume you did something wrong. This belief results in needless guilt and erodes self-esteem.

---

bored? Do the foods you eat require preparation or some ritual? If so, this could be your way of relieving boredom. Plan even a short activity for this time of day to change the pace: Make a phone call, take a walk, play music, or stretch. You'll relieve the boredom without turning to food. Do you eat in front of the television at night? Again, this could be a sign of boredom or tension. Try some nonfood activity such as riding a stationary bicycle, taking a hot bath, or writing letters. Even just increasing your awareness of why you are eating might help.

Slip Management

The more aware you are of when and why you eat, the more capable you will be of developing an eating plan tailored to your moods, your food preferences, and your lifestyle. However, even the best-laid plans can go awry. The secret is not to let a minor slip progress to a major relapse.

A slip is any time you get sidetracked from efforts to reach your goals. It might be a day when you do not follow the Feeling Good Diet or a week when you don't exercise. It might even be something as simple as eating a forbidden food.

A slip is not bad. In fact, it is normal and expected whenever a person is changing habits. How that slip is managed, however, could make or break the best intentions. If not addressed immediately and effectively, a series of slips will lead to discouragement, irrational thinking, and eventually a major relapse during which you return to previous bad habits. In short, a slip does not inevitably result in a relapse, but every relapse begins with a slip.

To effectively manage a slip and fend off a relapse, identify those situations when you are most vulnerable, such as when you have certain thoughts or emotions, are ill, have an upset in routine including travel or a change in sleep habits, or feel a lack of support. Plan ahead how you will handle these situations. Weigh the short-term benefits of emotional eating (it temporarily makes you feel good) against the long-term consequences (mood swings, poor sleep habits, poor physical health, weight gain). Determine how to avoid the triggers of emotional eating or learn new ways to respond to them.

If a slipup just sneaks up on you, then learn from it. Treat the situation as an opportunity to grow. What caused the slip? How can it be avoided in the future? What will you do next time? Focus on the long term. How does this slip compare to your overall efforts? Avoid indulging in negative thoughts, such as the "all-or-nothing" belief (refer again to Table 11.2, "Some Irrational Beliefs," on page 263).

Curbing your emotional eating is more than just a food issue, however. A healthful lifestyle is essential for healthy emotions and healthful eating. For example, daily exercise helps prevent (and lessen the symptoms of) depression, anxiety, and other feelings associated with emotional eating. Developing a personal community of supportive and loving family members, friends, and coworkers also is essential to a healthful lifestyle. Learning effective ways to cope with emotions that do not include food is a necessity. Finally, remember to keep eating and food in perspective. Food should taste good, look and smell appealing, and be good for you. It should nourish your body, your moods, and your mind. (See Table 11.3, "Tried-and-True Tricks for Healthy Eating," below.)

Table 11.3   Tried-and-True Tricks for Healthy Eating

Along with the countless suggestions throughout this book, here's a list of additional tried-and-true, painless tricks to help you drop a few pounds and feel a lot healthier, without a hint of effort.

1. *Include two fruits and/or vegetables at every meal and snack:* You'll meet your daily quota of five to nine servings, feel full, and automatically cut back on fat and calories. It's as simple as adding blueberries and a glass of OJ along with cereal for breakfast; a salad and a glass of V8 juice to accompany a turkey sandwich at lunch; two steamed vegetables at dinner; and a few pieces of fruit for snacks.

2. *Have a specific plan:* Approach all food-related situations with a specific plan as to what and how much you will eat, how you will refuse unwanted food offers, and what you will do instead of overeating.

3. *Include your favorite foods:* If you love a glass of wine in the evening or a cookie at the mid-morning break, then drop something else during the day or walk an extra mile at lunch.

4. *Drink water:* Meet your daily quota of six to eight glasses, curb your appetite, and possibly avoid late-night cravings by keeping bottled water in the refrigerator or filling a container with eight glasses of water and drinking one glass every one to two hours.

5. *Eat slowly:* It takes up to twenty minutes for signals from the stomach to reach the brain; if you are wolfing down food, you could be stuffed before those signals hit. Instead, put the fork down between bites, focus more on the conversation, take small bites, or wait fifteen minutes before going back for seconds.

6. *Cut 100 calories each day:* Lose one pound a month by simply replacing that candy bar with an orange and a banana, the one-half cup granola with two cups of Cheerios, or one-half cup of frozen broccoli in cheese sauce with one-half cup steamed fresh broccoli.

7. *Lose weight gradually:* You are more likely to lose fat weight and maintain the loss if you take it slow: no more than two pounds a week. Better yet, forget the scale and monitor your weight by how your clothes fit or by the notch on your belt.

8. *Focus on your health, not your waistline:* Eat for health and you automatically adopt the best weight-management diet in the world. Successful diets fit easily into your daily routine and nourish your body, soul, and taste buds.

9. *Use time-savers:* Buy precut and bagged lettuce for a salad, baby carrots for a stew, precut fruit for a snack, premade hummus for a dip or sandwich spread; or steam frozen plain vegetables for dinner.

10. *Eat consciously:* Don't nibble while cleaning up the kitchen, taste-test while cooking, eat from the serving bowl, or graze from someone else's plate.

11. *Throw it out:* If those brownies or homemade cookies beckon to you, get rid of them … now! Drown them in water, dump them down the disposal, or bury them under garbage in the trash.

12. *Brush your teeth.* This can stop the cravings or uncontrollable grazing from the refrigerator by eliminating the taste of food from the mouth and signaling the body that eating is over.

13. *If you can't live with it, don't buy it:* "Just say no" to tempting foods at the grocery store if they are likely to beckon you to indulge at home. Also, store tempting foods out of sight.

14. *Taste, don't gorge:* When preparing food, take one or two half-teaspoon tastes to adjust seasonings. If you taste repeatedly and in tablespoon doses, you easily could be consuming 200 or more calories before you sit down to eat. Drink ice water when cooking—it helps curb the desire to taste-test.

III.

NUTRITION KNOW-HOW
FOR FEELING YOUR BEST

CHAPTER TWELVE

The Feeling Good Diet

What you eat could be at the root of how you feel. Granted, there are no magic diet pills, nutrition potions, or herbal remedies to painlessly, effortlessly, and immediately make a troublesome mood go away. However, a few simple changes in your diet might be all it takes to improve your mood, boost your energy level, or help you sleep through the night. In some cases, the problem is too little of one or more nutrients. In other cases, the problem is too much of something, such as sugar or caffeine. In still other cases, it is not what but when you are eating that has contributed to the emotional downhill spiral.

The good news is it takes only minor adjustments in your current eating pattern to produce improvements in your mood—sometimes dramatic ones. Even if your diet requires a major face-lift, the process can be relatively painless if you make small, progressive changes in what and when you eat. The Feeling Good Diet helps you put your diet and your mood back on track. However, it is not a "diet" in the true sense of the word; rather, it is an eating plan that slowly adapts your food preferences to help you feel your best. (See Table 12.1, "The Feeling Good Diet Philosophy," on page 270.)

Table 12.1   The Feeling Good Diet Philosophy

The goals of the Feeling Good Diet are to:

1. Slowly reduce dietary fat to 20 to 25 percent of total calories; refined and added sugars to 10 percent or less of total calories; and caffeine to no more than two servings of caffeinated beverages each day.
2. Gradually increase naturally occurring carbohydrate-rich foods, such as fruit, vegetables, whole-grain breads and cereals, nonfat milk products, and legumes, so that you consume at least three fruits, four vegetables, seven whole-grain breads and cereals, three servings of nonfat milk or yogurt, and one serving of legumes each day. For the mood-boosting fats, consume at least two servings of fish each week.
3. Evenly disperse calories and nutrients into five or six mini-meals throughout the day.
4. Ensure optimal nutrient intake by consuming at least 2,000 calories from a variety of nutrient-packed foods each day and choosing a moderate-dose multiple vitamin and mineral supplement.

The Un-Diet

Quick-weight-loss diets don't work. They produce temporary results, but the weight inevitably is regained; often people gain back even more weight as a result of dieting. On the other hand, low-fat diets are difficult for people to stick with, so people often abandon them in despair and return to familiar foods. Even the best low-fat or weight-loss diet was not designed to help you feel your emotional best or to improve your mental health. In fact, most strict diets aggravate mood and behavior problems.

For all people—from those struggling with mood, sleep, or energy problems to those who just want to feel a little better—the Feeling Good Diet is a breath of fresh air. It promotes mental, emotional, and physical health over counting calories, measuring fat grams, or calculating spoonfuls of sugar. It embraces the sensory delights of a good meal, yet is based on commonsense dietary guidelines to help you feel your best. And it promises results from realistic efforts.

The Feeling Good Diet: Step I

Gradually progress from your current food intake to this initial stage of the Feeling Good Diet:

1. Divide food intake into four servings a day.
2. Limit caffeine—from coffee, tea, and colas—to no more than three servings daily.
3. Drink at least two glasses of water a day.
4. Include the following foods in your daily menus:*

AT LEAST

- Two servings of fruit (at least one serving should be a high–vitamin C selection)
- Two servings of vegetables and beans (at least two servings should be dark green or orange)
- Four servings of grains (at least two servings should be whole-grain varieties)
- Two servings of nonfat or low-fat milk or milk products (if you choose a fattier selection, then deduct the extra fat from the fats and oils allotment below)

NO MORE THAN

- Two servings of extra-lean red meat, chicken, or fish
- Two servings of nutritious fatty foods, such as avocados, full-fat cheeses, ice cream, luncheon meats, nuts, peanut butter, fatty cuts of meat, or fried foods
- Five tablespoons of fats and oils, such as vegetable oil, butter, margarine, shortening, cream cheese, mayonnaise, and salad dressing (used in cooking or added to foods)
- Three small servings of sugary foods, such as angel food cake, a cookie, sherbet, maple syrup, jam, honey or sugar, or fruit-flavored gelatin

5. Take a moderate-dose multiple vitamin and mineral supplement.

* See the appendix for information on specific foods and serving sizes.

In a Nutshell

The Feeling Good Diet is a stepping-stone to healthful eating. First, you keep track of what, how much, and when you eat, by maintaining a food diary for one week. (A sample diary, "Worksheet 12.1," can be found on page 282.) From the eating patterns and food choices noted in the diary, you gradually adapt your current eating habits to meet the nutrition goals of Step 1 in the Feeling Good Eating Plan. When the Step 1 dietary guidelines become habit, you move on to Step 2, and finally to Step 3 (see "The Feeling Good Diet: Step 1," on page 271).

The dietary guidelines help you make the gradual transition from an eating plan that interferes with feeling your best to an eating style that helps you maximize your energy, good mood, and thinking ability. When used with the specific dietary advice outlined in each chapter, from food cravings, fatigue, and PMS to depression, stress, and sleep, the Feeling Good Diet combines the latest research and dietary advice into an eating plan that helps you feel your best.

The Rationale

As you read this and the following chapter, the rationale underlying the Feeling Good Diet eating guidelines will become clear. A brief explanation is provided here to summarize the basic nine components of this nutrition plan.

1. *Listen to your cravings.* They're telling you something. In many cases, cravings for sweets are an unconscious effort to raise serotonin or NPY levels; a desire for creamy or fatty foods, from ice cream to steak, might be a basic need to satisfy galanin levels. These appetite-control chemicals are very powerful, and trying to use willpower to make them go away is, in many cases, like trying to give up breathing. So work with them instead. If by midafternoon you crave something sweet, turn to fig bars, graham crackers with peanut butter, or a raisin bagel with all-fruit jam. If your "weakness" is chocolate in the evening, dip two cups of oranges, bananas, and strawberries in one-fourth cup fat-free chocolate syrup, or indulge in three to four chocolate Hershey's Kisses, not the entire bag. As you adopt the Feeling Good Diet, your food cravings will dwindle—and they might even vanish.

2. *Make changes slowly.* Quick-weight-loss diets, dramatic changes in dietary habits, skipping meals, erratic eating habits, and stress are all eating patterns that upset brain chemistry and often result in the pendulum swinging from abstinence to binge. The Feeling Good Diet takes you systematically through a change in eating habits that

slowly shifts your food intake while gradually coaxing your brain chemistry into balance.

3. *Eat several small meals and snacks.* People who divide their total day's food intake into mini-meals and snacks evenly distributed throughout the day maintain a more even temperament; are less prone to fatigue, insomnia, and depression; maintain a more desirable weight; and are less susceptible to disease, as compared to people who eat most of their day's food intake in a few large meals. The body also is better able to absorb and use nutrients and maintain stable levels of blood sugar and nerve chemicals when supplied with frequent, moderate-sized meals than when confronted with the feast-and-famine scenario characteristic of the three-square-meals plan.

On the other hand, nibbling can lead to cravings and gorging if a person uses the mini-meal recommendations as an excuse to eat continuously all day. Ideally most people should eat a moderate-sized meal or snack approximately every four hours. Gradually increase the number of meals and snacks from three to at least five. If you already are eating too often, set a personal goal to reduce the number of times you eat to no more than six times each day.

4. *Eat breakfast.* People who skip breakfast struggle more with weight problems and low energy later in the day than do people who take time to eat. As discussed in chapter 4, eating breakfast boosts your energy for the rest of the day, breaks the fast-and-feast cycle, prevents fatigue, and helps improve your mood.

5. *Cut back on sugar and caffeine.* These quick-fix solutions to lagging energy and poor mood fuel your fatigue and depression and aggravate food cravings. You can achieve the same neurotransmitter "fix," but provide your body with a sustained energy boost and mood elevation, by switching to fiber-rich carbohydrates, such as breads, rice, pasta, low-sugar cereals, and starchy vegetables. Coffee is a mixed bag. One to two cups a day boosts energy and mood, but more than that—especially in people who are unknowingly sensitive to caffeine—can fuel the fatigue spiral. Never consume sugar and caffeine together, and include the occasional sweet treat with a meal—don't eat sweets alone.

6. *Eat more fish.* The omega-3 fatty acids in fish help reduce depression

and boost mental power. Replace other meats with fish at least twice a week.

7. *Increase your water intake.* Water is the most important nutrient to general health and emotional well-being. However, it is often ignored or forgotten. Water is essential for all body processes. It surrounds, fills, and nourishes all cells and tissues, helps regulate body temperature, and transports oxygen and nutrients to all the tissues. Water helps maintain the proper acidity of the body, which in turn helps stabilize the nerves and tissues. Chronic low-grade dehydration that results from drinking a little, but not enough, water is one of the most common causes of fatigue.

8. *Follow Steps 1, 2, and 3 in the Feeling Good Diet.* These progressive steps slowly wean you off of sugar and fat and reprogram your taste buds to enjoy the nutrient-packed vegetables, fruits, grains, and other nutritious foods that boost your energy level and help you feel your best.

9. *Take supplements.* Even the best diet is likely to fall short of one or more nutrients when your daily energy intake is less than 2,500 calories. Some nutrients, such as vitamin E, are needed in amounts too large to obtain from diet alone. Therefore, a responsible supplementation program offers safe and potentially beneficial nutritional insurance. (See chapter 14 for guidelines on how to select a supplement. See "The Feeling Good Diet: Step 2," on page 275.)

The Tortoise and the Hare

"But, I want to feel good right now! Why can't I just move ahead to Step 3 and skip all the in-between dietary advice?"

It is not dieting per se but how you adopt new eating habits that determines how successfully you will stick with a new eating plan. Rapid weight loss, radical changes in food intake or dietary habits, and other dramatic alterations in your life-long eating patterns wreak havoc with brain chemicals that regulate appetite, body weight, and even basic survival instincts. The more strict the diet and the more rapid the changes, the more aggressive are your brain chemicals in trying to reestablish the old order.

On a more practical note, remember that it took years to develop your current

---

The Feeling Good Diet: Step 2

Congratulations: You've made it to the next step in the Feeling Good Diet. In this step, you'll focus on breakfast; more mini-meals, fruits, vegetables, and whole grains; and less coffee and sugar.

1. Eat something for breakfast.
2. Divide food intake into four to five mini-meals and snacks throughout the day.
3. Limit caffeine—from coffee, tea, and colas—to no more than two servings a day.
4. Increase your daily water intake to four glasses.
5. Include the following foods in your daily menus:*

AT LEAST

- Three servings of fruit (at least one serving should be a high–vitamin C selection)
- Three servings of vegetables and beans (at least two servings should be dark green or orange)
- Six servings of grains (at least three servings should be whole-grain varieties)
- Two servings of nonfat or low-fat milk or milk products (if you choose a fattier selection, then deduct the extra fat from the fats and oils allotment below)

NO MORE THAN

- Two servings of extra-lean meat, chicken, or fish
- Two servings of nutritious fatty foods (see Step 1 for examples)
- Three tablespoons of fats and oils (see Step 1 for examples)
- Two small servings of sweets

6. Take a moderate-dose multiple vitamin and mineral supplement.

* See the appendix for information on specific foods and serving sizes.

---

eating habits. You are accustomed to extra cheese in your lasagna and you expect creamy gravy on your pot roast. To assume you can reprogram your taste buds overnight so they delight in a black bean and couscous casserole is asking more than the typical taste bud can deliver. Without the cooking skills or the taste for the new low-fat or less-sweet fare, it is easy to feel overwhelmed, unhappy, deprived, or resentful of a new eating plan. Already burdened by depression, a sleep disorder,

The Feeling Good Diet: Step 3

Hurrah! You're almost there! In Step 3, you'll perfect your eating plan by improving breakfast choices, drinking more water, and consuming more vegetables, whole grains, nonfat milk, and fish while cutting back a bit more on fats and sweets.

1. Eat a breakfast that includes at least one grain, one fresh fruit, and one low-fat milk product.
2. Divide food intake into five to six mini-meals and snacks throughout the day.
3. Limit caffeine—from coffee, tea, and colas—to no more than two servings a day.
4. Increase your daily water intake to six glasses.
5. Include the following foods in your daily menus:*

AT LEAST

- Three servings of fruit (at least one serving should be a high–vitamin C selection)
- Four servings of vegetables (at least two servings should be dark green or orange)
- Seven servings of grains (at least five servings should be whole-grain varieties)
- Three servings of nonfat or low-fat milk and milk products

NO MORE THAN

- Two servings of extra-lean meat, chicken, or fish (one serving should be cooked dried beans and peas, and two or more servings a week should be fish)
- One serving of nutritious fatty foods (see Step 1 for examples)
- Two tablespoons of fats and oils (see Step 1 for examples)
- One serving of sweets

6. Take a moderate-dose multiple vitamin and mineral supplement.

* See the appendix for information on specific foods and serving sizes.

low energy, or other mood problems, you will soon begin wondering why you are bothering with this—yet another—diet.

By following the Feeling Good Diet gradually, you'll gently reprogram your taste buds while you learn new cooking skills. This step-by-step approach works with, rather than against, your appetite-control and mood-altering brain chemicals, so you are more likely to feel and be successful. (See "The Feeling Good Diet:

Step 3," on page 276.) Check the appendix (Food Groups and Serving Sizes in the Feeling Good Diet) for specific information on foods and portions.

In most cases, only minor changes in fat, sugar, and caffeine intake make dramatic differences in how you feel. For example:

- Eating something for breakfast, when typically you have skipped this meal, might be all it takes to boost your otherwise dwindling midmorning energy level.
- Replacing a sugary snack, such as a granola bar or piece of pie, with a bagel and fat-free cream cheese might soothe afternoon doldrums that otherwise have resulted in uncontrollable food cravings.
- Reducing the butter on your morning toast from 1 tablespoon to 2 teaspoons (a difference of only 1 teaspoon) can decrease the meal's fat calories by as much as 10 percent and help you overcome cravings for fat.
- Replacing two beef tacos with two chicken tacos for lunch decreases the fat from 46 percent to 33 percent of calories, and keeps you more alert after lunch.
- Switching from oil-packed to water-packed tuna reduces the fat content by almost 20 percent, thus leaving more room for nutrient-packed foods.
- Replacing a soda pop with a glass of orange juice decreases your intake of refined sugar by nine teaspoons and helps avoid the blood-sugar roller coaster that can undermine mood.

As you wean yourself off fat and sugar, the quantity and nutritional quality of the diet increases to make up for the lost calories. In short, you eat more food for less calories! For those concerned about weight or figure, a bonus of the Feeling Good Diet is that you might lose a few pounds without really trying. (See "A Word of Caution," on page 278).

Reprogramming Your Taste Buds

A light meal of pasta and salad can sound like a death penalty if you are used to meals planned around meat; foods cooked or served with gravies, cream sauces, or butter; generous servings of desserts; fast-food lunches; or meals of only a bag of potato chips. Don't despair—you can reprogram your taste buds to enjoy low-fat, high-carbohydrate fare.

A Word of Caution

Fat and sugar should be reduced, but they shouldn't be eliminated. Fat is needed to help absorb the fat-soluble vitamins (A, D, E, and K), supply the essential fat called linoleic acid, and add variety to the diet. The natural fats found in seeds, nuts, avocados, and olives also provide phytochemicals, health-enhancing compounds that lower disease risk. The fats in fish, flaxseed meal, and walnuts supply the omega-3 fatty acids that help prevent depression and age-related memory loss. The body needs some salt (sodium) to regulate muscle and nerve function and maintain its natural fluid balance. Sugar adds taste and pleasure to a meal or snack. This dynamic trio is reduced, but you still can find desserts, nuts, salmon, and chocolate in the Feeling Good Diet.

Researchers at the Cancer Prevention Research Center in Seattle surveyed 448 women who had participated in nutrition classes to lower their fat intake. More than half of the participants reported that their love for fatty foods changed to a growing dislike for the creamy, greasy taste the longer they remained on a low-fat diet. More than 60 percent said they actually felt physical discomfort after eating high-fat foods. "The women had been consuming very high-fat diets, as high as 60 percent fat calories," says Elizabeth Burrows, M.S., R.D., researcher at the Cancer Prevention Research Center. Over the course of three to six months, they lowered that fat intake to 20 percent. "They would go out to eat at a restaurant or friend's house, eat two or three fatty foods, and find they not only did not like the taste, but they had difficulty digesting the food," says Ms. Burrows. The secret is to make the adjustment gradually and avoid feeling deprived.

The Feeling Good Diet does just that. It slowly reduces the day's fat intake from the typical 37 percent of total calories to approximately 20 to 25 percent and gradually lowers sugar and caffeine, two dietary ingredients that contribute to mood swings, sleep problems, and fatigue. In addition, several tricks of the trade incorporated into this eating plan help satisfy your taste buds without adding fat and sugar. Meal-planning tips are discussed in detail in chapter 13.

It is the entire day's fat, sugar, and caffeine intake that is important. Consequently, some meals can be higher in fat or sugar than other meals while remaining within the guidelines of the Feeling Good Diet. In short, don't sweat the small stuff. Minor fluctuations in fat, sugar, and caffeine have little or no impact on the total day's food intake, or on most people's moods. Fat intake can vary a few percentage points, and a teaspoon of sugar one way or the other is not important. Your goal is not a food-by-food inventory but rather an overall daily and weekly reduction in fat, sugar, and caffeine and an even distribution in food intake throughout the day.

Tailor-made for Good Health

The Feeling Good Diet avoids the "canned menu" plans of other dieting methods—guidelines that leave many people feeling defeated before they even start. Restrictive fad diets are an artificial fix for a lifelong challenge of attaining and maintaining emotional well-being. A healthful eating style gradually tailored to your preferences, tastes, and time demands can do wonders for your mental, emotional, and physical well-being while providing a plan you can stick with.

You have two options with the Feeling Good Diet. If you need structure, at least when starting out, then follow the guidelines in Steps 1, 2, and 3 (see pages 271, 275, and 276). Menus based on these guidelines can be found in chapter 13, and specific foods and portions are listed in the appendix at the back of this book. Follow these guidelines until they are habits, and remember to take it slow. Even tailoring your diet to the Step 1 guidelines can take weeks or months, depending on how different these guidelines are from your current diet and on your level of commitment. The pace is entirely up to you. When the Step 1 guidelines are habit, then progress in a similar fashion to Step 2, and then to Step 3.

A less-structured option is to design your own three-step program based on the goals of the Feeling Good Diet that are outlined on page 270. You may want to use some of the guidelines in Steps 1 through 3, but personalize them to meet your specific needs. For example, you already might have reduced your dietary intake of fats from meats and added oils, while your main dietary goal is to reduce the sweet-and-creamy cravings for chocolate and ice cream that are contributing to your mood swings. Therefore, you already might be following Step 3 when it comes to fats and oils, meat and legumes, and low-fat milk products, but you need a program for reaching the goals of Step 1 for desserts. After reading the chapter on insomnia, you might decide that caffeine is of primary concern, in which case you could focus your dietary goals on reaching the Step 3 guidelines for caffeine and tackle other dietary goals at a later date.

This second option requires more time and organization on your part but gives you the opportunity to tailor a plan specifically to your dietary needs. In both cases, read the chapters in the book that pertain to your health concerns and use the additional dietary information provided there to further clarify what dietary changes will produce the best results for you.

Quiz 12.1 Are You Ready and Willing to Make a Change?

Changing dietary habits, even when the steps are small, requires a commitment to stick with it. Before you take the plunge, be sure you are ready and willing to do what it takes to feel your best. In short, is this the best time for you to take charge of your diet?

Using a scale of 1 to 5 (1 = not at all; 5 = more so than ever), answer the following questions:

1. Compared to attempts in the past to change your eating habits, how motivated are you to stick with it this time? _____
2. How determined are you to stick with the Feeling Good Diet until you reach your dietary goals? _____
3. Eating right when you're feeling down requires effort. How willing are you to take the time and make the effort to reach your goals? _____
4. Making dietary changes should be gradual. If you tackle too many dietary changes too fast, you're likely to fail. Are you willing to take it slowly—possibly taking a year or more to reprogram your taste buds and redesign your diet—if the end result is having more energy and feeling your best? _____
5. How much support for your nutrition efforts can you expect from friends, family, coworkers, and other people around you? _____
6. Learning new eating habits is like developing any new skill: It requires time. How much time do you have to make permanent changes in your life? _____

Scoring:
6 to 16: Reflects a low commitment to making dietary changes and a high likelihood of failure in the long run. Wait and try another time.
17 to 23: Reflects a moderate commitment to make dietary changes that will help you feel, think, and sleep better. However, you still need to work on motivation.
24 or higher: Reflects high motivation. This could be the best time to venture down the dietary road to feeling your best.

Before You Begin

The first step to feeling better is to assess whether now is the best time for you to make a change. Make sure you are ready and willing to take the time and make the effort. The quiz on page 280 is one way to measure your motivation and commitment to feeling your best.

Making Changes in Your Life

In addition to the genes you were born with, lifestyle habits are the most powerful shapers of your mood. These habits didn't begin yesterday. Day in and day out, year in and year out, you have repeated the same patterns and routines in your life. So telling yourself to "eat right" or "exercise more" won't make those lifelong habits go away. You need a realistic plan, a few basic skills in changing behavior, and a plan for staying motivated through the tough times. You must identify lifelong habits that have contributed to your mood problems; set realistic goals; and practice effective tactics for developing new habits.

The Feeling Good Diet has taken some of the guesswork out of setting goals and designing strategies. If you move gradually through the three-step program, you will slowly reprogram your taste buds without feeling deprived or overwhelmed. In short, your goals will be realistic, achievable, and specific. However, you might choose to further divide these goals into weekly minigoals, such as planning to replace your high-sugar midmorning snack with a piece of fruit. These minigoals work within the framework of the Feeling Good Diet and further increase your chances for success in making dietary changes.

The Food & Mood Journal (see Worksheet 12.1, on page 282) and other record-keeping forms and self-assessments in this book are essential for making these dietary changes. You can't change behavior until you know what behaviors you need to change. Keeping a diary or written record of your actions is the only way to accurately identify what behaviors are contributing to your mood problems. Since memory is inaccurate and often biased, writing down information such as when, what, why, and how you feel before and after eating provides invaluable and accurate feedback on habits.

Keep detailed records for at least one to two weeks and you will note patterns. Everything you do is triggered by something, so watch for the thoughts, moods, events, or circumstances that trigger an eating episode or the foods eaten just before a change in mood. (See chapter 11 for more information on the ABCs of behavior.) These patterns are clues about the conditions, thoughts, and feelings that cause you to eat inappropriately, and can help you identify how foods affect how you feel. From these clues you can develop strategies for making changes in your habits.

Worksheet 12.1   The Food & Mood Journal

It is essential that the information on this worksheet be specific and be filled out promptly, honestly, and completely. Fill in the day/date and complete each column of the worksheet whenever you eat or drink, including meals, snacks, a glass of water, or a stick of gum.

Use a scale from 0 to 5 for the Hunger column: 0 = not hungry; 5 = very hungry. Use a different color pen or mark all foods and beverages that contain sugar or caffeine. Use this sheet as a master for making additional copies.

DATE: _____

TIME	FOOD/AMOUNT BEVERAGE	HUNGER	WHERE?	WITH WHOM?	DOING WHAT ELSE?	FEELINGS BEFORE? AFTER?

Granted, keeping records takes time and commitment, but it is one of the most important skills you will learn!

Look for high-risk situations where you are likely to overeat, eat sugary or sweet-and-creamy foods, or experience low energy and moods. A high-risk situation is anytime you are tempted to waver from the Feeling Good Diet. It might be a depressing moment, another person, a particular place, a specific event, a time of day or a season of the year, a high-stress period, or the easy availability of tempting foods such as coffee or desserts. High-risk situations also can include discouraging thoughts or excuses we find for why it is all right to slip from the Feeling Good Diet. Feelings such as fatigue, happiness, loneliness, or anxiety trigger problem eating, but remember that your nutritional needs are greatest during these emotionally stressful times, and poor eating habits will only make the situation worse.

Once you have set realistic goals, identified the eating or exercise behaviors you want to change, and learned what triggers these inappropriate habits, the next step is to develop tactics that will encourage new eating habits. These tactics are as varied as the people who use them, and include:

- Shopping from a list.
- Discarding problem foods currently in the kitchen.
- Eating at regular times.
- Planning snacks.
- Sending leftover desserts home with guests.
- Asking for the salad dressing on the side at restaurants.
- Taking a walk to calm yourself when you can't avoid a stressful situation.
- Replacing negative thoughts, beliefs, and attitudes with positive, encouraging ones.

Refer to chapter 13 for more information on tactics useful in applying the Feeling Good Diet to shopping, preparing foods at home, and ordering foods in restaurants. For further tips on how to begin your new regime, see Table 12.2, "Getting Started," on page 284.

How you think and feel about making dietary changes influences how much you eat or whether you stick with a new eating plan. It is important to understand and untangle the link between eating and feelings. Certain beliefs or attitudes can cause problems. For example, the "all-or-nothing" belief that you must never eat a forbidden food can lead to feelings of failure. This type of thinking weakens your control. Examine your beliefs, attitudes, and thoughts and counteract any negative ones

Table 12.2   Getting Started

Here is a step-by-step guide for incorporating the Feeling Good Diet into your life:

1. Copy one week's worth of Worksheet 12.1, "The Food & Mood Journal," on page 282. Keep an accurate record of what foods, how much, when and where you ate, how you felt before and during the one hour following eating, and any other related information that will help you recognize food-and-mood patterns, high-risk situations where you are likely to overeat or eat the wrong foods, situations that trigger snack attacks, or even how much you are eating. Be specific, accurate, thorough, and honest in your record keeping.

2. Review your Food & Mood Journal and complete Worksheet 12.2, "A Look at Your Food & Mood Journal," on page 285.

3. Familiarize yourself with the Feeling Good Diet, its philosophy, and the three steps.

4. Compare your eating style, based on information obtained from your journal and the self-assessment, with the Feeling Good Diet and specific dietary information presented in the chapters pertinent to your mood problems. Choose the dietary changes you want to make to feel better. This could be as simple as adopting the dietary guidelines in Step 1 of the diet, choosing to mix and match these recommendations to better suit your food and mood needs.

5. Refer to chapter 13 for sample menus and tips on shopping, food preparation, and ordering meals in restaurants.

6. Practice new eating habits until they become habit. (This step can take one week to one year or longer. If you adhere to the Feeling Good guidelines, you should begin feeling better within a few weeks. It could take twelve weeks or more to reprogram your taste buds.)

7. Graduate to Step 2 in the Feeling Good Diet and practice these new eating habits until they become habit.

8. Graduate to Step 3 in the Feeling Good Diet and practice these new eating habits until they become habit.

9. Enjoy your new energy, improved mood, sound sleep, and reduced stress.

with more realistic and positive ones. (See chapter 11 for more information on how emotions affect food choices.)

Remind yourself that it took a long time to develop the habits you have. Be patient with yourself as you take the steps to identify and replace old patterns with new eating habits that help you feel your best. Set realistic goals, keep records, plan

Worksheet 12.2   A Look at Your Food & Mood Journal

Complete this self-assessment after keeping your Food & Mood Journal for at least one week. Look for patterns and trends that will help you design a personalized eating plan.

1. What times of the day and night did you most frequently eat? What patterns do you see?

2. What patterns do you see in your food and beverage intake? How did snacks, skipping a meal, or unplanned eating affect your caloric intake? How did portion sizes affect your intake? Does caffeine or sugar affect your food intake?

3. How did you feel before eating and during the hour after eating? Do you see any patterns?

4. What moods and feelings are associated with eating? Do you eat more or less when you are calm, relaxed, agitated, stressed, tired, angry, etc.?

5. What was your most frequent reason for eating? What patterns do you notice between foods eaten and feelings before and after you ate?

6. Where did you eat most frequently? What connections do you see between the locations and your food intake?

7. Who do you eat with? Did you tend to eat more or less with certain people?

8. What activities were most strongly linked with eating?

9. Describe the consequences linked with your eating. Do you see any patterns?

10. If you kept a journal for more than two weeks, did you notice any cyclical changes in your food intake or mood—for example, did you crave foods more during certain times of the month?

and practice new behaviors until they become habit, and develop a reward system that keeps you motivated. It doesn't matter if you slip off your eating plan. What matters is that you plan to do something about it to prevent the slip in the future.

You're Worth It

Eating the right foods at the right time and in the right amounts could be a simple answer to your lack of energy, depression, sleep problems, stress-related problems, or inability to concentrate. But even if how you feel stems from factors other than nutrition, eating well is the foundation for getting well. You don't have to feel this way. There is hope. That hope lies in making a lifelong commitment to be the best and healthiest you. Set a realistic image in your mind's eye of how you want to feel and look, and then make small, daily adjustments in your lifestyle to reach those goals, based on the dietary guidelines outlined in the Feeling Good Diet. This plan requires a lifetime commitment to modify your eating habits so they support your mental and emotional health. But, you're worth it, don't you think?!

CHAPTER THIRTEEN

Putting the Feeling Good Diet into Practice

- Is organic produce better than regular produce?
- Which is more nutritious: fresh or frozen vegetables?
- When is a loaf of whole wheat bread really a loaf of white bread in disguise?
- Chicken and turkey are lower in fat than red meat, right?
- Which fish is safe to eat? What about pesticides and mercury?

Putting know-how into practice requires some supermarket and restaurant survival skills. Grocery stores stock tens of thousands of different foods: Many of them undermine your mood; even more of them are nutritious mood boosters. You just need to know what to look for.

The Shopping Tour

The healthful meals and snacks in the Feeling Good Diet begin with healthful ingredients. In general, most of the nutritious foods are found on the periphery of the store, including the produce section, the bakery, the dairy case, and the meat or seafood department. Venture down the aisles in the middle only to purchase minimally processed items such as beans, grains, and low-fat canned goods. Here are the easy rules for shopping:

- Check the percentage of fat indicated on the label and purchase only products that contain 30 percent or less fat calories. This is the equivalent of no more than 3 grams of fat for every 100 calories. To check a product's fat content, multiply the grams of fat in a serving by 9, divide by the total number of calories, and multiply by 100. For example, suppose a label states that a serving supplies 4 grams of fat and 150 calories. So, 4 grams $\times$ 9 calories/gram = 36 calories divided by 150 calories = .24 $\times$ 100 = 24 percent fat calories.
- Check the sugar content. Since many products do not list refined sugar directly, read the ingredients list and avoid any product that lists sugar as one of the first three ingredients or that lists sugar (or any related sweeteners, including fructose, corn syrup, and honey) more than once for every five ingredients.
- Buy minimally processed foods. Choose 100 percent whole wheat bread rather than white bread; 100 percent fruit juice rather than a fruit juice blend; plain rather than processed meats; plain fresh or frozen vegetables rather than vegetables frozen in sauces; low-fat or nonfat plain yogurt rather than fruited-yogurt; and whole fresh potatoes rather than scalloped or French-fried potatoes.

Now let's take a shopping tour for more nutritious food purchases.

Produce Potpourri: Fresh, Frozen, Canned, and Organic

Left untouched by food manufacturers, there is no such thing as a bad vegetable or fruit. However, some are better than others. It's the colorful produce you want in your diet. Dark green leafy vegetables, blueberries, oranges, apricots, broccoli, tomatoes, and kiwi are a few of the superheroes when it comes to vitamin, mineral, phytochemical, and fiber content. Purchase enough rainbow-colored fruits and vegetables to supply at least two servings at meals and snacks. If a lack of time is your excuse for not eating more vegetables and fruits, look for prewashed and chopped vegetables, shredded cabbage, bags of bite-sized carrots, peeled and cored pineapple, jars of minced garlic, and prepared fresh fruit salads in the produce department. Frozen berries and melons also add variety without adding time to meal preparation.

Which is Best—Fresh, Frozen, or Canned?

If you are fortunate enough to have access to produce straight from the farm, then fresh is best. However, the longer that fruits and vegetables sit in a warehouse or grocery store, the more vitamins they lose. When selecting fresh produce, always choose crisp, plump, firm, and unbruised items. (To tell whether a fruit is ripe, smell it at room temperature. If it smells the way you want it to taste, then it probably is ripe.) Buying produce in season is one way to ensure freshness and reduce cost. Remember to purchase only quantities that you can eat within a few days.

If superfresh produce is not available, then your next best bet is frozen vegetables. Frozen vegetables have been processed immediately after harvest and are a better choice when superfresh produce is unavailable. Canned vegetables are the last resort. The heating process used in canning destroys much of the vitamin C and folic acid as well as some other vitamins, and salt and sugar often are added to canned fruits and vegetables.

Your best bets for canned fruits and vegetables are those very difficult or impossible to obtain fresh, such as water chestnuts, bamboo shoots, and baby corn. Artichoke hearts (canned in water) and hearts of palm add variety and taste to salads. Canned corn, beets, tomato paste and sauce, and pumpkin also are nutritious selections that add quick vegetables to a meal. Fruits canned in their own juice, such as pineapple, cherries, mandarin oranges, pears, and peaches, or pureed fruit, such as plain applesauce, are nutritious foods to keep on hand for quick meals and snacks.

Is Organic Produce Healthier?

Organic produce has made it into mainstream America, sitting side by side with conventional produce in grocery stores and restaurant menus. But is it worth the extra cost? It makes sense that since organic soil is healthier, the produce grown in it would be more nutritious. But, as yet, there is little research to support this claim. One study found that organic foods contained more calcium, magnesium, manganese, zinc, and other minerals than conventional produce. But other studies have found only minimal differences in nutritional quality between organic and conventional produce, concluding that ". . . seasonal variations in the weather have a greater influence on plant production than the source and amount of compost applied." A better way to maximize the vitamin and mineral content of your produce—conventional or organic—is to buy vine-ripened, very fresh produce, or grow your own.

Certified organic produce does contain lower levels of pesticides. Consumers Union tested one thousand pounds of unrinsed produce (tomatoes, bell peppers, apples, and peaches) for more than three hundred pesticides. Only 25 percent of the organic produce contained residues, compared to 77 percent of the conventional produce. Moreover, the residues on the organic produce were less toxic. Three-quarters of Americans say that the 566 million pounds of pesticides dumped on food crops each year are a major health concern. So, cutting back on pesticides whenever possible might be a priority for many people. (See below for more information on pesticides.)

The other consideration is price, both to your pocketbook and to the environment. Organic produce costs between two and three times more than conventional produce. That can be a deterrent to someone on a limited budget. On the other hand, organic farming is much less harmful to the environment than conventional farming methods, reducing both the pesticide residues in food and the land, as well as reducing the contamination of our water supplies. Conventional farming pollutes water with pesticide runoff, degrades topsoil, and uses nonrenewable energy resources. In contrast, organic farming releases few chemicals into the environment, enhances soil quality, and encourages biodiversity of crops, thus protecting our natural resources. So, while organic produce is more costly on an immediate and personal level, it is very cost-effective for future generations.

What About Pesticides?

Our daily food supply is laced with thousands of pesticides and pesticide residues with ominous names like polychlorinated naphthalenes (PCNs), polychlorinated biphenyls (PCBs), dibenzo-p-dioxins (PCDDs), 2-2-2-trichloroethane (DDT), 2,2-bis(4-chlorophenyl)-1,1,-dichloroethylene (DDE), and hexachlorobenzene (HCB). Are these chemicals harmful to our health? To be honest, nobody really knows at what level they are a health risk.

There is a scarcity of well-designed, long-term epidemiological studies to investigate the effects of pesticide exposure on our health. We know that some pesticides already have affected the health and reproductive functions of numerous wildlife and their offspring; however, most researchers doubt that the low levels of environmental pesticides are sufficient to produce similar health effects in humans. But that's an educated guess. The Environmental Protection Agency (EPA) reports that approximately seventy pesticides now in use are "probable" or "possible" cancer-causing agents. For example, researchers at Mount Sinai School of Medicine and New York University Medical Center analyzed blood samples of women with and without breast cancer. They found that women who had the highest levels of DDE in their blood (a breakdown product of the pesticide DDT, banned from use more than a decade ago) were four times as likely to develop breast cancer as women with low levels of the pesticide residue.

Many researchers believe the pesticide scare is overrated. Dr. Bruce Ames at the University of California, Berkeley, states that eliminating the small amount of synthetic chemicals in our diets would have no effect on cancer rates, while more than two hundred studies show that eating lots of fruits and vegetables with or without pesticides lowers cancer risk. According to Dr. Ames, exposure to pesticides is nowhere near as important a health concern as smoking, excessive alcohol consumption, being overweight, or consuming too much saturated fat.

There's no getting rid of pesticides, but you can reduce exposure by following these guidelines:

- While regulations on pesticide use are enforced somewhat in the United States, in other countries, regulations (if there are any) might not be enforced. Consequently, produce coming into the United States from other countries can contain illegal residues or levels of pesticides not allowed in this country. These foods are the ones to limit or avoid, if possible. Buy United States–grown organic produce, milk, and other products when possible.
- If you can't find organic, look for "green" or Integrated Pest Management (IPM) labels.
- Wash fruits and vegetables with a mild soap solution. Rinse well.
- Eat a low-fat diet of minimally processed foods. Keep in mind that pesticide residues also are found in meat, poultry, fish, butter, grains, and other foods. You can cut down on your risk by removing the fat, since that's where some pesticides are concentrated.
- Include soy products in the daily menu. Consuming soy foods daily can reduce the hormonelike effects of some pesticides by up to 50 percent.

The bottom line is that regardless of the pesticide controversy, fresh fruits and vegetables are the most nutritious foods in the diet and should be consumed in greater quantities.

The Grain Exchange: Whole Grains
Versus Refined

Along with fresh fruits and vegetables, whole grains have top billing in the Feeling Good Diet. In essence, you can't tell a grain by its name. A bread labeled "Light Whole-Grain Sourdough" might sound like a 100 percent whole-grain product, but it actually contains mostly white flour with only a dusting of whole-grain flour. Some commercial breads with "Twelve Grain" or "multigrain" in the name have little more fiber than white bread.

When selecting products made from grains, ignore the name and go straight to the ingredients list. Purchase those products that list whole wheat flour (not wheat flour), brown rice, oats, or another whole grain or grain product as the first ingredient. If the label on a loaf of bread, a box of crackers, a bag of cookies, or a package of frozen pancakes does not read 100 percent whole wheat flour, assume the item is made primarily from refined flour. (A slice of white bread has a fraction of the chromium, selenium, and several other nutrients found in a slice of whole wheat bread.)

Where's the Fat and Sugar?

Check the fat and sugar content on food labels. By nature, whole grains are almost fat- and sugar-free. In general, the more processed a grain product is, the more likely it will be high in fat, sugar, and/or salt. Your best bet is to select only those cereals, crackers, and breads that contain 1 gram of fat or less for every 100 calories; at worst, select those with no more than 3 grams of fat for every 100 calories. Avoid products that have fatty additions, such as cheese, put into some crackers. Read the label and steer clear of any grain product—especially ready-to-eat cereals—that lists sugar (under any of its names) in the top three ingredients (see Table 13.1, "Sweet Without Sugar," on page 293).

The Meat and Seafood Market

It takes only 3 ounces a day of extra-lean meat (roughly the size of a deck of cards) to maximize all of its nutritional benefits. Consume any more and the increased intake of saturated fat, protein, and cholesterol will compromise your health by increasing your risk of developing heart disease, cancer, and other degenerative diseases. Too

Table 13.1   Sweet Without Sugar

Apple juice concentrate and pureed fruits such as bananas, apples, and prunes can be used to replace some of the fat and sugar in recipes. When you omit or reduce the sugar, honey, or other sweeteners, you can add sweetness with one of the following spices or with extracts that provide a sweet flavor, such as vanilla, almond, and cherry.

- *Allspice.* Use to season baked products such as muffins and breads; also vegetables such as carrots, winter squash, and sweet potatoes.
- *Anise.* These seeds give breads and desserts a unique licorice flavor.
- *Cardamom.* The unique flavor of this spice is good in curries or to flavor winter squash, sweet potatoes, breads, cakes, and cookies.
- *Cinnamon.* Use the sticks to give a spicy flavor to hot beverages; use ground cinnamon in baked goods, fruit sauces, stews, and puddings; also with carrots, sweet potatoes, and baked apples.
- *Cloves.* The most aromatic spice, it adds flavor to hot beverages, beets, carrots, sweet potatoes, winter squash, baked goods, meats, stews, and soups.
- *Coriander* (also called *cilantro*). Fresh coriander has a sharp, citrus-rind flavor that is good in salads and spicy casseroles, soups, and stews. The ground seeds impart a nutty flavor to rice, dried beans, shellfish, poultry, vegetables, salsa, and salads.
- *Ginger.* The fresh root is peeled and grated to add spice to marinades and with steamed vegetables, chicken, or fish. Use ground ginger in baking and marinades, rice dishes, and soups, and in preparing carrots, beets, and squash.
- *Mace.* Similar in taste to nutmeg but milder (it is the fibrous covering on the nutmeg seed), this spice enhances the flavor of broccoli, carrots, cauliflower, brussels sprouts, baked goods, and puddings.
- *Mint.* Choose from more than thirty types of mint (fresh is most flavorful and sweet) to enhance grains, vegetable and fruit salads, iced teas, peas, corn, beans, cucumbers, carrots, and potatoes.
- *Nutmeg.* A nutty, versatile spice that brings out the best in spinach, broccoli, cauliflower, carrots, brussels sprouts, onions, beans, and sweet potatoes; excellent in sauces, pasta, stews, and low-fat desserts.
- *Pumpkin pie spice.* A blend of nutmeg, cinnamon, cloves, and ginger that adds a sweet flavor to winter squash, sweet potatoes, and carrots, as well as to fruit desserts such as baked apples.

much saturated fat also upsets the balance of fats, increasing your risk for developing depression. In fact, you could eliminate meat from your diet and replace it with more servings of legumes and fish with no harm—and much benefit—to your nutritional status.

If you do choose to eat meat, make sure it is extra-lean. Don't assume that ground chicken or turkey is low in fat. Purchase only ground meat with a fat content of 7 percent or less by weight. Cast a wary eye at the meat department, and don't assume anything. For example:

- Chicken and turkey were not created equal; chicken is one and one-half times as fatty as turkey.
- Chicken also is not always leaner than beef. For example, a 4-ounce serving of chicken thigh meat contains more fat than an equal serving of fat-trimmed sirloin or chuck pot roast.

When it comes to poultry, stick to white meats such as chicken and turkey breast. Assume a processed meat product contains high-fat poultry parts unless the label states that it is made entirely from breast meat.

Is Fish Safe to Eat?

Although fish deserves a healthy round of applause, the waters in which they swim are not so pure. Many of the chemicals, pollutants, and pesticides used on land leach into the lakes, rivers, streams, and coastal waters where they are ingested by simple forms of marine life. These life-forms, in turn, are consumed by medium-sized fish, which then are consumed by larger fish. Each step of this food chain—from plankton to trout—further concentrates chemical contaminants in fish tissues.

The chemicals of biggest concern include mercury and pesticides such as DDT and dioxin, and polychlorinated biphenyls (PCBs). Their use was discontinued in the 1970s after evidence showed they caused cancer, low birth weights, and developmental problems. DDT also causes liver tumors and affects reproduction in laboratory animals, and was banned in the United States in 1972. Yet eleven years later, this pesticide was found in 334 of the 386 samples of domestic fish tested. While levels gradually receded in the United States, DDT still is used in other countries, and its wide distribution in the environment and slow disintegration means that DDT and its breakdown products will be around for decades to come.

"PCB and DDT contamination is as much a problem today as it was in 1992 because there has been no significant cleanup of the waters where fish swim," says Caroline Smith DeWaal, director of food safety at the Center for Science in the Public Interest in Washington, D.C. Some fish, however, contain more than others. In a 1992 *Consumer Reports* investigation, 50 percent of lake whitefish and 25 percent of swordfish sampled contained PCBs, while flounder and sole were almost PCB-free. Catfish, carp, and lake trout contained the most DDT. Pacific Coast fish are less contaminated with PCBs than fish caught in the Atlantic or Great Lakes. "Large, fatty fish [such as bluefish] are the biggest concern because these fish bioaccumulate chemicals such as PCBs over time," says David Harvey, agricultural economist for the U.S. Department of Agriculture.

But is the relative risk of DDT and PCB exposure that big of a concern? According to Harvey, "Most trout and catfish purchased in grocery stores or eaten in restaurants are purchased from fish farms where the fish are raised on grain-based diets and don't bioaccumulate pesticide residues to anywhere near the levels found in the wild."

DeWaal disagrees. "Farm-raised trout and catfish are no guarantee of safety," she says. "Granted, some farms are stellar operations, but many were built on old agricultural lands where years of pesticide use and contaminant runoff resulted in high levels of residues that now leach into the waters used for raising fish." According to DeWaal, for consumers who want to avoid these chemicals, the less trout, bluefish, and inland lake fish they eat, the better; women who might become or are pregnant should probably avoid these fish altogether.

Swordfish, shark, and fresh tuna also are suspect, especially for pregnant women. These fish concentrate mercury in their tissues, which is known to cause birth defects, psychomotor retardation, and severe cerebral palsy, especially in children whose mothers consumed large amounts of mercury-contaminated fish or grain during pregnancy. However, a recent study from the University of Rochester proposes that although mercury has not been exonerated, it might not be as dangerous as once thought. "We studied 700 children who were prenatally exposed to varying levels of mercury when their mothers consumed up to 12 servings of fish each week. We examined neurological, developmental, and psychological factors and found no adverse associations between mercury exposure and test outcomes through 5½ years of age," reports Gary Myers, M.D., a principal investigator in the study and professor of neurology and pediatrics at the University of Rochester in New York. However, since other research has shown a benefit to restricting mercury during pregnancy, it is probably wise to limit swordfish, shark, and fresh tuna to one serving a month (and avoid all fish caught in the Great Lakes) if you are considering becoming or are pregnant.

Despite these concerns, fish and shellfish still remain one of the healthiest, low-calorie sources of many nutrients, such as the B vitamins (especially vitamin B_2, niacin, vitamin B_6, and vitamin B_{12}), fluoride, iodine, and iron. Canned salmon and sardines eaten with the bones are excellent sources of calcium. Oysters are the best dietary source for zinc (one large oyster supplies an entire day's requirement for this trace mineral) and a good source of copper. Fish and shellfish also provide high-quality protein: a 3½-ounce serving of baked flounder, sole, halibut, or cod supplies one-third of a person's daily need for protein, but only about 10 percent of his or her calorie allotment. Even the fattiest types of fish contain less fat and cholesterol than most cuts of red meats, and the type of fat is healthier to the heart—for example, oily fish contains one-fifth to one-half the fat content of beef.

In short, there is no need to stop eating seafood; just avoid the high-risk selections. In fact, most seafood is still a healthy alternative to beef and pork, especially since your risk for heart disease far outweighs your risk for seafood poisoning. To avoid the contamination issue, purchase lean or Pacific-caught fish, buy very fresh, keep it cold, and cook it thoroughly.

The Dairy Case

The "purchase minimally processed food" rule does not apply to the dairy case. Left untouched, most dairy products contain more fat, especially saturated fat, than any other food except red meat. However, when some of the fat is removed, many items in the dairy case take on a new look. Low-fat milk (2 percent fat) has 1 teaspoon of fat for every cup; this is only a slight reduction from whole milk's 1½ teaspoons. On the other hand, 1 percent low-fat and nonfat milk and yogurt are low-fat nutritional powerhouses. Go easy on the fruited-yogurts, however, since some contain more sugar than a candy bar. Your best bet is to purchase low-fat or nonfat plain yogurt and mix it with fresh fruit or a small amount of all-fruit jam. Use the label guidelines on page 288 when choosing low-fat cheese. Also check out the new soy cheeses: Many are low-fat, taste great, and cook well.

Select only fat-free versions of cream cheese and sour cream. Even the "light" version of cream cheese—touted as half the fat of regular cream cheese—contains 75 percent fat calories, and a low-fat version of sour cream contains up to 51 percent

Table 13.2   The Feeling Good Shopping List

Use this sheet as a master copy. Keep a copy posted in the kitchen to circle needed items, then take the list with you when you shop.

THE PRODUCE SECTION

(vitamin C–rich selections are marked with an asterisk before the item)
Fruit: Apples/Apricots/Bananas/Berries/*Cantaloupe/Casaba melon/Cherries/
*Grapefruit/Grapes/*Kiwifruits/Kumquats/*Honeydew melon/Nectarines/*Oranges/
*Papayas/Peaches/Pears/Pineapple/Plums/Pomegranates/Quince/*Tangerines/Watermelon
Other: _____

(beta-carotene–rich vegetables are marked with an asterisk)
Vegetables: Artichokes/*Asparagus/Bean sprouts/Beets/*Broccoli/Brussels sprouts/Cabbage/
*Carrots/Cauliflower/Celery/Cucumbers/*Chard/*Collards/Corn/*Dandelion greens/
Eggplant/Green beans/*Kale/Leeks/Lettuce/Mushrooms/*Mustard greens/Okra/Onions/
Parsnips/Peas/Peppers/Potatoes/Pumpkin/Rhubarb/Rutabaga/Snow peas/*Spinach/Summer
squash or zucchini/*Sweet potatoes/Tomatoes/*Turnip greens/Winter squash/Yams
Other: _____

BAKED GOODS

Bread: Whole wheat/Pumpernickel/Pita/Rye/Oat
Crackers: Ry-Krisp/Graham/Akmak/Saltines
Other: Bagels/English muffins/Rice cakes/Corn tortillas
Other: _____

DAIRY CASE

Nonfat milk/Nonfat plain yogurt/Buttermilk/Low-fat and nonfat cheeses
Egg substitute/Fat-free sour cream/Fat-free cream cheese
Other: _____

MEAT AND FISH DEPARTMENT

Beef, extra-lean cuts only/Veal, extra-lean cuts only/Chicken/Turkey/Seafood/Luncheon meats, 95 percent fat-free/Ground turkey breast

Other: _____

DRY GOODS

Powdered buttermilk/Powdered nonfat milk/Whole wheat flour/Dried beans and peas/Pasta/ Brown rice/Wheat germ

Other: _____

CANNED GOODS

Applesauce, no sugar added/Apricots, canned in own juice/Artichoke hearts, water-packed/ Kidney, black, garbanzo beans/Carrot juice/Evaporated nonfat milk/Fruit cocktail, canned in own juice/100% fruit juices/Mandarin oranges, juice-packed/Peaches, canned in own juice/ Peanut butter/Pears, canned in own juice/Pineapple chunks, canned in own juice/Salmon/ Soups, low-fat/Spaghetti sauce, fat-free/Tomato juice/Tomato paste/Tomato sauce/Tuna, water-packed

Other: _____

BREAKFAST CEREALS

Cooked: Oatmeal/Barley/Farina
Ready-to-eat: Grape-Nuts/Shredded wheat/Nutri-Grain

Other: _____

FROZEN FOODS

Desserts: Frozen fruit ice/Ice cream, fat- and sugar-free/Sherbet/
Sorbet/Blueberries/Strawberries
Other: Vegetables/Whole wheat waffles

Other: _____

SNACK ITEMS

Dried fruit/Nuts and seeds/Popcorn, plain/Potato chips, oven-baked, fat-free/Pretzels/Tortilla chips, oven-baked, fat-free

Other: _____

DESSERTS

Angel food cake, no frosting/Sponge cake, no frosting/Animal crackers/Vanilla wafers

Other: _____

HERBS, OILS, AND CONDIMENTS

Active dry yeast/All-fruit jam/Baking powder/Baking soda/Catsup/Cornstarch/Herbs and spices/
Lemon juice/Mustard/No-fat salad dressing/Olive or canola oil/Salsa/Unflavored gelatin/
Vanilla/Vinegar

Other: _____

fat calories. Not much to rave about!

Remember: Butter is all fat. If you purchase butter, freeze three or four sticks. You will be using this fat sparingly, and it is likely to turn rancid if left for long periods in the refrigerator. When choosing margarine, select tub versions that are trans fatty acid–free. Better yet, select the fat-free butter alternatives available in the dairy case.

Feeling Good About Grocery Shopping

One of the main premises of the Feeling Good Diet is to make dietary changes slowly. That also applies to shopping. Set small goals for yourself, such as scouting out certain sections of the grocery store each month, practicing label reading, or substituting a new, minimally processed food for a familiar high-fat or high-sugar food. Make copies of Table 13.2, The Feeling Good Shopping List, on pages 297–299 and keep a copy on the refrigerator, where you can mark down needed items. Shopping can be fun without being time-consuming if you plan ahead and focus on meeting your mental and physical health needs with nutrient-packed, wholesome foods.

Planning Your Meals and Snacks

Eating right does not begin at the stove or at the table. It starts with a plan. But the best-laid plans are worthless if they don't fit your activities and food preferences. Follow the three steps of the Feeling Good Diet to plan the upcoming week. For examples and inspiration, review the sample menus beginning on page 306. These menus help translate the guidelines into real meals and snacks. The menus might not be a perfect fit for your tastes, so feel free to tailor them to your needs.

Planning your menus means more than just thinking about what you will eat; it means writing down your food choices on a day-by-day basis. The process should not feel overwhelming. If it does, reconsider the Feeling Good Diet step you selected; perhaps you are making too many changes too quickly. Even so, in the beginning all this menu planning might feel odd or cumbersome. Remind yourself that any new skill, whether riding a bicycle or driving a car, will seem uncomfortable at first, but gets easier with practice. Eventually you will develop several sets of menus that suit your preferences and lifestyle.

Five Simple Guidelines

Learning to eat right to feel your best initially takes some extra time and mental energy, but food preparation can be easy if you follow some easy guidelines:

1. Make nutritious foods readily available. For example, clean and store enough raw vegetables to supply meals and snacks for up to three days. (Or purchase vegetables already washed and cut.) Freeze an extra loaf of whole wheat bread, stock extra cans of kidney beans, or purchase several cans of nonfat evaporated milk for use in recipes in case you run low on regular low-fat milk.

2. Concentrate on food preparation only once or twice a week. Plan one evening on the weekend and/or one evening during the week to cook enough foods to last the rest of the week. Soups, stews, and casseroles can be portion-packed, stored in the refrigerator or freezer, and reheated in the microwave. Also, cook enough of certain foods to use in more than one meal. For example, rice, dried peas and beans, pasta, potatoes, and marinara sauce are easy to prepare in large quantities. Chicken can be cooked, then used in sandwiches, pasta dishes, and snacks. Store the leftovers in the freezer in the appropriate serving sizes for use in everything from burritos and side dishes to main meals.

3. Keep it simple. Unless you are a gourmet cook who loves to spend hours in the kitchen, avoid complicated recipes that require time, a lengthy list of ingredients, and fancy equipment. You can prepare

nutritious meals and snacks that take no more than five to thirty minutes. Have a set of simple meals that can be prepared in a flash. Almost all of the recipes provided at the back of this book require minimal amounts of ingredients and require less than thirty minutes of preparation time.

4. Make your meals attractive. Consider eye appeal and the three T's: taste, texture, and temperature. Eating should be a pleasurable experience, not a medical one.

5. Include two fruits and/or vegetables in every meal. Rather than 6-ounce pieces of beef and an iceberg lettuce salad, stir-fry strips of extra-lean beef with lots of vegetables and serve over instant brown rice with a leaf lettuce salad. Or add vegetables to your meals as follows:

- Spaghetti and pizza sauce: Stir in grated carrots, onions, mushrooms, peppers.
- Lasagna: Add a layer of broccoli or spinach in place of all or some of the meat and cheese.
- Casseroles: Add green peas, carrots, celery, onion, bell peppers, squash, or sweet potatoes to the mixture.
- Baked beans, chili, meat loaf: Include grated carrots, extra tomato sauce, canned tomatoes, or green beans in the recipe.
- Potato salad: Add carrots, peas, peppers, red onions.
- Canned soups: Include extra vegetables such as potatoes, corn, beans, peas, carrots, squash.
- Baked potato: Stuff with spinach and low-fat yogurt; broccoli, mushrooms, and part-skim ricotta cheese; or nonfat cottage cheese and salsa.
- Corn bread and muffins: Put grated carrots, zucchini, corn, or green chilies into the batter.
- Shish kebab: Skewer at least twice as many vegetables—including mushrooms, carrots, eggplant, cherry tomatoes, zucchini, onion, or potato—as extra-lean meat, chicken, or shellfish.
- Tortillas: Fill with ricotta or cottage cheese and spinach sprinkled with nutmeg; black beans, plain nonfat yogurt, and salsa; grated carrot and zucchini, low-fat cheese, and green chili peppers; nonfat refried beans, cilantro, tomato, and grated carrot.

- Salads: Try carrot-raisin, Waldorf (apples, celery, green pepper, and nuts), spinach and orange slices, or marinated vegetables.
- Burgers: Try grilling a Portobello mushroom (marinated in olive oil, balsamic vinegar, minced garlic, and salt) as an alternative to beef patties.
- Vegetables: Rather than always steaming your vegetables, try grilling or roasting them, which accents their flavors and sweetness.

The Right Pro-Portion

The best of eating plans are undermined when portion size expands. And with Americans accustomed to elephant-sized portions, that often is the case. For example, Step 3 of the Feeling Good Diet includes at least seven servings of grains. That might seem like a lot, but in reality, most Americans are eating much more than that because of supersized portions. Here are a few examples of how too much of a good thing could undermine your mood, health, and weight goals:

- A muffin should weigh about 1½ ounces, but bakeries sell 6- to 8-ounce muffins. That's a half pound's worth and up to five servings of grain in this one muffin!
- A bagel for breakfast can weigh 6 ounces. The recommended serving is one-half of a 2-ounce bagel, so this breakfast supplies six servings.
- The recommended serving size for pasta is ½ cup, or the size of a tennis ball. That is about four twirls of a fork. A more typical portion is three and a half times larger than this. If you had that oversized muffin or bagel for breakfast, this dinner will bring your grand total for grains up to twelve to fourteen, and that's not counting the grains you got at lunch or snacks. (See Table 10.3, "Size Matters," on page 249 for more information on portion size.)

The same holds true for meat. A recommended serving of chicken, red meat, or fish is 2 to 3 ounces. That's the size of the palm of your hand or a deck of cards. But Americans typically consume two to four times that amount. It is not unusual for a deli sandwich to contain up to a pound of meat, or two and a half days' worth of your protein needs in one meal.

Here are a few additional tips for improving your portion awareness:

- Ask the butcher at the meat counter to weigh your meat purchases so you know exactly what portions you are buying.
- Use measuring cups and spoons to portion out your food until your awareness improves.
- Consider making simple 2-, 3-, and 4-ounce food models from sponges or cardboard to make comparisons easier. Even when you are confident enough not to measure anymore, periodically check your accuracy.

Satisfying Snacks

Snacks play an important role in the Feeling Good Diet. When properly selected, snacks help control hunger by eliminating surges in your appetite-control chemicals. But before you race to the vending machine with a license to snack, keep in mind that healthful nibbling means following a few simple rules.

Rule 1: Keep it simple. A nutritious snack must be convenient; that is, it must be readily available, take little time to prepare, and taste great.

Rule 2: Include at least one fruit or vegetable at each snack, plus a nutritious second food, such as a whole grain, nuts and seeds, a nonfat milk product, cooked dried beans and peas, or extra-lean meat. For example, fruit slices dipped in nonfat yogurt with cinnamon or raw vegetables with a curried bean dip.

Rule 3: Minimally processed foods should outnumber highly processed snack items.

The Dining-Out Dilemma

Most restaurants are willing to prepare a meal that meets the Feeling Good Diet guidelines if you ask for exactly what you want. If a restaurant will not or cannot accommodate your needs, go elsewhere. Your primary strategies for dining out are the same ones you use when dining at home:

1. Limit or avoid fat. Choose foods that have been broiled, poached, roasted, or steamed. Select items described as "garden fresh"; "in a tomato base"; "in broth"; or cooked "in its own juice." Avoid foods that are described as crisp, braised, buttered or buttery, creamed,

scalloped, fried, à la mode, au gratin, au fromage, or refried; cooked in a butter, cheese, or cream sauce; served with gravy; or pan-fried, breaded, or sautéed.

2. Emphasize whole grains, vegetables, and fruits, and use meat, chicken, fish, and dairy foods as condiments.

3. Choose foods that are as close to their original form as possible; for example, order a plain baked potato rather than fried potato skins topped with cheese.

4. Have only the foods you intend to eat brought to your table. Ask the waiter to bring extra bread sticks, but not to bring the buttered garlic bread or the dessert tray.

5. Learn to eyeball accurate portions, and stick to them!

In addition, you can choose restaurants that specialize in healthful foods. Look for establishments that have salad bars with a wide assortment of fresh produce; that serve low-fat pasta dishes and fresh fruit for dessert; and that poach, broil, or steam fish, seafood, chicken, and other meats. Avoid restaurants that serve tempting but unhealthy foods such as baskets of fried tortilla chips at Mexican restaurants, gourmet chocolate desserts, or homemade cinnamon rolls and specialty coffees.

Ask whether special requests are honored before you make reservations. If you are not familiar with the restaurant, ask to see a menu so you can choose your meal and order it mentally before going to the restaurant. Request additional information about portion sizes, ingredients, preparation techniques, and accompaniments, such as side dishes or other items served with the entrée. Then frequent restaurants where you have had success ordering the meal you want; you will know the menu, and the servers will know your tastes.

At the restaurant, decide what you will order before you open the menu, or order without looking at the menu. Certain foods might be available but not listed on the menu, such as baked fish or chicken, nonfat milk, a baked potato, or a steamed vegetable plate. You should be able to assemble a low-fat meal from the appetizer, salad, and side-dish sections on the menu. For example, order two salads and split an entrée with your dining partner. Order first to avoid being influenced by other diners at your table.

When ordering, always ask and never assume anything. A food described as grilled could be grilled with butter. When you order, specify how you want your food prepared: broiled instead of fried; grilled without butter; plain vegetables instead of the creamed version; no sugar for your tea; or fresh fruit instead of syrup for pancakes.

Specify what you don't want. Learn to say, "Hold the butter, margarine, cream, or cheese." Ask for salad dressing, gravy, sugar, jam, or syrup on the side. Rather than rely on willpower after the food arrives, ask that tempting foods be left in the kitchen. Send back anything that is prepared incorrectly. If there are droplets of oil on your vegetables, they were probably sautéed in oil rather than steamed. If your muffin tastes too sweet or leaves a slippery feel on your fingertips, it probably is high in sugar and/or fat.

When the meal is served, before you start to eat, put any foods or portions you are not going to eat in a doggie bag or on a side plate, and ask that they be removed. If necessary, bring your own low-fat or fat-free salad dressing packets in case low-fat dressings, vinegar, lemon, salsa, or other no-fat options are unavailable at the restaurant. If you want chicken, but a skinless entrée is not available, remove the skin yourself when it is served.

Avoid drinking alcoholic beverages before and with your meal, or make selections very carefully. Alcohol stimulates the appetite and also can weaken your commitment to follow your diet when tempting foods are available.

Skip dessert unless it is fresh fruit, a low-sugar sorbet, or low-fat frozen yogurt. Split a dessert with a friend, or ask for a half-portion. Order tea or fruit juice.

There are also steps you can take beyond these food choices. For example:

- Go out for lunch rather than dinner; lunch entrées are smaller and less expensive.
- Don't starve yourself in anticipation of a big restaurant meal. A regular pattern of breakfast, lunch, and snacks will prevent overindulging at the restaurant.
- Start meals with volume (water, sparkling water, salad, raw vegetables, or clear soup) or have a snack before leaving home.
- Take a break halfway through the meal. It takes about twenty minutes for the brain to receive the message that you are full. Push back from the table for a few moments to help your body attune to its signals.
- Focus on the people during the meal, not on the food. In other words, make dining a social event rather than an eating event.

Feeling Good Menus

The following seven days of menus are based on Step 3 of the Feeling Good Diet, with detailed suggestions for Steps 1 and 2. Keep in mind these are only examples. You can follow these menus exactly or use them as a guide for developing your own eating plan, tailored to your food preferences and habits. Recipes for items marked with an * can be found in the "Recipes for Feeling Your Best" at the back of this book.

DAY 1:

Breakfast:

1 cup cooked oatmeal (cooked in nonfat milk)

1 cup orange juice

1 slice whole wheat raisin toast
   topped with 1 teaspoon butter

1 cup herb tea

A vitamin and mineral supplement

Midmorning Snack:

1 mango, peeled and sliced
   topped with 1 teaspoon fresh lime juice

2 cups sparkling water

Lunch:

PITA POCKET SANDWICH:

   1 whole wheat pita pocket bread filled with:

   1 ounce Jalapeño cheese, grated

   1 diced fresh tomato

   2 tablespoons grated zucchini

   ½ can canned kidney beans, drained

1 apple

2 cups water

Midafternoon Snack:

2 cups fat-free microwave popcorn

2 cups water

Dinner:

4 ounces Spicy Grilled Salmon with Ginger*

GREEN MASHED POTATOES:

   1 boiled potato, mashed and mixed with:

   ⅓ cup chopped, cooked chard

   ½ cup 1 percent low-fat milk

   1 tablespoon Parmesan cheese, grated

   Salt and pepper to taste

1½ cups steamed asparagus

CARROT-RAISIN-APPLE SALAD:

   1 cup grated carrot

   1 tablespoon raisins

   ½ apple, chopped

   2 tablespoons mayonnaise

   Lemon juice, salt, and pepper to taste

Evening Snack:

1 cup frozen seedless grapes

1 cup 1 percent low-fat milk, heated and flavored

   with almond extract

Nutritional information:
2,059 calories; 25 percent fat (57 grams); 59 percent
carbohydrates; 16 percent protein.

Step 1: Include at least two servings each of the fruits and vegetables; two servings of the milk and cheese; and at least two grains (oatmeal, toast, pita bread, or popcorn), which should be whole grains. The salmon at dinner fills one of the two requirements for meat; you can add an additional serving at lunch if you desire. You can include caffeinated beverages, sweets, and additional oils and fats, but cut back on these when you can. For example, you might choose to have a cup of coffee instead of herb tea at breakfast; substitute a dessert for the frozen grapes as an evening snack; or use more fats in cooking, such as butter on your breakfast toast, regular popcorn instead of fat-free, sautéed asparagus not steamed, and/or more mayonnaise when preparing the carrot-raisin-apple salad.

Step 2: Include at least three servings each of the fruits and the vegetables; two servings of the milk and cheese; and at least three grains (oatmeal, toast, pita bread, or popcorn), which should be whole grains. The salmon at dinner fills one of the two requirements for meat; you can add an additional serving at lunch if you desire. You still have some leeway on caffeinated beverages, sweets, and additional oils and fats, but cut back on these when you can. For example, you might choose a coffee latte for a beverage at lunch instead of water, cookies and milk for a midafternoon snack, or mayonnaise on your sandwich at lunch and butter when preparing the mashed potatoes at dinner.

DAY 2:

Breakfast:
1 whole-grain muffin with raisins and nuts
　　topped with 1 tablespoon cashew butter
1 cup fresh pineapple chunks
2 cups herb tea
A vitamin and mineral supplement

Midmorning Snack:
5 fat-free whole wheat crackers, topped with Peanut
　　butter candy:
　　　1 tablespoon chunky peanut butter mixed with:
　　　1 tablespoon wheat germ
　　　2 teaspoons honey
1 cup 1 percent low-fat milk
2 cups water

Lunch:
GRILLED CHEESE SANDWICH:
　　2 slices whole wheat bread

1 ounce cheddar cheese

mustard to taste

1 serving Zucchini Torte*

1 tomato, sliced

1 orange

2 cups sparkling water

Midafternoon Snack:

1 whole wheat bagel

topped with 2 teaspoons nonfat cream cheese and

2 teaspoons all-fruit jam

2 cups herb iced tea

Dinner:

½ roast chicken breast

1 cup steamed peas and carrots

½ acorn squash

filled with 1 teaspoon honey and 2 teaspoons

sherry

½ cup Wild Greens Topped with Pears, Blue

Cheese, and Walnuts*

1 cup 1 percent low-fat milk

1 cup water

Evening Snack:

FRUIT FONDUE:

½ cup strawberries

1 kiwi, peeled and sliced

½ banana, sliced

dunked in ¼ cup fat-free chocolate syrup

2 cups water

Nutritional information:
2025 calories; 25 percent fat (57 grams); 57 percent
carbohydrates; 18 percent protein.

Step 1: Include at least two servings each of the fruits and vegetables; two servings of the milk and cheese; and at least two grains (muffin, crackers, wheat germ, bread, or bagel), which should be whole grains. The chicken at dinner fills one of the two requirements for meat; you can add an additional serving at lunch if you desire. You can include caffeinated beverages, sweets, and additional oils and fats, but cut back on these when you can. For example, you might choose to have a cup of coffee instead of herb tea at breakfast, have a dessert at lunch or after dinner instead of fruit, or use more fats in cooking, such as butter on your breakfast muffin instead of cashew butter, regular cream cheese on the bagel and regular dressing on the salad, and/or gravy with the chicken at dinner.

Step 2: Include at least three servings each of the fruits and vegetables; two servings of the milk and cheese; and at least three grains (muffin, crackers, wheat germ, bread, or bagel), which should be whole grains. You can add an additional serving of meat at lunch or a larger serving at dinner, if you desire. You still have some leeway on caffeinated beverages, sweets, and additional oils and fats, but cut back on these when you can. For example, you might choose coffee or tea at breakfast or a cup of coffee at lunch, a chocolate dessert rather than the fruit fondue, or additional fats, such as whole milk instead of low-fat, grilling the cheese sandwich in butter, and/or sautéed chicken breast instead of roasted.

DAY 3:

Breakfast:
½ cup egg substitute, scrambled with salt and
    pepper
2 slices whole wheat toast
1 tomato, sliced
6 ounces fresh-squeezed orange juice
2 cups water
A vitamin and mineral supplement

Midmorning Snack:
1 slice whole wheat raisin bread

dunked in 6 ounces low-fat cinnamon-apple
yogurt
2 cups sparkling water

Lunch:

1 large tomato, cut partially through into quarters
    and filled with tuna salad:
    4 ounces tuna packed in water, drained
    ¼ cup celery, chopped
    1 teaspoon mustard
    2 tablespoons mayonnaise
    Salt, pepper, and dill to taste
4 fat-free whole wheat crackers
1 cup 1 percent low-fat milk
2 cups water

Midafternoon Snack:

½ whole wheat English muffin
    topped with 2 teaspoons fat-free cream cheese and
    1 kiwi, peeled and sliced
1 cup nonfat milk
1 cup water

Dinner:

1½ cups Chicken-Apricot Curry with Rice* (if you
    cook extra chicken here, you can use it for the
    couscous salad tomorrow!)
⅓ cup extra rice
½ cup Spicy Garlic Spinach*
TOSSED SALAD:
    1 cup mixed leaf lettuce
    2 tablespoons mandarin oranges
    ⅓ avocado, sliced
    Fat-free vinaigrette dressing
2 cups sparkling water, with lemon

Evening Snack:

1 slice Frozen Vanilla Yogurt Pie with Berries*

Nutritional information:
2005 calories, 25 percent fat (55 grams), 52 percent
carbohydrates, 23 percent protein.

Step 1: Include at least two servings each of the fruits and vegetables; two servings of the milk and yogurt; and at least two grains (toast, bread, crackers, English muffin, or rice), which should be whole grains. You can add an additional serving of meat at lunch or increase the serving size at dinner, if you desire. You can include caffeinated beverages, sweets, and additional oils and fats, but cut back on these when you can. For example, have a cup of coffee or tea at breakfast, regular cake instead of angel food cake, and include more fats such as butter on the morning toast, additional mayonnaise in preparing the lunch salad, and/or sautéed not steamed spinach.

Step 2: Include all three of the fruits; at least three of the vegetables; two servings of the milk and cheese; and at least three grains (toast, bread, crackers, English muffin, or rice), which should be whole grains. You can add an additional serving of meat at lunch or a larger serving at dinner, if you desire. You still have some leeway on caffeinated beverages, sweets, and additional oils and fats, but cut back on these when you can. For example, you can include more coffee at breakfast or midmorning, a noncaffeinated soda pop at the midafternoon snack, and/or more fats, such as tuna packed in oil for the lunch salad, and/or regular crackers, cream cheese, or salad dressing.

DAY 4:

Breakfast:

2 whole wheat frozen waffles, toasted
    topped with 3 tablespoons fat-free sour cream and
    ⅔ cup strawberries (fresh or thawed)
1 cup grapefruit juice
1 cup 1 percent low-fat milk
A vitamin and mineral supplement

Midmorning Snack:

1 papaya
    filled with 6 ounces low-fat lemon yogurt
    1 teaspoon fresh mint, chopped
2 cups water

Lunch:

1 generous cup Southwest Couscous Salad*
SPINACH SALAD:
    1½ cups spinach, washed and stemmed
    2 tablespoons mushrooms, sliced
    2 tablespoons red raspberries
    2 tablespoons fat-free raspberry vinaigrette
    dressing
2 cups sparkling water

Midafternoon Snack:

20 large low-fat tortilla chips
¼ cup fat-free refried beans (as a dip)
2 tablespoons salsa
2 cups water

Dinner:

SEAFOOD PASTA:
    1 cup linguini noodles, cooked
    Sauce: Sauté in 1 tablespoon olive oil the
    following: ½ cup chopped onion, 8 ounces stewed
    tomatoes, 2 teaspoons chopped fresh parsley,
    2 minced garlic cloves, ½ teaspoon marjoram,
    and salt and pepper to taste. Simmer in nonstick
    skillet until onion is tender. Add ¼ pound fresh
    steamer clams and cook for 10 minutes over
    medium-high heat.
    Pour over pasta.
1 cup broccoli, steamed

TOSSED SALAD:

    1 cup romaine lettuce, chopped

    ½ cup cucumber, sliced

    3 tablespoons mushrooms, sliced

    1 tablespoon low-calorie cucumber dressing

2 cups water

Evening Snack:

½ cup Cheerios

2 tablespoons dried mixed fruit

1 tablespoon semisweet chocolate chips

Nutritional information:
2,024 calories; 23 percent fat (52 grams); 58 percent
carbohydrates; 19 percent protein.

Step 1: Include at least two servings each of the fruits and vegetables; two servings of the milk and yogurt; and at least two grains (waffles, couscous, tortilla chips, linguini), which should be whole grains. This menu already includes two servings of meat (chicken at lunch and clams at dinner), which fills the quota for this food group. You can include caffeinated beverages, sweets, and additional oils and fats, but cut back on these when you can. For example, add a cup of coffee or tea at breakfast and/or lunch, a piece of pie for an evening dessert, and/or additional servings of fat, such as whole-fat sour cream for the breakfast waffle, regular salad dressing at lunch and dinner, and/or sautéed broccoli instead of steamed.

Step 2: Include at least three servings each of the fruits and vegetables; two servings of the milk and yogurt; and at least three grains (waffles, couscous, tortilla chips, linguini), which should be whole grains. Your meat allotment is met, so don't add any more meat to this day's menu. You still have some leeway on caffeinated beverages, sweets, and additional oils and fats, but cut back on these when you can. For example, include a cup of coffee in the morning, additional chocolate chips in the evening, and/or a few extra fat servings, such as regular tortilla chips and regular refried beans instead of low-fat versions.

DAY 5:

Breakfast:
BREAKFAST BURRITO:
  1 8" flour tortilla heated and filled with
  ½ cup scrambled egg substitute and 1 ounce
  grated cheddar cheese, topped with
  2 tablespoons salsa
6 ounces grapefruit juice
2 cups water
A vitamin and mineral supplement

Midmorning Snack:
1 soft, whole wheat pretzel
6 ounces low-fat strawberry-kiwi yogurt mixed with
  1 kiwifruit, chopped
2 cups water

Lunch:
1 cup Vegetable Beef Soup*
1 whole wheat roll
1 cup 1 percent low-fat milk
1 cup water

Midafternoon Snack:
1 mango, cubed and seasoned with 1 tablespoon
  lime juice
1 cup 1 percent low-fat milk

Dinner:
3 ounces baked halibut, seasoned with mustard, salt,
  and dill
½ cup whole wheat pasta topped with ½ cup
  Eggplant Caponata*
1 cup fresh green beans, steamed

2 whole wheat bread sticks

2 cups water

Evening Snack:

1 piece Lemon Chiffon Pie*

Nutritional information:
1,961 calories; 21 percent fat (45.7 grams); 61 percent
carbohydrates; 18 percent protein.

Step 1: Include at least two servings each of the fruits and vegetables; two servings of the milk, yogurt, and cheese; and at least two grains (tortilla, pretzel, wheat roll, pasta, or bread sticks), which should be whole grains. You can add an additional serving of meat at lunch or increase the serving size at dinner, if you desire. You can include caffeinated beverages, sweets, and additional oils and fats, but cut back on these when you can. For example, add coffee or tea at breakfast or a diet cola at lunch, add cookies to the sorbet or a dessert at lunch, and/or add additional servings of fat, such as butter on the roll at lunch, fried rather than baked halibut, butter for the bread sticks, or additional olive oil in preparing the pasta.

Step 2: Include at least three servings each of the fruits and vegetables; two servings of the milk, yogurt, and cheese; and at least three grains (tortilla, pretzel, wheat roll, pasta, or bread sticks), which should be whole grains. You can add an additional serving of meat at lunch or increase the serving size at dinner, if you desire. You still have some leeway on caffeinated beverages, sweets, and additional oils and fats, but cut back on these when you can. For example, add a cup of coffee at breakfast, increase the serving of sorbet, and/or add additional servings of fat (scramble the eggs in butter or oil, use whole-milk yogurt, and/or have extra vegetables with a sour cream dip).

DAY 6:

Breakfast:

2 pancakes, made with low-fat Bisquick, nonfat
   milk, eggs, and 1 tablespoon wheat germ per
   pancake. Topped with:
   2 tablespoons fat-free sour cream
   ¼ cup apricots, canned in own juice and drained
   1 banana, peeled, sliced
1 cup herb tea
2 cups water
A vitamin and mineral supplement

Midmorning Snack:

3 fig bars
1 cup warmed nonfat milk flavored with almond
   extract and sprinkled with nutmeg

Lunch:

1½ cups Vegetable Lentil Soup*
1 piece jalapeño corn bread (2½" × 2½" × 1½" piece)
1 ounce cheddar cheese
1 cup tomato or vegetable juice, seasoned with a
   dash of Tabasco
2 cups water

Midafternoon Snack:

1 fresh nectarine, sliced
3 graham crackers
2 cups water

Dinner:

4 ounces Paprika and Red Pepper Chicken*
1 baked potato, topped with:
   2 teaspoons butter

2 tablespoons fat-free sour cream

1 cup zucchini, sautéed in chicken stock and
   seasoned with thyme, salt, and pepper

1 large tomato, sliced and topped with:
   1 tablespoon fresh basil leaves, chopped
   2 teaspoons olive oil
   2 teaspoons red wine vinegar
   salt and pepper to taste

2 cups water

Evening Snack:

1 fresh peach, peeled, sliced, and sprinkled with
   nutmeg

1 cup 1 percent low-fat milk

Nutritional information:
2,030 calories; 57 grams fat (25 percent); 55 percent
carbohydrates; 20 percent protein.

Step 1: Include at least two servings each of the fruits and vegetables; two servings of the milk and cheese; and at least two grains (pancakes, wheat germ, cornbread, graham crackers), which should be whole grains. You can add an additional serving of meat at lunch or increase the serving size at dinner, if you desire. You can include caffeinated beverages, sweets, and additional oils and fats, but cut back on these when you can. For example, add coffee or tea at breakfast and/or lunch, have dessert instead of peaches after dinner, and/or add extra servings of fat, such as butter on the pancakes, whole milk instead of nonfat milk, fried or sautéed fish instead of broiled fish, and/or more olive oil on the tomato salad at dinner.

Step 2: Include at least three servings each of the fruits and vegetables; two servings of the milk and cheese; and at least three grains (pancakes, wheat germ, corn bread, graham crackers), which should be whole grains. You can add an additional serving of meat at lunch or increase the serving size at dinner, if you desire. You still have some leeway on caffeinated beverages, sweets, and additional oils and fats, but cut back on these when you can. For example, add a cup of coffee at breakfast, a fruited-yogurt for a snack or a dessert at dinner, and/or extra servings of fat, such as regular sour cream instead of fat-free sour cream at breakfast, more butter on the baked potato, or potato chips for a snack.

DAY 7:

Breakfast:
⅔ cup low-fat granola
    topped with 2 tablespoons dried-fruit bits
    ⅔ cup 1 percent low-fat milk
½ cantaloupe
2 cups herb tea
A vitamin and mineral supplement

Midmorning Snack:
6 ounces low-fat vanilla yogurt mixed with:
    1 sliced banana, ½ cup fresh pineapple chunks,
    and 1 teaspoon fresh mint leaves
2 cups water

Lunch:
1 piece Veggie Flat Bread Pizza*
10 baby carrots
KIWI-PEAR SALAD:
    1 kiwi, peeled and sliced
    1 pear, sliced
    1 teaspoon honey
    1 teaspoon lemon zest
2 cups sparkling water

Midafternoon Snack:
2 small bran muffins
½ cup 1 percent low-fat milk
1 cup water

Dinner:

1 serving of Shepherd's Pie*

SAUTÉED MUSHROOMS:

    10 mushrooms, washed and sautéed with:

    1 teaspoon olive oil

    3 garlic cloves, diced

    ¼ cup white wine

    Salt and pepper to taste

Evening Snack:

4 vanilla wafers

½ cup 1 percent low-fat milk

1 cup water

Nutritional information:
2,026 calories; 24 percent fat (54 grams); 63 percent
carbohydrates; 13 percent protein.

Step 1: Include at least two servings each of the fruits and vegetables; two servings of the milk, yogurt, and cheese; and at least two grains (granola, pita bread, muffins, pie crust), which should be whole grains. You can add an additional serving of meat at lunch, if you desire. You can include caffeinated beverages, sweets, and additional oils and fats, but cut back on these when you can. For example, add coffee or tea at breakfast or a diet cola at lunch, have a dessert at lunch or increase the number of cookies in the evening, and/or use 2 percent milk, butter or cream cheese on the muffins, or more olive oil in preparing the mushrooms.

Step 2: Include at least three servings each of the fruits and vegetables; two servings of the milk, yogurt, and cheese; and at least three grains (granola, pita bread, muffins, pie crust), which should be whole grains. You can add an additional serving of meat at lunch, if you desire. You still have some leeway on caffeinated beverages, sweets, and additional oils and fats, but cut back on these when you can. For example, add a cup of coffee at breakfast, have a fruited-yogurt or a decaffeinated soda pop for a snack, and/or add a few more servings of fat to the menu, such as cheese with hummus and pita bread at lunch, or a small serving of ice cream or two small chocolate chip cookies instead of the vanilla wafers.

CHAPTER FOURTEEN

Do You Need Supplements to Feel Good?

Movie stars, politicians, and physicians do it. Athletes, Ph.D.s, and dietitians do it. In fact, according to the Council for Responsible Nutrition (the professional branch of the supplement industry), as many as 50 percent of Americans are popping nutritional supplements—that makes supplements the most popped pills in America. One out of every two nonsupplementers would pop a vitamin pill if they were convinced it would do some good.

Every day at health food stores, grocery stores, pharmacies, and discount department stores people face a wall of vitamin and mineral supplements. A simple decision to take a supplement becomes a nightmare when you try to choose from thousands of powders, pills, potions, capsules, tablets, multiples, single nutrients, and "day packs." How do we know if the $6 to $10 billion worth of supplements sold in this country every year are doing us any good? Would we be just as well, or better off, without them, or would everyone benefit from a daily vitamin pill? Even if supplements are a good idea, how do you know what and how much to take, what to avoid, and how to even read those labels? What's USP, anyway? Is natural better than synthetic? What about time-released and chelated? This chapter will answer all those questions and more. (See "The Most-Asked Questions About Supplements," on pages 322–323.)

The Most-Asked Questions About Supplements

1. *How much should I pay for a supplement?*
You shouldn't pay more than ten dollars a month for any or all of your supplements. You can find quality multiple vitamin and mineral supplements that cost under ten cents a day, or three dollars a month. Add another one to three dollars a month for a good calcium-magnesium supplement, and about the same for an antioxidant or vitamin E capsule.

2. *What do the letters "USP" mean on a supplement label?*
United States Pharmacopeia, or USP, is a nongovernmental standard-setting body. This seal of quality means the supplement should dissolve within the digestive tract, is made from pure ingredients, and contains the amount of nutrients listed on the label. While the USP seal is definitely a plus and is found on supplement brands, such as Essential Balance, not all companies who follow high standards, such as One-A-Day, choose to put this seal on their products.

3. *Are "women's" or "men's" formulas better than just a general multiple?*
Women's nutritional needs are different from men's, so theoretically a special formula would more closely match their needs. But most products are formulated more on marketing than on science, falling far short of optimal and costing much more than well-formulated multiples. You're better off following the guidelines on pages 327–329 than you are selecting a supplement because of its name.

4. *Where's the best place to buy my supplements?*
In terms of quality, it doesn't make much difference. Most supplement companies purchase the raw ingredients from the same national manufacturers, like Hoffman-La Roche or Eastman Chemical Company. You'll probably pay less at a pharmacy or grocery store, because supplements here are less likely to contain expensive frills, such as herbs or bioflavonoids, which more often are found in products at health food stores or through mail order.

5. *Can I trust the claims on the label?*
Usually not. Claims that a product is "complete"; "balanced"; "high potency"; or "specially formulated" or that it contains "extra antioxidants" or is a "multivitamin or multimineral" have little to do with the real formulations. Claims that a supplement will cure, treat, or even prevent any health condition are more hype than fact. Ignore the packaging and go straight to the nutritional information on the back of the label. Again, the USP seal on a label is the only accepted guarantee of quality.

6. *The ingredients list of my supplement contains starch, methylcellulose, FD&C Yellow No. 5* *dye, and other extras. Are any of these harmful and why are they there in the first place?*

Vitamins and minerals are basic ingredients, but an effective supplement is a work of art. Nutrients don't just stick together, so manufacturers use binders, stabilizers, fillers, and other so-called "inert" substances to make a product that not only stays together in the bottle, but flows through the machinery at the manufacturing plant, protects ingredients from rancidity, keeps a pill from sticking to your throat, and makes the tablet or pill a recognizable size. According to David Kropp, manager of regulatory and legal affairs at Pharmavite Corporation, the parent company of NatureMade vitamins, "There are relatively few additives in supplements and most of these inert ingredients, including one of the most common ones, dibasic calcium phosphate, have been used safely in pharmaceuticals for a long time."

Even the ones that on rare occasions cause side effects, such as FD&C Yellow No. 6 dye, lactose, or fructose, are unlikely to be a problem at the minuscule doses found in a supplement. For example, the possibility of an allergic reaction to the refined starch used as a filler is extremely rare; the amount of lactose in a supplement is a few milligrams, but it takes grams of lactose to produce a reaction.

In Search of the Balanced Diet

If there is a first commandment in nutrition, it is, "Thou shalt meet all your nutritional needs from a balanced diet." In essence, you eliminate all nutritional worries if you eat daily at least five to nine fresh fruits and vegetables, six to eleven whole grains, three glasses of low-fat milk, and two servings of extra-lean meat, chicken, fish, or legumes. Sounds reasonable, but there's a catch: finding people who do that. The irony is most of us think we're eating pretty well. In a 1994 Nielsen survey, 78 percent of respondents said they were eating healthier than in the past. A Gallup poll conducted by the American Dietetic Association found that 90 percent of women surveyed said their diets were healthful.

Most of those people must be fooling themselves, at least according to every national nutrition survey. As far back as the 1960s, reports on Americans' eating habits repeatedly show that Americans are eating too much fat and too few fiber-rich fruits, vegetables, whole grains, and legumes. The most recent findings from the U.S. Department of Agriculture's (U.S.D.A.) Continuing Survey of Food Intakes by Individuals (CSFII) show that only one out of every one hundred people meets even minimum standards for dietary adequacy: Only one-third of Americans meet the recommendations for grains (and hardly ever are they whole grain). People average only two to three servings of vegetables, not the more optimal five, and only one and one-half servings of fruit compared to the recommended two to four servings. Three out of every four people consume far too few milk products; many don't consume any at all. No wonder so many of us battle energy and mood problems!

This isn't the first time researchers have exposed our poor eating habits. When scientists at the U.S.D.A. developed the Healthy Eating Index, which ranked dietary intakes on a scale from 0 to 100, they found that most Americans barely passed with a "D" average of 63.9; less than 2 percent of the diets received an "A" rating. According to the National Health and Nutrition Examination Survey (NHANES), which has gathered information on Americans' eating habits for decades, people are more likely to go for doughnuts than whole wheat bagels, soft drinks than nonfat milk, hot dogs than split pea soup, and iceberg lettuce rather than spinach.

So What?

Okay. So most people aren't eating exactly perfectly; but most of us feel pretty healthy, look all right, and have enough energy to get through the day. So we must be getting enough vitamins and minerals, right? Sorry.

"It's possible that people's diets could be nutritionally adequate if they ate really well at every meal; unfortunately, most people aren't doing that," says Walter Willett, M.D., D.P.H., professor of nutrition at Harvard School of Public Health in Boston. Americans haven't been doing that for some time. In the 1980s, the Food and Drug Administration's Total Diet Study found that diets were low in calcium, magnesium, iron, zinc, copper, and manganese, increasing our risks for developing a variety of complaints, from PMS and fatigue to memory loss and sleep problems. Ten years later, Americans' diets weren't any better: The Nationwide Food Consumption Survey in 1992 reported that only 22 percent of adults met even two-thirds of their requirements for fifteen vitamins and minerals, and only 2 percent of diets were both low in fat and nutritionally adequate. Then there's the NHANES data that showed people are consuming as little as one-half their requirements for many essential nutrients; only one out of every ten people consumes optimal amounts of calcium, iron, and zinc. Consumption of other essential nutrients, such as chromium and vitamin K, which are essential in blood-sugar regulation and bone health, is also suspected to be low. Folic acid is of particular concern, since the average woman consumes only half the optimal dose. Low folic acid intakes increase the risk for neural tube defects, cancer, heart disease, depression, and memory loss. According to Dr. Willett, vitamin B$_6$, vitamin D, and vitamin E also are typically low in many people's diets.

Sixty-two Cups of Spinach

In all fairness to those struggling to eat well, even the balanced diet doesn't deliver all that it promises. When nutritionists designed forty-three menus based on the U.S. Dietary Guidelines, most of those diets were low in zinc, vitamin B$_6$, folic acid, and iron. If trained nutrition professionals can't design perfect diets, it's unrealistic to expect the rest of us to do much better! Even the best of "balanced" diets can't realistically provide optimal amounts of certain nutrients. Take, for example:

- Vitamin E: You need at least 100 IU of this vitamin daily to lower your risk for heart disease and possibly improve your immune response. Most people aren't eating eight cups of almonds, three-fourth cup of safflower oil, or sixty-two cups of fresh spinach every day to meet this need.
- Calcium: The latest calcium recommendations for adults are 1,000 to 1,200 milligrams daily, which is easy enough if you drink three to four glasses of milk daily. For those people who don't drink milk, meeting this quota means consuming six ounces of tofu, a can of salmon with the bones, and two cups of black bean soup every day, food intakes that are highly unlikely.
- Folic acid: To reach the daily goal of 400 micrograms, people must double or even triple their current intakes of fruits and vegetables. That means at least two servings of dark green leafy vegetables, such as spinach, romaine lettuce, or kale, a day. But when Gladys Block, Ph.D., at the University of California, Berkeley, analyzed data from three major national surveys, she found that 86 percent of women fail to eat even one dark green leafy vegetable, the best dietary source of folic acid, on any one of four days!
- Vitamin D: You are hard-pressed to meet your need for this essential nutrient if you don't drink four glasses of milk or a bowl or two of fortified cereal (which is just a supplement in food form) every day or

frequently spend time in the sun (without sunscreen lotion). Otherwise, it takes an eight-egg-yolks omelette to meet even minimum amounts of this bone-building nutrient.

The Supplement Controversy

Despite the wealth of research showing that people's diets are anything but "balanced," many nutrition experts still resist recommending supplements. "Many people think they are under a vitamin security blanket because they take supplements; consequently, they are more likely to let their eating habits slide," says JoAnn Hattner, R.D., M.P.H., spokesperson for the American Dietetic Association and clinical nutritionist at Stanford University in Palo Alto, California. But Jeffrey Blumberg, Ph.D., professor of nutrition at the U.S.D.A. Human Nutrition Research Center at Tufts University in Boston, counters by saying there is no evidence that this happens; in fact, just the opposite is true. Compared to nonsupplementers, people who supplement take better care of themselves, eat better, maintain better mental and physical health, and are more health conscious. Preliminary studies show they also might be at lower risk for developing heart disease, cancer, osteoporosis, hypertension, depression, and stress-related problems.

In addition, many studies report that certain vitamins and minerals in amounts greater than current recommendations might help prevent premature aging and age-related disorders, including memory loss, mood swings, cancer, and heart disease. Medication use, illness, and stress also increase nutrient needs to levels difficult to obtain from even the best diet. For example, birth control pills might increase a woman's need for vitamin B_6, while stress raises requirements for magnesium, vitamin C, and zinc. Intense exercise also raises nutrient needs above what normal sedentary people require.

Despite this growing body of research showing that people do not consume even recommended, let alone optimal, levels of certain nutrients, many nutrition advocates in the past considered vitamin and mineral supplements quackery. "Until recently, someone who took supplements was considered suspect," says William Pryor, Ph.D., Boyd professor of chemistry and biochemistry at Louisiana State University. "Solid research supporting increased nutrient requirements has replaced the unscientific testimonials of the past, so people now are coming out of the closet and admitting they take supplements."

Including a balanced supplement with good eating habits could stack the deck in favor of a better mood and clearer mind. Researchers at the University College Swansea in the United Kingdom measured mood in 129 healthy adults, then asked them to take daily multiple-vitamin supplements. As a result, blood levels of vitamins increased within three months, and mood improved within one year of supplementation. Men and women reported that they felt "more agreeable"; the women also felt more composed and generally in better mental health when taking daily supplements.

Supplements + Diet

"The 'balanced diet' is increasingly recognized as narrow-minded. Nutrition and supplements are not an either-or issue, but rather the two enhance each together. You can't always get optimal amounts of all the vitamins and minerals from food, just as pills don't contain everything that food has to offer," recommends Dr. Blumberg. For one thing, supplements can replace the vitamins and minerals, but they never will supply the thousands of other health-enhancing phytochemicals in chin-dribbling strawberries, crunchy carrots, or a crispy sprig of broccoli. Although the research is too new to know if these phytochemicals affect mood, there is evidence that they reduce the risk for developing most chronic diseases, such as cancer and heart disease. Secondly, while a well-chosen supplement can improve some of the nutritional shortcomings of a good diet, it can't compensate for bad dietary habits. "You can't live on French fries and hamburgers, then take a vitamin E supplement and think you're doing fine," says Dr. Blumberg.

In short, the problem is not whether or not some people might benefit from supplements, but rather how do you sift through the supplement quagmire to find a worthy product.

The Guidelines: As Simple as 1, 2, 3

Even if you are following the Feeling Good Diet to the letter, you should consider taking one to three supplements.

1. Take a well-balanced multiple vitamin and mineral supplement. A multiple supplies a balance of nutrients while avoiding secondary deficiencies that result when you take too much of one nutrient and crowd out another. For example, a woman who takes only iron to

prevent anemia might become zinc deficient. A man who supplements his diet with only calcium could increase his risk for developing a magnesium deficiency. Many nutrients work as teams and should be provided as a group in the proper ratio for maximum effectiveness. For example, the B vitamins, including vitamin B_1, vitamin B_2, niacin, pantothenic acid, and biotin, work together to convert food components into energy. Supplementing with only one is unlikely to improve overall mental and emotional health. Finally, if your diet is low in one nutrient, it probably is low in others. Foods provide a mixture of nutrients. A person who avoids meat is at risk for consuming inadequate amounts of iron, zinc, and the B vitamins. You are likely to be low in beta carotene, vitamin C, folic acid, and some trace minerals if you don't consume at least two servings daily of dark green leafy vegetables and two servings of citrus fruits.

Select a broad-range multiple vitamin *and* mineral supplement. Look for one that contains vitamins A, D, and K, all of the B vitamins (vitamins B_1, B_2, B_6, B_{12}, niacin, and folic acid), and the trace minerals (chromium, copper, manganese, selenium, and zinc). Children, teenagers, and women during the childbearing years should take a multiple that contains iron; men and postmenopausal women don't need supplemental iron unless blood tests show they are iron deficient.

Ignore chloride, pantothenic acid, biotin, potassium, choline, and phosphorus, since the diet either already supplies optimal levels of these compounds or supplements contain too little to be useful. Also ignore nickel, iodine, vanadium, and tin, since it's not clear whether they're essential for people. Read the column titled "Daily Value" on the label. Look for a multiple that provides approximately 100 percent, but no more than 300 percent, of the Daily Value for all nutrients provided. You want a "balanced" supplement, not one that supplies 2 percent of one nutrient, 50 percent of another, and 600 percent of another.

2. Take extra calcium and magnesium. Most one-dose multiples don't contain enough of these two minerals, which help prevent the mood swings associated with PMS and improve a person's ability to cope with stress, not to mention lowering risk for developing osteoporosis, heart disease, hypertension, and colon cancer. Unless you con-

sume at least three servings daily of low-fat milk products or other calcium-rich foods and lots of magnesium-rich soybeans, nuts, bananas, dark green leafy vegetables, and wheat germ, you might consider an extra supplement of these two minerals. The best ratio for calcium and magnesium is 2:1. Find a supplement that provides at least 100 milligrams of magnesium for every 200 milligrams of calcium, with a maximum intake of 500 milligrams of magnesium and 1,000 milligrams of calcium.

3. Take extra antioxidants. If your multiple doesn't contain ample amounts of one or more antioxidants, especially vitamin C or vitamin E, consider taking a third supplement that supplies between 250 and 1,000 milligrams of vitamin C and/or between 100 and 400 IU of vitamin E. Beta carotene also is a potent antioxidant. If you don't consume several deep orange or green vegetables every day, consider taking a supplement that contains between 10 and 30 milligrams of beta carotene. A mixture of carotenoids is even better, if you can find a supplement that contains them. Smokers should consult their physicians before supplementing with beta carotene.

When's the best time of day to take a supplement? The time of day is not as important as what you take them with. Most nutrients are best absorbed when taken with meals. Nutrients are best absorbed when taken in small doses throughout the day. For example, the body absorbs only about 100 milligrams of magnesium at one time. Doses greater than this are likely to be excreted. Multidose multiples also provide flexibility: You can reduce the number of tablets on days when your diet is optimal and increase the number of tablets on days when you didn't have time to eat right. But the inconvenience of taking divided doses might make a one-pill-a-day product more appealing. For maximum absorption, take a multiple with iron at a different meal than your calcium supplement, since these two minerals compete for absorption. (See Table 14.1, "What to Look For: A Sample Supplement Program," on page 331.)

Avoid the Glitz

Although the debates continue over what is best, when it comes to supplements, your best bet usually is to stick with the basics and avoid the glitz. Here's a crash course on label lingo.

Time-released vitamins: Theoretically, these supplements should raise and maintain blood levels of a vitamin better than regular supplements. In reality, most time-released tablets dissolve too slowly to be completely absorbed. Time-released forms of niacin are well absorbed, but might be more toxic to the liver than a similar amount of a non–time-released brand; you should be monitored by a physician if you are taking large doses of niacin to lower blood cholesterol.

Chelated minerals: A chelated mineral is chemically bound to another substance, usually an amino acid (the building blocks of protein). Examples include iron/amino chelate or chromium proteinate. Although manufacturers propose that chelation improves the absorption of a mineral, there is little proof that chelated minerals are any better absorbed than other supplements.

Synthetic versus natural nutrients: The terms "organic" and "natural" might have a wholesome aura, but in reality these products are more likely to tax your pocketbook than improve your health. In most cases, the body cannot distinguish a natural from a synthetic nutrient. In addition, many products labeled as natural are actually synthetic vitamins mixed with small amounts of "natural" vitamins. For example, a natural vitamin C supplement contains mostly laboratory-made ascorbic acid with a small amount of vitamin C from rose hips or acerola berries.

Selenium, chromium, and vitamin E are exceptions to the rule. The "organic" forms of the trace minerals selenium and chromium are called selenium-rich yeast or L-selenomethionine and chromium-rich yeast, chromium nicotinate, or chromium picolinate. They are better absorbed and used by the body than the synthetic sodium selenite and chromic chloride and, therefore, are your best bets. Body tissues prefer the "natural" form of vitamin E, called d-alpha-tocopherol, to the synthetic counterpart, called dl-alpha- or all-rac-alpha-tocopherol. In these three cases, a slightly more expensive "natural" source of the nutrient might be your best bet.

In short, supplements support and reinforce the Feeling Good Diet, but they can't replace it. They cannot grant immunity to disease for a body that is otherwise unhealthy. Supplements are just that: They supplement a good diet and provide a safe and convenient form of nutritional insurance that fills in the gaps when eating habits fall short of perfect. (See Table 14.2, "Fifteen Essential Nutrients You Can't Do Without," on pages 332–335.)

Table 14.1   What to Look For: A Sample Supplement Program

Put together your own supplement program, based on the following optimal intakes. You should be able to meet these needs by taking two to four tablets (a multiple, antioxidants, and calcium, magnesium, or calcium-magnesium tablets) daily with meals.

	OPTIMAL AMOUNT	% OF DAILY VALUE
Vitamin A (retinol)	2,500 IU	50
Beta carotene	15 milligrams	*/**
Vitamin D	400 IU	100*
Vitamin E (d-alpha tocopherol)	200 IU	600*
Vitamin B_1 (thiamin)	1.5 milligrams	100
Vitamin B_2 (riboflavin)	1.7 milligrams	100
Niacin (niacinamide)	20 milligrams	100
Vitamin B_6 (pyridoxine)*	2 milligrams	100*
Vitamin B_{12} (cobalamine)*	6 micrograms	100*
Folic acid (folacin)	400 micrograms	100
Pantothenic acid	10 milligrams	100
Vitamin C	250 to 1,000 milligrams	400+
Calcium (calcium carbonate)	1,000 milligrams	100
Chromium (chromium-rich yeast, picolinate, or nicotinate)	200 micrograms	**
Copper	2 milligrams	100
Iron (ferrous fumarate)#	18 milligrams	100
Magnesium (magnesium citrate)	500 milligrams	125
Manganese	5 milligrams	**
Molybdenum	75–250 micrograms	**
Selenium (L-selenomethionine)	200 micrograms	**
Zinc	15 milligrams	100

* Requirements for these nutrients increase above these amounts with age and during mental or emotional stress.

** No Daily Value has been established for these nutrients. The amounts listed are based on the Food and Nutrition Board's Safe and Adequate daily amounts.

Iron supplements are recommended only for women during the childbearing years. Men and postmenopausal women should take iron supplements only with approval from their physicians.

Table 14.2   Fifteen Essential Nutrients You Can't Do Without

Here's a brief glance at some of the nutrients needed for health, and what you should look for when choosing a supplement.

Nutrient: Vitamin A/Beta carotene
How Much? The Daily Value of 5,000 IU for vitamin A is a safe dose, especially for women who might become or are pregnant; higher amounts might cause birth defects in fetuses. Better yet, choose beta carotene, which is relatively nontoxic at doses of 10 to 30 milligrams, and can be converted to vitamin A in the body. Smokers should consult their physicians before supplementing with beta carotene, since one preliminary study concluded that beta carotene supplements might increase lung cancer risk in people who are heavy smokers.
What Should You Look For? A mixture of vitamin A and beta carotene. Most forms of vitamin A, such as retinyl palmitate or acetate, are well absorbed.
Why Do You Need It? Strengthens immunity; maintains healthy epithelial tissues, such as skin, mucous membranes, urinary tract, and the lungs; aids in bone and tooth formation; and maintains normal vision.

Nutrient: Vitamin D
How Much? The Daily Value of 400 IU is a safe dose. Only seniors might need more than this (600 IU to 800 IU).
What Should You Look For? Vitamin D or cholecalciferol.
Why Do You Need It? Aids in calcium absorption and deposition into bones. Might help lower the risk for colon cancer and depression.

Nutrient: Vitamin K
How Much? The RDA* is 65 micrograms, but you're lucky if you find 25 micrograms in most multiples.
What Should You Look For? Usually listed as vitamin K, vitamin K_1, or phylloquinone.
Why Do You Need It? Essential for normal blood clotting and helps maintain strong bones, thus aiding in the prevention of osteoporosis.

Nutrient: Folic acid
How Much? The Daily Value is 400 micrograms (or 0.4 milligram). Don't take more than 800 micrograms without physician approval.
What Should You Look For? Folic acid or folate.

---

* The Recommended Dietary Allowance (RDA) is used here when no Daily Value has been established. These values won't appear on labels.

Why Do You Need It? Aids in the growth and development of all normal cells, prevents anemia and birth defects, and possibly helps reduce the risk for heart disease, colon or cervical cancer, depression, mood swings, fatigue, and memory problems.

Nutrient: Vitamin C
How Much? The RDA is 60 milligrams. You might need up to 250 milligrams to saturate your body's tissues. To reduce the severity and duration of a cold, you might need closer to 1,000 milligrams.
What Should You Look For? Vitamin C, ascorbic acid, or calcium ascorbate.
Why Do You Need It? Maintains connective tissue, promotes wound healing, helps manufacture nerve chemicals such as dopamine, strengthens the immune response, and, as an antioxidant, prevents damage to tissues, possibly strengthening the body's defenses against cancer, heart disease, cataracts, memory loss, and stress-related diseases.

Nutrient: Vitamin E
How Much? The Daily Value is 30 IU, but doses of 100 IU to 400 IU are safe and possibly beneficial. Few multiples contain this much, so a separate supplement is worth considering.
What Should You Look For? D-alpha tocopherol is the natural form of vitamin E and appears to be slightly better used by the body than the synthetic dl-alpha tocopherol; however, the extra cost might not be worth the minor benefit.
Why Do You Need It? It is an antioxidant that protects tissues from damage, possibly lowering the risk of developing heart disease, cancer, and stress-related disorders. Also strengthens the immune system and protects nerve and brain tissue from free-radical damage.

Nutrient: Vitamin B_6
How Much: The Daily Value is 2 milligrams. Women on birth control pills and people as they age or who are under stress might need slightly higher amounts. However, doses in excess of 200 milligrams might cause neurological problems.
What Should You Look For? Vitamin B_6 or pyridoxine hydrochloride (HCl).
Why Do You Need It? Aids in the manufacture of all body proteins, including hormones; hormonelike compounds called prostaglandins that regulate blood pressure; enzymes; nerve chemicals such as serotonin; and hemoglobin in red blood cells. Also aids in muscle contraction and heart function, mental function, and fends off depression, insomnia, and seasonal affective disorder (SAD).

Nutrient: Vitamin B_{12}
How Much? The Daily Value is 6 micrograms. People as they age or who are under stress might need slightly higher amounts.
What Should You Look For? Vitamin B_{12} or cobalamin.

Why Do You Need It? Prevents anemia and maintains nerve function, normal cognition, and neurotransmitter production. Helps prevent insomnia and depression, and increase mental function.

Nutrient: Boron
How Much? No Recommended Dietary Allowance (RDA) or Daily Value has been set for boron. Typical daily intakes range from 0.5 to 7.0 milligrams, and studies showing a health benefit often use 3 milligrams daily.
What Should You Look For? Boron, sodium borate.
Why Do You Need It? Boron probably helps prevent bone loss associated with osteoporosis, and might help maintain mental function, hand-eye coordination, attention span, and memory.

Nutrient: Calcium
How Much? The Daily Value is 1,000 milligrams. No one-tablet-daily multiple contains this much, so you might consider taking a separate supplement, such as a combination calcium and magnesium. The safe Upper Limit (UL) is 2,500 milligrams.
What Should You Look For? Most forms of calcium are well absorbed. Calcium carbonate and calcium citrate contain the most calcium per tablet. Calcium gluconate or lactate contain less calcium, so more tablets must be taken. "Natural" calcium from oyster shell, bonemeal, or dolomite might contain lead.
Why Do You Need It? Reduces the risk of osteoporosis and possibly colon cancer. Aids in blood clotting, blood pressure regulation, muscle contraction, and nerve transmission, and might prevent depression, premenstrual syndrome (PMS), and insomnia.

Nutrient: Chromium
How Much? The Safe and Adequate Range* is 50 to 200 micrograms. There's no evidence that amounts greater than this are of any health benefit, except possibly during times of stress or for people with diabetes.
What Should You Look For? Chromium nicotinate, chromium-rich yeast, or chromium picolinate appear to be absorbed better than chromium chloride.
Why Do You Need It? Aids in blood sugar regulation.

Nutrient: Copper
How Much? The Daily Value is 2 milligrams.
What Should You Look For? Copper gluconate, oxide, or sulfate, or cupric oxide.
Why Do You Need It? Aids in nerve transmission and brain function, heart function, red blood cell formation, and normal hair and skin color. Helps protect cells from damage, and assists in blood sugar regulation.

* No RDA has been established for this mineral, only a range of intakes considered both safe and probably adequate. These values won't appear on labels.

Nutrient: Iron

How Much? The Daily Value is 18 milligrams, which is a safe amount for premenopausal women. Postmenopausal women and men should not take supplemental iron or should limit intake to 10 milligrams.

What Should You Look For? Iron is best absorbed in the "ferrous" form, such as ferrous fumarate or ferrous sulfate.

Why Do You Need It? To replace iron losses from menstruation and to prevent fatigue, improve exercise and cognitive performance, strengthen immunity, and help prevent depression, PMS, and sleep problems.

Nutrient: Magnesium

How Much? The Daily Value is 400 milligrams. No one-tablet-daily multiple contains this much, so you might consider taking a separate supplement, such as a combination calcium and magnesium. Doses of 600 milligrams or more might cause diarrhea.

What Should You Look For? Magnesium oxide, citrate, or hydroxide.

Why Do You Need It? Aids in muscle relaxation, heart function, nerve transmission, blood pressure regulation, and bone formation and maintenance. Helps prevent depression, insomnia, PMS, and effects of stress.

Nutrient: Selenium

How Much? The RDA* is 55 micrograms for women, and 70 micrograms for men. Don't take more than 200 micrograms, since this mineral can be toxic.

What Should You Look For? Selenomethionine or selenium-rich yeast are possibly better absorbed than sodium selenate or selenite.

Why Do You Need It? As an antioxidant, selenium might reduce the risk for developing heart disease, depression, rheumatoid arthritis, and the tissue damage associated with the development of cancer.

Nutrient: Zinc

How Much? The Daily Value is 15 milligrams. Doses greater than 50 milligrams might suppress immune function.

What Should You Look For? Zinc gluconate, picolinate, oxide, or sulfate.

Why Do You Need It? Aids in wound healing and in the immune system; reducing the effects of depression, PMS, stress, and eating disorders such as anorexia; the prevention of birth defects; and possibly maintaining strong bones.

---

* The Recommended Dietary Allowance (RDA) is used here when no Daily Value has been established. These values won't appear on labels.

Appendix:
Food Groups and Servings Sizes in the
Feeling Good Diet

The following are groups of foods, based on their calorie and nutrient content. This is only a sampling of foods, but provides structure and specific examples when you first begin adapting your eating style to the Feeling Good Diet. As you become more comfortable with the dietary guidelines, branch out from these food groupings to include other favorite foods.

Fruit

Each fruit and its amount stated below is equivalent to one serving of fruit in the Feeling Good Diet. Each serving provides approximately 100 calories and 25 grams of carbohydrates. These foods, in general, also are excellent sources of vitamin C, beta carotene, trace minerals, phytochemicals, and fiber. The dark orange varieties are especially good sources of beta carotene, while orange juice also is a good source of the B vitamin folic acid. Consume at least one serving daily of the vitamin C–rich fruits marked with an *.

ITEM	SELECTION SIZE
Apple	1 small
Applesauce	¾ cup
Apricots	6 fresh

ITEM	SELECTION SIZE
Apricots, canned, without syrup	6 halves
Banana	One 6-inch, medium
Berries:	
Blackberries	1¼ cup
Blueberries	1¼ cup
Boysenberries	1½ cup
Raspberries	1½ cup
*Strawberries	2 cups
*Cantaloupe	2 cups
Casaba melon	2 cups
Cherries	20 large
Dates	4 medium
Figs	2 dried
Fruit cocktail, canned, without syrup	¾ cup
Fruit Roll-Ups	2 rolls
Fruit salad, fresh	¾ cup
*Grapefruit	1 medium
Grapes	1 cup
*Kiwi	2 small
Kumquats, raw	8 medium
*Honeydew melon	½ medium or 2 slices
Juices:	
apple cider	¾ cup
apple juice	1 cup
apricot nectar	¾ cup
*grapefruit	1 cup
grape	¾ cup
*orange	1 cup
papaya nectar	6 ounces
peach nectar	6 ounces
pear nectar	⅔ cup
pineapple juice	1 cup
prune	½ cup

ITEM	SELECTION SIZE
*Mandarin oranges, juice-packed	1 cup
Nectarine	1 large
*Orange	1 large
*Papaya	1 medium
Peach	2 medium
Peaches, canned, without syrup	¾ cup
Pear	1 large
Pears, canned, without syrup	3 halves
Pineapple	1 cup packed
Pineapple chunks	¾ cup
Plum	3
Pomegranate, raw	1 medium
Prunes	5 medium
Quince, raw	2 medium
Raisins	3 tablespoons
*Tangerine	2 large
Watermelon	2 cups

Vegetables

Each vegetable and its amount listed below is equivalent to one serving in the Feeling Good Diet. One serving provides approximately 50 calories, 10 grams of carbohydrates, and 4 grams of protein. These foods also are excellent sources of the antioxidant nutrients (i.e., beta carotene and vitamin C), other vitamins, minerals, phytochemicals, and fiber. Dark green leafy vegetables are particularly rich sources of beta carotene and the B vitamin folic acid. (One serving is equivalent to 1 cup cooked, 2 cups raw, or the amount listed.) Consume daily a minimum of one (preferably at least two) servings of the beta carotene–rich vegetables marked with an *.

ITEM	SELECTION SIZE
Artichoke	1
Artichoke hearts, water-packed	
*Asparagus	
Bean sprouts	1½ cups
Beans, green	
Beets	
*Broccoli	
Brussels sprouts	
Cabbage, raw	3 cups
cooked	1½ cups
*Carrots, whole	1½ large or 2 medium
*Carrot juice	½ cup
Cauliflower, cooked	1½ cups
*Chard, cooked	1½ cups
*Collards, cooked	1½ cups
*Dandelion greens, cooked	1½ cups
Eggplant	
*Kale	
Leeks	
*Mustard greens, cooked	1½ cups
Okra	¾ cup
Onions, raw	¾ cup
cooked	⅔ cup
Parsnips, cooked	⅓ cup
Pea pods	¾ cup
Peas, green, cooked	½ cup
Rhubarb, frozen, raw	2 cups
Rutabaga	
Tomato	2 medium
Tomato juice	1 cup
Tomato paste	4 tablespoons
Tomato sauce	⅔ cup
*Turnip greens, cooked	2 cups
V8 juice	1 cup

Grains and Starchy Vegetables

Each bread, cereal, starchy vegetable, rice, and pasta and its amount stated below is equal to one serving in the Feeling Good Diet and provides approximately 75 calories, 15 grams of carbohydrates, and 3 grams of protein. The whole-grain selections also are good sources of trace minerals, vitamins, phytochemicals, and fiber, while the starchy vegetables, such as the sweet potato or baked potato, are sources of either beta carotene or vitamin C.

ITEM	SELECTION SIZE
Bagel	½ medium
Bread: whole wheat, rye, white	1 slice
Cereal, cooked: oatmeal, barley, farina	½ cup
Cereal, cold:	
Grape-Nuts	⅓ cup
shredded wheat	1 large biscuit or ½ cup of bite-sized biscuits
puffed	½ cup
Cheerios or cornflakes	¾ cup
Corn kernels	½ cup
Corn-on-the-cob	½ a cob
Crackers:	
Ry Krisp	4
graham	3 2½-inch square
saltines	6
Dinner roll	1 small
English muffin	½
Flour	2½ tablespoons
Hamburger bun	½
Hot dog bun	½
Noodles or pasta	½ cup
Lima beans	½ cup
Pita bread	½
Popcorn, plain, air-popped	2 cups

ITEM	SELECTION SIZE
Potato:	
boiled/baked	1 small
mashed, plain	⅓ cup
Pumpkin	1½ cups
Pretzels:	
thin sticks	40
three-ring style	3
Rice	⅓ cup
Rice cakes	2 large (9 grams each)
Squash: acorn, butternut, hubbard, winter	¾ cup
Succotash	⅓ cup
Sweet potato, plain	½ cup
Tortilla, corn (not fried)	1, 6 inches across
Wheat germ	3 tablespoons
Yam, plain	½ cup

The following breads and cereals contain some fat. Reduce your intake of fat from other sources if one or more of these foods is included in your Feeling Good Diet plan. (Each serving contains approximately 1 teaspoon of fat.)

Bread stuffing	¼ cup
Corn bread	One 2-inch square
Crackers:	
Wheat Thins	15
Pancake	2
Taco shell, corn	2
Waffle	4 ½-inch square
Tortilla, flour	One, 8 inches across

Milk Products

Each food listed below is equal to one serving of a calcium-rich milk product in the Feeling Good Diet and provides approximately 100 calories, 15 grams of carbohydrates, and 9 grams of protein. These foods, in general, also are excellent sources of magnesium, vitamin B_2, and other vitamins and minerals. Fortified milk is the only reliable dietary source of vitamin D.

ITEM	SELECTION SIZE
Buttermilk, made from nonfat milk	1 cup
Evaporated nonfat milk	½ cup
Powdered nonfat milk	⅓ cup
Nonfat yogurt	¾ cup
Nonfat milk	1 cup

The following milk products also contain approximately 1 teaspoon of fat and an additional 45 calories per serving. Cut back on fatty foods if you choose one of these selections.

Calcimilk (lactose-reduced low-fat milk)	1 cup
Cottage cheese, low-fat 2%	¾ cup
Lactaid (lactose-reduced low-fat milk)	1 cup
Low-fat milk, 2%	1 cup
Low-fat yogurt, 2%	1 cup
Soymilk (calcium-fortified)	1 cup

The following milk products contain just shy of 2 teaspoons of fat and an additional 60 calories, for a total of 160 calories per serving. Cut back even further on fatty foods if you choose one of these selections.

Canned or evaporated milk	½ cup
Cheese:	
cottage cheese, creamed	¾ cup
grated Parmesan	⅓ cup
low-fat cheeses with less than 150 calories per 2-ounce serving	⅓ cup

Goat milk	1 cup
Whole milk, 3.5%	1 cup
Yogurt, whole, plain	1 cup

Meat and Legumes

The following meats (or the equivalent amount in legumes or eggs) cooked without fat or oil are equal to one serving in the Feeling Good Diet and provide approximately 150 calories, 21 grams of protein, and two teaspoons or less of fat. These foods also are excellent sources of trace minerals, such as iron and zinc, and the B vitamins.

ITEM	SELECTION SIZE
Cooked dried beans and peas	1½ cups
Beef—chipped beef, flank steak, London broil, round steak, stew meat, tenderloin, filet mignon, top round roast	3 ounces
Veal—chop, steak, roast	3 ounces
Pork—boiled ham, Canadian bacon (high in salt), tenderloin	3 ounces
Poultry—chicken without skin, Cornish game hen, pheasant, quail, turkey without skin	3 ounces
Fish—bass, catfish, flounder, halibut, red snapper, sole, turbot	4 ounces
Cod	5 ounces
Shellfish—clams, crabs, shrimp	4 ounces
Scallops	5 ounces
Tuna, canned in water	4 ounces

ITEM	SELECTION SIZE
Turkey luncheon meat (95% fat-free)	5 slices
Eggs (high in cholesterol)	2
Egg substitute	⅓ cup

Nutritious Fatty Foods

Each of the following foods is a good source of two or more nutrients, but comes with a high-fat price tag. Each serving provides approximately 100 calories and between 1½ and 2 teaspoons of fat. Ideally, these foods should be limited to no more than two selections per day.

ITEM	SELECTION SIZE
Avocado	¼
Beef—ground beef, sirloin steak, porterhouse, rib roast, ribs, T-bone steak	1 ounce
Cheeses—full-fat hard cheeses, including American, Cheddar, Brie, feta, Gouda, Swiss	1 ounce
Ice cream	⅓ cup
Lamb—breast, crown roast, chop, shoulder, rib roast	1 ounce
Luncheon meats—bologna, hot dogs, turkey hot dogs, Italian sausage, salami, Spam	1 ounce
Nuts:	
almonds	2 tablespoons
Brazil, medium	5 teaspoons
cashews, medium	2 tablespoons
filberts	2 tablespoons

ITEM	SELECTION SIZE
macadamias, medium	6
peanuts, large	2 tablespoons
peanuts, Spanish	2 tablespoons
pecans, large	8 halves
pistachios	2 tablespoons
walnuts	8 halves
Peanut butter	1 level tablespoon
Pork—ribs, spareribs, drained sausage, steak	1 ounce
Seeds:	
pumpkin seeds	⅓ cup
sesame seeds	2 tablespoons
sunflower seeds	2 tablespoons

Fats and Oils

The following servings of fats in the Feeling Good Diet provide approximately 100 calories and 2 or more teaspoons (10+ grams) of fat. These foods should be kept to a minimum when planning menus, preparing food, and when ordering foods in restaurants.

ITEM	SELECTION SIZE
Bacon	2 strips
Butter	1 tablespoon
Chocolate, unsweetened	⅔ square or ⅔ ounce
Coconut	½ ounce
Coffee whitener:	
liquid	½ cup
powder	8 teaspoons
Cream cheese	2 tablespoons
Cream, heavy	2 tablespoons
Cream, sour	3 tablespoons

Margarine:
   regular   1 tablespoon
   diet   4 teaspoons
Mayonnaise   1 tablespoon
Oil   2 teaspoons
Olives, black   20
Salad dressing:
   low-calorie   varies, check label
   regular   2 tablespoons
Tartar sauce   4 teaspoons

Guiltless Desserts

Desserts add pleasure and fun to the day's menu and, when chosen from the following selections, can even be low-fat and nutritious. Each of the following guiltless desserts and "sweets" provides approximately 100 calories with no fat. Serving sizes are moderate to limit sugar intake. Fruits also make excellent desserts.

ITEM	SELECTION SIZE
Cake (no frosting):	
angel food	2-inch slice
sponge	2-inch slice
Cookies:	
animal crackers	20
vanilla wafers	5
Fruit ice	½ cup
Gelatin, fruit-flavored	⅔ cup
Honey	1½ tablespoons
Jam or jelly	2 tablespoons
Molasses	2 tablespoons
Sherbet	⅓ cup
Sugar: brown or table	2 tablespoons
Syrup: corn or maple	2 tablespoons

Freebies

The following foods contain negligible calories and can be included in the diet without affecting the calorie content, while still providing small amounts of vitamins, minerals, and fiber.

Celery

Cucumbers

Endive

Green onions

Lettuce

Mushrooms

Parsley

Peppers—green, red, or chili

Radishes

Spinach

Summer squash

Zucchini

Catsup (limit to 1 tablespoon a day)

Club soda

Decaffeinated coffee

Gelatin, unflavored, plain

Herbs and spices

Lemon juice

Mustard

～ Recipes for Feeling Your Best ～

BEVERAGES

1. The Zinger Smoothie

Ingredients:

4 apricot halves, canned and drained

1/2 cup nonfat plain yogurt

1/2 cup fresh orange juice

1/4 cup toasted wheat germ

1/2 banana

Dash of nutmeg

Directions:

Place all ingredients in blender and blend until smooth. Pour into glass and sprinkle with nutmeg.

Makes one 15-ounce serving.

Nutritional information per serving:
337 calories; 10 percent fat (3.8 grams); 71 percent
carbohydrates; 19 percent protein; 5.7 grams fiber.

2. The PMS Smoothie

Ingredients:

4 dried apricots, soaked in 1/2 cup
        apple juice

1/2 cup nonfat milk

2 tablespoons orange juice
        concentrate

1 banana

2 kiwifruits, peeled

3 tablespoons wheat germ

Ice (optional)

Directions:

Remove apricots from juice. Combine all ingredients in a blender and blend for 3 minutes or until thoroughly mixed.

Makes two 8-ounce servings.

Nutritional information per serving:
205 calories; 8 percent fat (1.9 grams); 79 percent
carbohydrates; 13 percent protein; 5.7 grams fiber.

3. Brain Teaser

Ingredients:

4 carrots, peeled

1 medium apple, quartered and
    seeded

1 tablespoon fresh ginger, sliced

1/2 red pepper, seeded

Dash of Tabasco sauce

Lemon zest

Directions:

Juice all ingredients in a juicer. Pour into tall glass and top with lemon zest.

Makes one 16-ounce serving or two 8-ounce servings.

Nutritional information for the 16-ounce serving:
220 calories; 4 percent fat (.2 grams); 89 percent
carbohydrates; 6 percent protein; 6 grams fiber.

4. Pumpkin Pie Smoothie

Ingredients:

2 cups fat-free vanilla frozen yogurt

3/4 cup canned pumpkin

3/4 cup nonfat milk

1/2 teaspoon pumpkin pie spice

Directions:

Place all ingredients in blender, cover, and blend on high until well blended.

Makes 3 servings.

Nutritional information per serving:
169 calories; 2.5 percent fat (.484 grams); 76 percent
carbohydrates; 21 percent protein; 1.7 grams fiber.

5. Gazpacho Smoothie Over Ice

This vegetable drink has body, since the vegetables are blended, not juiced.
It also keeps in the refrigerator for up to twenty-four hours.

Ingredients:

One 14¹/2-ounce can plum
   tomatoes, drained

1 cup cucumber, peeled and diced

¹/4 cup roasted red peppers

¹/4 cup green onion, sliced

1 cup orange juice

¹/4 teaspoon hot pepper sauce

Directions:

Combine all ingredients in a blender, cover, and puree until smooth. Pour gazpacho over ice in tall glasses. Garnish with a celery stalk.

Makes 3 servings (approximately 1 cup each).

Nutritional information per serving:
70 calories; 6 percent fat (.5 grams); 83 percent
carbohydrates; 11 percent protein; 2.3 grams fiber.

APPETIZERS, SNACKS, AND QUICK FIXES

1. Cranberry-Orange Relish

Ingredients:

One 12-ounce bag fresh cranberries

1¹/2 cups orange juice

1 cup sugar

2 tablespoons fresh ginger, peeled
   and finely chopped

Directions:

Combine all ingredients in heavy, large saucepan. Bring to boil over high heat, stirring until sugar dissolves. Reduce heat to a low simmer until relish is thick, stirring often and mashing berries slightly (about 15 minutes). Transfer relish to small bowl. Cover and chill. (Can be prepared up to 1 month ahead. Keep refrigerated.)

Makes 3 cups or twelve ¼-cup servings.

Nutritional information per serving:
93 calories; 1 percent fat (.126 grams); 98 percent
carbohydrates; 1 percent protein; 1.27 grams fiber.

2. *Veggie Flat Bread Pizzas*

This flavorful snack is a garlic-lover's dream. The vegetable mixture also is good packed into pocket bread as a sandwich.

Ingredients:

Two 6-inch diameter whole wheat
  pita breads, cut horizontally
  in half
2 teaspoons olive oil
1 tablespoon minced garlic (about
  3 large cloves)
1 tablespoon balsamic vinegar

2 large tomatoes, chopped
2 cups fresh spinach, washed,
  stemmed, and chopped
1 cup red onion, thinly sliced
1/2 teaspoon red pepper flakes
1 teaspoon dried oregano
1 teaspoon dried basil
1/3 cup feta cheese, crumbled

Directions:

Preheat oven to 450 degrees Fahrenheit. Place 4 bread halves on baking sheets and bake until crisp and slightly brown, about 4 minutes. Cool.

Combine oil, garlic, vinegar, tomatoes, spinach, onion, and seasonings in a large bowl. Stir until thoroughly mixed.

Divide vegetable mixture evenly and heap onto bread halves. Sprinkle with feta cheese and bake for 5 minutes. Cut into wedges and serve.
Makes 8 servings.

Nutritional information per serving:
91 calories; 36 percent fat (3.6 grams); 48 percent
carbohydrates; 16 percent protein; 2.4 grams fiber.

3. *Savory Cilantro Dip with Baked Tortilla Chips*

Ingredients:

1 8-ounce container of fat-free sour
  cream (Choose a firm brand;
  otherwise, dip is runny.)
1/4 cup nonfat mayonnaise
1/2 cup fresh cilantro, chopped
1 tablespoon honey

1/2 teaspoon cumin
1/4 teaspoon red pepper flakes
2 tablespoons fresh lime juice
1/2 cup salsa
12 corn tortillas
Salt, cayenne, or garlic powder

Directions:

DIP:

In a medium bowl, combine first 7 ingredients; mix well. Cover and refrigerate 1 to 2 hours or overnight. When ready to serve, pour ½ cup salsa over dip. Serve with chips, or a few veggies!

CHIPS:

Preheat oven to 375 degrees Fahrenheit. Stack tortillas and cut in half, then into thirds. Place wedges on ungreased cookie sheets and sprinkle with salt, cayenne, or garlic powder, as desired. Bake about 10 minutes, or until wedges are crisp.

Makes 6 dozen chips. Serves 8.

Nutritional information per serving:
135 calories; 7 percent fat (1.1 grams); 80 percent
carbohydrates; 13 percent protein; 2.5 grams fiber.

4. Baked Apples

These spicy apples taste great warm from the oven, or let them cool, slice them into 1-inch slices, and serve as a sweet snack.

Ingredients:

½ cup raisins or dried cranberries

¼ cup brown sugar

½ teaspoon cinnamon

½ teaspoon nutmeg

Pinch of cardamom

6 medium red cooking apples, cored with top half peeled

2 tablespoons reduced-fat margarine

½ cup apple juice concentrate mixed in ½ cup water

Directions:

Preheat oven to 350 degrees Fahrenheit. Combine raisins and next four ingredients; stir. Spoon raisin mixture evenly into cavity of each apple. Place apples in a baking dish. Top each apple with 1 teaspoon margarine. Pour apple juice over apples, cover, and bake for 50 minutes or until apples are tender (cooking time will vary with type of apple). Baste with juice occasionally.

Makes 6 servings.

Nutritional information per serving:
244 calories; 9 percent fat (2.6 grams); 89 percent
carbohydrates; 2 percent protein; 5.2 grams fiber.

5. Black Bean and Cheese Roll-Ups

These tasty burritos can be eaten as a snack, or cut into 1-inch rounds and served as appetizers along with the Savory Cilantro Dip (see recipe on page 351).

Ingredients:

One 16-ounce can black beans, drained

One 4-ounce can chopped green chilies

2 tablespoons salsa

6 teaspoons fat-free sour cream

4 tablespoons fresh cilantro, chopped

6 tablespoons low-fat Monterey jack cheese

Six 10-inch whole wheat or chili tortillas

Directions:

In a medium bowl, combine beans, chilies, and salsa. Add sour cream, cilantro, and cheese. Evenly divide mixture and spread evenly on each tortilla to within 2 inches of edges. Tuck in one end and tightly roll each tortilla. Tightly wrap each roll-up in plastic wrap and refrigerate until ready to eat.

Makes 6 roll-ups.

Nutritional information per 1 roll-up:
301 calories; 17 percent fat (5.6 grams); 65 percent
carbohydrates; 18 percent protein; 5.9 grams fiber.

SALADS

1. Southwest Couscous Salad

Ingredients:

2 cups canned low-salt chicken broth

1/4 teaspoon salt

1 1/4 cup couscous

1/2 teaspoon cumin

1/4 cup orange juice

1/3 cup red wine vinegar

2 tablespoons olive oil

1 teaspoon grated orange rind

1 1/2 cups shredded cooked chicken

2 green onions, sliced

1/4 cup minced fresh cilantro

1 medium tomato, diced

Directions:

In a medium saucepan, bring chicken broth and salt to a boil. Stir in couscous and remove from heat. Cover and let stand 5 minutes. Fluff with fork and cool slightly.

In a large bowl, combine cumin, orange juice, vinegar, oil, and orange rind. Mix in couscous. Refrigerate until well chilled. Add chicken, green onions, cilantro, and tomato and stir until thoroughly mixed.

Makes 5 to 6 servings (1 generous cup each).

Nutritional information per serving:
214 calories; 29 percent fat (6.8 grams); 43 percent
carbohydrates; 28 percent protein; 2.75 grams fiber.

2. Wild Greens Topped with Pears, Blue Cheese, and Walnuts

Ingredients:

2 fresh pears, peeled and chopped
    into 1/2-inch pieces

One 16-ounce bag of prewashed
    continental salad blend or fresh
    salad mix, washed and drained

1/4 cup walnuts, coarsely chopped

1/4 cup blue cheese, crumbled

1/2 cup bottled fat-free raspberry
    vinaigrette dressing

Directions:

Arrange greens on large platter or in salad bowl. Evenly place pears on top of greens. Add chopped walnuts and blue cheese. Drizzle with salad dress-

ing. (Can make 2 hours before serving. Cover salad with moist paper towel and refrigerate. Add dressing just before serving.)
Makes 1 generous cup (8 servings).

Nutritional information per serving:
75 calories; 40 percent fat (3.3 grams); 46 percent
carbohydrates; 14 percent protein; 2.4 grams fiber.

3. Cold Curried Chicken Salad with Cranberries

Ingredients:
2 cups cubed, cooked chicken
   breast meat
1/2 cup celery, finely chopped
1 cup apples, chopped
1 teaspoon fresh ginger, finely grated
1 teaspoon curry powder

1/8 teaspoon cayenne
1/3 cup low-fat mayonnaise
3 tablespoons cranberry-orange
   relish (bottled with other relish
   or fresh in deli section)
2 cups mixed baby greens

Directions:
In a large bowl, combine all the above ingredients, except the greens. Toss well, cover, and chill for 15 minutes (or, make the day before). To serve, divide chicken salad in half and place each serving on a bed of greens.
Serves 2.

Nutritional information per serving:
426 calories; 30 percent fat (14 grams); 28 percent
carbohydrates; 42 percent protein; 3 grams fiber.

4. Sliced Tomatoes with Low-fat Mozzarella and Fresh Basil

Ingredients:

4 large tomatoes, sliced 1/2 inch thick

4 ounces low-fat mozzarella cheese,
    best if fresh (Buffalo-Mozzarella)

4 tablespoons of red wine vinaigrette

1/4 cup chopped packed fresh basil
    leaves

1 teaspoon sugar

Basil leaves

Directions:

Place sliced tomatoes on platter, then place cheese slices on top of each tomato. Combine red wine vinaigrette, basil, sugar; mix well. Pour the above mixture over the tomato and cheese slices. Chill; allow to marinate at least 1 hour. (You might want to add a little more red wine vinaigrette over tomatoes once chilled.) Garnish with whole fresh basil leaves.
Serves 4.

Nutritional information per serving:
131 calories; 34 percent fat (5.0 grams); 39 percent
carbohydrates; 27 percent protein; 2.5 grams fiber.

5. Crunchy Pea and Shrimp Salad

This is a crunchy salad for all seasons. Kids like it, too! For variety, add water chestnuts.

Ingredients:

One 10-ounce package frozen baby
    peas, thawed

1 cup celery, diced

1 cup cauliflower, finely chopped

1/4 cup green onion, diced

1/3 cup fat-free sour cream

2 tablespoons ranch dressing
    seasoning (from package)

1 pound small shrimp, cooked

Directions:

Combine all ingredients. Chill for 1 hour.
Makes 6 servings (approximately 2/3 cup each).

Nutritional information per serving:
135 calories; 11 percent fat (1.59 grams); 30 percent
carbohydrates; 59 percent protein; 3.1 grams fiber.

SOUPS AND STEWS

1. Cajun Shrimp and Corn Bisque

Ingredients:

4 cups nonfat milk

2 cups potato, peeled and diced

1/4 cup celery, finely chopped

1/4 teaspoon black pepper

1 teaspoon Cajun seafood seasoning

1/2 can chopped green chilies (a
   41/2-ounce can)

2 cans of creamed-style corn

1 pound of medium-large peeled
   and deveined shrimp

Dash of nutmeg

Directions:

Combine the first 5 ingredients in a large Dutch oven. Bring to boil, then reduce heat and simmer for 10 minutes, stirring occasionally. Stir in chilies and corn and bring to boil. Add shrimp. Reduce heat to medium and cook for 2 minutes, or until shrimp is done. Sprinkle with nutmeg.

Serves 6 (serving size approximately 1 1/2 cups).

Nutritional information per serving:
276 calories; 15 percent fat (4.5 grams); 48 percent
carbohydrates; 37 percent protein; 2.0 grams fiber.

2. Vegetable Lentil Soup

Ingredients:

1 large onion, chopped (1 cup)

2 teaspoons chili powder

1 teaspoon salt

1 teaspoon ground cumin

3 cloves of garlic, chopped

1 can (13 ounces) spicy tomato juice

4 cups water

1 cup dried lentils, sorted and rinsed

1 can (28 ounces) tomatoes, diced
and undrained

1 can chopped green chilies,
undrained (4 ounces)

2 small carrots, thinly sliced

1 cup fresh whole kernel corn
(frozen corn will work if fresh is
unavailable)

2 small zucchini, diced (2 cups)

Directions:

In a 3-quart saucepan, heat onion, chili powder, salt, cumin, garlic, and tomato juice to boiling; reduce heat. Cover and simmer for 5 minutes. Stir in water, lentils, tomatoes, and chilies. Heat to boiling; reduce heat, cover, and simmer 30 minutes. Stir in carrots and corn and simmer 10 minutes. Stir in zucchini, cover, and simmer another 5 minutes or until lentils and zucchini are tender, but not mushy.

Makes 6 servings (1½ cups each).

Nutritional information per serving:
200 calories; 5 percent fat (1.2 grams); 71 percent
carbohydrates; 24 percent protein; 9.23 grams fiber.

3. Curried Squash Soup

Ingredients:

4 medium carrots, peeled and sliced

1 hubbard squash (approximately
4 pounds), peeled, seeded, and
cut into cubes

2 baking potatoes (approximately
1 pound), peeled and cut
into cubes

1 medium onion, chopped

One 49-ounce can chicken broth

2 cups 1 percent low-fat milk

3 teaspoons salt

7 teaspoons curry powder

4 tablespoons lemon juice

4 tablespoons brown sugar

1 large jar roasted red peppers

1/4 teaspoon cayenne pepper

Salt

Directions:

Soup: In a large steamer, place carrots and steam for 5 minutes. Add squash, potatoes, and onion. Steam until tender. In a blender or food processor, add the vegetable mixture in small batches with enough broth in each batch to thoroughly blend. When the entire vegetable mixture is creamy, place in large saucepan, and add milk, salt, curry, lemon, and sugar. Over medium heat, stir to heat and blend seasonings.

Makes eight 2-cup servings.

Topping: Blend roasted red peppers, cayenne, and salt in a blender. Drizzle in a zigzag pattern across each bowl of soup, then run a fork through the drizzle.

Nutritional information per serving:
276 calories; 12 percent fat (4 grams); 65 percent
carbohydrates; 23 percent protein; 8.38 grams fiber.

4. Vegetable Beef Soup

Ingredients:

Vegetable cooking spray

2/3 pound extra-lean stew beef, cut
    into 1/2-inch cubes

2 large carrots, cut into 3-inch
    chunks

1 large onion, cut into quarters

10 cups water

2 whole allspice

2 bay leaves

2 teaspoons butter

1 1/4 cup onion, chopped

1/2 cup celery, chopped

3 cloves garlic, finely chopped

1 1/2 pounds mushrooms, washed
    and thickly sliced

One 14 1/2-ounce can of stewed
    tomatoes

1 1/4 cup fresh green beans, cut into
    1-inch strips

1/4 cup pearl barley

1 carrot, cut into thin strips

1/3 cup fresh parsley, chopped

1 cup white wine

Salt and pepper to taste

Directions:

Spray a large Dutch oven with cooking spray and place over medium-high heat. Brown beef, carrots, and quartered onion for 5 minutes, remove from pan, and wipe pan to remove fat. Return beef mixture to pan, add 8 cups water, allspice, and bay leaves. Bring to boil, stirring occasionally. Cover, reduce heat, and simmer for 1½ hours. Remove from heat.

Strain mixture. Reserve liquid. Place beef and carrots aside and discard onion, allspice, and bay leaves. Melt butter in Dutch oven over medium heat. Add chopped onions, celery, and garlic. Cover and cook for 10 minutes. While this mixture is cooking, cut cooked carrots into ¼-inch strips and shred beef. Set aside.

Add mushrooms to onion and celery mixture. Reduce heat and simmer for 10 minutes covered, stirring frequently. Add beef, cooking liquid, remaining 2 cups of water, tomatoes, green beans, barley, and sliced uncooked carrot. Cover and simmer for 35 minutes, then add the parsley and wine. Cook uncovered an additional 20 minutes. Add cooked carrots, salt, and pepper. Cook 5 minutes until heated through.
Serves 8.

Nutritional information per serving:
185 calories; 28 percent fat (5.8 grams); 47 percent
carbohydrates; 25 percent protein; 5.11 grams fiber.

5. Curried Turkey Vegetable Soup

Ingredients:

¼ cup chicken broth	3 tablespoons fresh parsley, chopped
2 medium onions, chopped	1 teaspoon poultry seasoning
2 tablespoons flour	½ teaspoon salt
1 tablespoon curry powder	2 cups cooked turkey (or chicken)
3 cups chicken broth	breast, cubed (about 1 pound)
1 cup red potatoes, chopped	One 10-ounce package frozen
½ cup celery, chopped	chopped spinach
1 cup carrots, sliced thin	1½ cups 1 percent low-fat milk
	Pinch of nutmeg

Directions:
Heat ¼ cup chicken broth in a large Dutch oven over medium heat. Add onions and sauté until tender, about 5 minutes. Stir in flour and curry, and cook 2 minutes. Add rest of chicken broth, potatoes, celery, carrots, parsley, and poultry seasoning. Bring to boil, then reduce heat and simmer for

10 minutes. Add turkey and frozen spinach and simmer for 10 minutes, or until spinach is thawed, soup is thoroughly hot, and vegetables are tender, but crisp. Add milk and nutmeg and serve.
Makes 8 cups.

Nutritional information for a two-cup serving:
396 calories; 23 percent fat (10 grams); 35 percent
carbohydrates; 42 percent protein; 5 grams fiber.

LUNCHABLES: BURRITOS, WRAPS, AND SANDWICHES

1. Roasted Pepper Focaccia Sandwich

Ingredients:

1 round loaf of whole wheat or
    white focaccia bread

VINAIGRETTE MIXTURE:

1/4 cup balsamic vinegar

1 1/2 tablespoons olive oil

1 teaspoon oregano

1 teaspoon basil

2 garlic cloves, minced

1 small jar of roasted yellow and red
    peppers

1/2 cup shredded low-fat mozzarella
    cheese

1/2 red onion, thinly sliced

1/2 cup arugula greens

Directions:

Preheat oven to 350 degrees Fahrenheit (or, preheat outdoor grill). Slice bread into 2 layers (a top and a bottom half). Combine vinaigrette mixture; mix well. Drain peppers. Pour 1 tablespoon vinaigrette mixture on bottom half of bread. Add a layer of peppers, cheese, onion, and greens. Sprinkle with more vinaigrette. Continue layering until all ingredients are used. Put top slice of bread on layered ingredients, cover with foil, and bake or grill for 20 minutes. Uncover for 10 minutes or until brown. Slice and serve.
Makes 8 servings.

Nutritional information per serving:
162 calories; 30 percent fat (5.5 grams); 55 percent
carbohydrates; 15 percent protein; 2.7 grams fiber.

2. Open-Faced Black Bean Burritos

This spicy dish is filling and takes only 5 minutes to prepare. It's also high in folic acid, vitamin B₁, calcium, iron, magnesium, potassium, and selenium. You can cut the fat grams even further by using low-fat or fat-free cheese.

Ingredients:

3 tablespoons water (optional)

3 cloves garlic, minced (optional)

1 can black beans, drained and
rinsed

2 tablespoons salsa

2 corn tortillas

1 ounce cheddar cheese, sliced into
strips

2 tablespoons fat-free sour cream

3 tablespoons fresh cilantro, washed
and chopped

Directions:

Heat water in a small pan over medium-high heat. Add garlic and cook until tender (about 5 minutes). Add beans and salsa and heat through. While beans are cooking, place cheese on top of tortillas and heat in microwave for one minute or until cheese melts. Place bean mixture on top of tortillas. Top with sour cream and cilantro.

Makes 1 serving.

Nutritional information per serving:
498 calories; 21 percent fat (11.9 grams); 57 percent
carbohydrates; 22 percent protein; 13.5 grams fiber.

3. Thai Wraps

Ingredients:

¼ cup chicken broth

1 tablespoon sesame oil

½ of a 16-ounce bag of
preshredded coleslaw mix
(cabbage and carrot mixture)

2 tablespoons bottled peanut sauce
(about 2½ grams of fat per
tablespoon) or hoisin sauce
(fat-free)

¼ cup fresh cilantro, chopped

One 4-ounce can sliced water
chestnuts

Four 8-inch tortillas (the chili-
tomato–flavored tortillas are
particularly good for this recipe)

Directions:

In a large skillet, heat broth and sesame oil on medium heat until it boils. Add coleslaw mix and quickly stir-fry for 1 to 2 minutes (vegetables should remain very crisp!). Add peanut or hoisin sauce, heat for 30 seconds, and remove from stove. Divide crispy coleslaw mixture into four portions and spread along the middle length of each tortilla. Sprinkle with cilantro and water chestnuts. Firmly roll each tortilla.
Makes 4 servings.

Nutritional information per serving:
217 calories; 32 percent fat (7.7 grams); 55 percent
carbohydrates; 13 percent protein; 3.2 grams fiber.*

4. Shepherd's Pie

This country meat pie is a classic "comfort food." It's rich in iron, B vitamins, and zinc, and goes well with a side of vegetables and a salad.

Ingredients:

1 single piecrust

2/3 pound ground turkey breast

1 cup onion, chopped

4 garlic cloves, chopped

2 cups frozen peas and carrots

1 packet Hunter sauce

1 tablespoon oil

2 cups mashed potatoes, made with
    nonfat milk and no
    butter/margarine

1/2 cup low-fat cheddar cheese,
    grated

Directions:

Preheat oven to 350 degrees Fahrenheit. Poke 6 to 8 holes in piecrust with a fork, then bake until golden brown (approximately 15 minutes). In a large cast-iron skillet, add turkey, onions, and garlic. Cook until meat is brown and onions are translucent. At the same time, in a medium saucepan, steam peas and carrots. Drain, if necessary, and add to turkey mixture. Set aside. Prepare Hunter sauce according to directions on package, except use only 1 tablespoon of oil. When thickened, add sauce to turkey and vegetable

* If made with peanut sauce. When made with hoisin sauce: 187 calories; 30 percent fat (6 grams); 57 percent carbohydrates; 12 percent protein; 3.2 grams fiber.

mixture and heat through. Pour turkey and vegetable mixture into pie-crust, top with potatoes, and sprinkle cheese over top. Heat in oven until cheese melts.

Makes 8 servings.

Nutritional information per serving:
295 calories; 41 percent fat (13 grams); 37 percent
carbohydrates; 22 percent protein; 3.5 grams fiber.

5. Grilled Chicken Salsa Wraps

You can make the filling ahead of time, store in the refrigerator, heat, and
roll into the tortilla for a quick lunch. Serve with a tossed salad or coleslaw.
For different flavors, try adding any of the following: fresh cilantro, garlic to
the marinade, chopped fresh tomatoes, sun-dried tomatoes, grated carrots,
or shredded fresh spinach.

Ingredients:

2 chipotle peppers, chopped

1/2 teaspoon salt

1 teaspoon white vinegar

12 ounces chicken breast, cut into strips

Vegetable cooking spray

1 green pepper, seeded and sliced
    into 1/4-inch strips

1 red pepper, seeded and sliced into
    1/4-inch strips

1 medium red onion, halved and cut
    into 1/2-inch strips

Salt and pepper

1/2 cup canned black beans, drained

1/2 cup corn kernels, cooked

4 tablespoons fat-free sour cream

4 tablespoons salsa

Four 10-inch flour tortillas

Directions:

In a large, shallow baking dish, mix chipotle peppers, salt, and vinegar. Rub chicken with mixture and place in dish. Cover and refrigerate to marinate for an hour or more. Grill on medium flame for 5 minutes per side, or until cooked through. Remove from heat and place in warm oven while preparing vegetables.

Coat a large skillet with vegetable spray and place over medium-high heat. When pan is hot, add green and red peppers and onions. Stir constantly to avoid burning and add a tablespoon of water as needed. Cook until onion strips are transparent and peppers are limp but crispy. Add salt and pepper to taste. Transfer to a platter and keep warm.

In the same skillet, add beans and corn and heat through, about 2 minutes.

When ready to serve, heat tortillas on a griddle or in the microwave, evenly divide chicken and vegetables and place in center of tortillas, top with 1 tablespoon each of sour cream and salsa. Tuck one end of tortilla and roll into a burrito.

Makes 4 servings.

Nutritional information per serving (1 wrap):
419 calories: 27 percent fat (12.5 grams); 47 percent
carbohydrates; 26 percent protein; 5.54 grams fiber.

BREADS, PASTA, AND RICE DISHES

I. Fettuccine à la Tomato and Basil

Ingredients:

1 12-ounce package of dried fettuccine noodles

4 cloves garlic, minced

Two 14$\frac{1}{2}$-ounce cans of Italian stewed tomatoes, drained

1 tablespoon olive oil

1 teaspoon butter

$\frac{3}{4}$ cup fresh basil leaves, torn

Salt and pepper to taste

$\frac{1}{3}$ cup freshly grated Parmesan cheese

Directions:

Pasta: Cook fettuccine in boiling, salted water until al dente, 15 to 20 minutes.

Sauce: Meanwhile in a nonstick, medium saucepan, cook garlic and tomatoes over medium heat until simmering, about 4 minutes. Stir in oil and butter until blended. Add basil and season with salt and pepper. Reduce heat and simmer, stirring occasionally, for 10 minutes.

Drain pasta and place in a large, warmed bowl. Pour sauce over the top and toss. Adjust seasoning with salt and pepper. Sprinkle with Parmesan cheese.

Makes 4 servings.

Nutritional information per serving:
452 calories; 17 percent fat (8.5 grams); 68 percent
carbohydrates; 15 percent protein; 9.4 grams fiber.

2. Linguini with Fresh Tomatoes, Capers, and Lemon

Ingredients:

5 vine-ripened tomatoes, chopped

3 large garlic cloves, minced

1 cup zucchini, shredded

1 small jar capers, drained

1/2 cup chicken broth

1/4 cup olive oil

2 tablespoons fresh basil, chopped

1 tablespoon fresh lemon juice

1 leek (white only), thinly sliced

16 ounces linguini (preferably fresh)

3 tablespoons Parmesan cheese, grated

4 tablespoons fresh parsley, chopped

Salt and pepper to taste

Directions:

In a large bowl, combine all the above ingredients except cheese, linguini, and parsley. Mix well. Cook linguini as directed on package (don't overcook). While pasta is cooking, pour mixed ingredients into a large skillet and heat over medium heat for approximately 2 minutes, or until hot. Drain pasta and place in a large pasta bowl or dish. Pour hot vegetable mixture on top and toss. Sprinkle with Parmesan cheese and parsley.

Makes 6 servings.

Nutritional information per serving:
348 calories; 28 percent fat (11 grams); 58 percent
carbohydrates; 14 percent protein; 4.5 grams fiber.

3. Apple-Raisin Stuffing

Ingredients:

2 tablespoons margarine	2 teaspoons poultry seasoning
1/2 cup apple juice	1/2 teaspoon cinnamon
1 1/2 cups onion, chopped	1 teaspoon salt
1 1/2 cups celery, diced	8 cups dried whole wheat bread
2 cups red apples with skin, chopped	cubes (12 slices, cubed and
1 cup raisins	dried overnight)
	1 cup chicken broth, as needed

Directions:

Melt margarine in large skillet over medium heat. Add apple juice and heat. Add onion and celery and cook until tender, not brown (about 7 minutes). Remove from heat. Add and mix well apples, raisins, poultry seasoning, cinnamon, and salt.

Place bread cubes in a large mixing bowl. Add the onion mixture. Drizzle with enough broth to moisten, tossing lightly. Stuff neck and body cavities of up to a 20-pound turkey. Roast immediately.

Makes sixteen ½-cup servings.

Nutritional information per serving:
133 calories; 22 percent fat (3.3 grams); 70 percent
carbohydrates; 8 percent protein; 4 grams fiber.

4. Wild Rice with Mushrooms

Ingredients:

1 cup wild rice	1/4 cup onion, minced
1 pound mixed mushrooms, washed	1/2 cup sliced almonds
and sliced	3 cups chicken broth

Directions:

Preheat oven to 325 degrees Fahrenheit. Rinse wild rice under running water using a strainer. Drain. Combine rice, mushrooms, onion, and almonds in large bowl. Add broth and stir thoroughly. Transfer to a 13" ×

9" × 2" baking dish. Cover with tin foil. Bake for 1½ hours or until rice is tender and liquid is absorbed.
Makes 8 servings.

Nutritional information per serving:
141 calories; 32 percent fat (5 grams); 49 percent
carbohydrates; 19 percent protein; 3.23 grams fiber.

5. Vegetable Tabbouleh

Ingredients:
I cup bulgur wheat
2 garlic cloves, minced
I teaspoon ground black pepper
1¼ cups hot water
½ cup lemon juice
½ cup red onion, chopped
I tablespoon olive oil

½ pound broccoli, chopped
½ cup fresh parsley, chopped
2 carrots, peeled and shredded
I large tomato, chopped
I can garbanzo beans, rinsed and
  drained
I tablespoon fresh mint, chopped

Directions:
In a large bowl, combine bulgur, garlic, pepper, and 1¼ cups hot water. Let stand until cool (approximately 15 minutes). Add lemon juice, onion, and oil. Let stand until bulgur is tender (approximately 20 minutes). Stir in vegetables, beans, and mint. Store in refrigerator. Stir before serving.
Makes 8 servings (approximately ½ cup each).

Nutritional information per serving:
202 calories; 22 percent fat (5.0 grams); 63 percent
carbohydrates; 15 percent protein; 8.5 grams fiber.

VEGETABLES AS A SIDE DISH OR MAIN COURSE

This tasty vegetable dish also is a great snack or lunch meal. Serve with Sliced Tomatoes with Low-fat Mozzarella and Fresh Basil (see recipe on page 356).

1. Zucchini Torte

Ingredients:

1 slice whole wheat bread, dried

2 tablespoons Parmesan cheese

2 cups egg substitute (equivalent of 2 eggs)

1/2 cup nonfat milk

1/4 teaspoon salt

1/4 teaspoon pepper

1 teaspoon finely chopped, fresh basil

1/8 teaspoon dried leaf oregano

1 teaspoon butter

2 medium zucchini, cut into 1/4-inch-thick rounds

1/2 cup chopped onion

2 tablespoons chopped fresh parsley

1 medium tomato, sliced

1 teaspoon chopped fresh basil

Directions:

Preheat oven to 350 degrees Fahrenheit. Break bread into several pieces and blend in blender to make crumbs. Place crumbs in small bowl. Stir in cheese and set aside. In a medium bowl, whip egg substitute with whisk until frothy. Stir in milk, salt, pepper, basil, and oregano; set aside. In a nonstick skillet, melt butter. Add zucchini and sauté over medium heat until tender, about 7 minutes, stirring frequently. Arrange sautéed zucchini in an ungreased 10-inch quiche pan or 9-inch piepan. Sprinkle onion and parsley over zucchini, then pour in egg mixture and sprinkle crumb mixture over the top. Add sliced tomato and sprinkle with 1 teaspoon basil. Bake in preheated oven about 30 minutes or until a knife inserted in the middle comes out clean. Let stand 5–10 minutes, then slice into 4 wedges. Makes 4 servings.

Nutritional information per serving:
138 calories; 30 percent fat (4.7 grams); 35 percent carbohydrates; 35 percent protein; 2.77 grams fiber.

2. Fresh Green Bean Bundles with Dill

Ingredients:

1 pound fresh young green beans, washed and stem ends removed

2 yellow squash, about 1 1/2 inches in diameter

2 tablespoons olive oil

2 cloves garlic, minced

2 teaspoons balsamic vinegar

1/2 teaspoon dried dill

Salt and pepper to taste

12 whole cranberries

Directions:

Arrange beans in 16 stacks (about 8 to 10 young beans in each stack). Cut squash into sixteen 1/2-inch-thick rounds. Hollow out the centers with a spoon to within 1/4 inch of the rind. Thread the bean stacks through the squash pieces (like a napkin ring). Place steamer basket in large stockpot or saucepan. Add 1 inch of water and place bean bundles in the steamer basket. Cover and bring to a boil over high heat. Steam 4 minutes or until beans turn bright green and are crisp but tender. Add water if necessary to prevent pan from boiling dry.

While beans are steaming, place oil in a small saucepan on medium heat. Add garlic and stir until hot, but not brown. Transfer bean bundles to a warmed serving plate, pour garlic oil over top, and sprinkle with balsamic vinegar and dill. Season with salt and pepper. Garnish with whole cranberries.

Makes 16 bundles (1 serving = 4 bundles).

Nutritional information per serving:
114 calories; 51 percent fat (6.5 grams); 40 percent
carbohydrates; 9 percent protein; 4.91 grams fiber.

3. Apricot-Glazed Carrots

Ingredients:

6 cups fresh baby carrots

3/4 cup water

1/4 teaspoon salt

1/3 cup apricot preserves

1/8 teaspoon curry

3 tablespoons fresh parsley, chopped

Directions:

In medium saucepan, combine carrots and water. Bring to boil. Reduce heat, cover, and simmer until carrots are tender, yet crisp. Drain. Stir in salt, preserves, and curry. Garnish with parsley.

Makes 8 generous ½-cup servings.

Nutritional information per serving:
84.6 calories; 2 percent fat (0.23 gram); 92 percent
carbohydrates; 6 percent protein; 3.86 grams fiber.

4. Eggplant Caponata

This delicious mix is a great vegetable side dish, or can be piled on top of thin slices of French bread as an appetizer or snack, or is even a good main entrée on top of pasta.

Ingredients:

2 tablespoons olive oil

1 pound eggplant, unpeeled and diced

1 medium onion, chopped

2 garlic cloves, minced

1 stalk celery, finely chopped

One 14½-ounce can stewed
    tomatoes, chopped

2 tablespoons red wine vinegar

2 tablespoons capers, drained

1 tablespoon canned roasted red
    peppers, diced

¼ teaspoon red pepper flakes

Salt and pepper to taste

Directions:

Heat olive oil in large skillet. Add eggplant and onion and cook uncovered over medium heat for 10 minutes or until tender. Stir in garlic, celery, tomatoes, vinegar, capers, peppers, and red pepper flakes. Bring to boil, reduce heat, and simmer for 15 minutes or until liquid is almost evaporated. Cool and chill or serve warm as a main dish.

Makes 6 servings.

Nutritional information per serving:
87.6 calories; 44 percent fat (4.3 grams); 48 percent
carbohydrates; 8 percent protein; 3.4 grams fiber.

5. Spicy Garlic Spinach

This flavorful side dish comes packed with folic acid (more than 25 percent of your daily need), iron (more than 2 milligrams), and potassium. It goes well with Spicy Grilled Salmon with Ginger (see recipe on page 378) or Chicken-Apricot Curry with Rice (see recipe on page 373). And, it takes less than 10 minutes to prepare!

Ingredients:

2 teaspoons olive oil

3 cloves garlic, minced

1/2 or a 7 1/2-ounce jar of roasted red
   peppers, chopped

1/4 teaspoon red pepper flakes

Pinch of salt

One 10-ounce bag fresh baby
   spinach

Directions:

In a large skillet, heat olive oil over medium heat. Add garlic and stir until garlic is heated through, but not toasted (approximately 3 minutes). Add peppers, pepper flakes, and salt and continue stirring for an additional minute. Add spinach and toss to coat with the garlic mixture. Cover and cook for 4 minutes, or until spinach is wilted. Serve immediately.

Makes four ½-cup servings.

Nutritional information per serving:
41 calories; 38 percent fat (2.2 grams); 33 percent
carbohydrates; 19 percent protein; 2.11 grams fiber.

ENTRÉES AND ONE-DISH MEALS

I. Chicken-Apricot Curry with Rice

Ingredients:

2/3 cup long-grain brown rice

1 tablespoon butter

2/3 cup chopped onion

1/4 cup diced celery or leeks

3 garlic cloves, minced

1 tablespoon curry powder

8 ounces skinless, boneless chicken
    breasts, cut into bite-sized
    pieces

1/3 cup apricot preserves or 1/4 cup
    apricot pepper jelly

1 medium apple, cored and cut into
    small pieces

1/3 cup water

1/4 cup golden raisins

1/2 teaspoon salt

1 1/2 cups plain, low-fat yogurt

2 tablespoons cornstarch

1/4 teaspoon hot pepper flakes

Directions:

While preparing curry sauce, cook rice according to package directions without using salt or butter/margarine. If rice is finished before sauce is ready, cover and keep warm.

In a large, nonstick skillet, melt butter over medium heat. Add onion, celery, garlic, and curry powder and cook for 1 minute. Push onion mixture to the side of the skillet and add chicken; cook and stir for 5 minutes or until chicken is no longer pink. Stir in onion mixture from the sides. Add and stir preserves, apple, water, raisins, and salt into chicken mixture. In a small bowl, blend yogurt and cornstarch; add and stir into chicken mixture. Cook until mixture is thickened and bubbly, stirring constantly over medium heat. Add pepper flakes. Simmer for 2 minutes, remove from heat, and serve over rice.

Makes 4 servings (1½ cups each).

Nutritional information per serving:
350 calories; 15 percent fat (6 grams); 61 percent
carbohydrates; 24 percent protein; 3.23 grams fiber.

2. Cornish Game Hen with Caramelized Onion

Ingredients:

SAUCE:

1/2 cup honey

2 cups white wine

1/2 cup sherry

2 cups chicken broth

ONIONS:

10 bunches green onions

2 tablespoons butter

2 cloves garlic, minced

1/2 cup water

2 tablespoons honey

GAME HENS:

4 Cornish game hens, cut in half, washed, and patted dry

Salt and pepper

Vegetable spray

2 bunches spinach, washed and trimmed (or 2 bags precut, fresh spinach)

Directions:

Sauce: Heat honey in medium-sized skillet over medium-high heat until honey darkens, stirring occasionally (about 3 minutes). Slowly add wine, sherry, and chicken broth (sauce will foam if added too fast). Boil mixture until reduced by half, about 30 minutes. (This part can be prepared ahead of time, covered, and refrigerated for use later.)

Onions: While sauce is boiling, cut off beard of onions and use white bulbs plus 1 inch of green (slices should be about 2½ inches in length). Discard remaining greens. Cut slices in half lengthwise to form onion slivers. Melt butter in medium-sized saucepan, add onions and garlic, and sauté until golden brown and almost tender, about 15 minutes. Add water and honey. Cover and simmer until onions are tender, about 10 minutes. Uncover and continue cooking until onions are caramelized, stirring occasionally, about 5 minutes. Remove from heat. (This part can be prepared ahead of time, covered, and refrigerated.)

Game Hens: While sauce is boiling, preheat oven to 425 degrees Fahrenheit. Season hen halves with salt and pepper on both sides. Place hen halves on a vegetable-sprayed baking sheet, skin side up. Bake until juices run clear when thighs are pierced, about 25 minutes. Keep warm.

About 10 minutes before hen halves are ready, place spinach in a large, nonstick frying pan and steam over medium heat until wilted. Drain. Season with salt and pepper. Reheat onions over medium heat, stirring occasionally. Add sauce and heat through.

Spread spinach on a large serving platter. Arrange hen halves on top of spinach. Pour sauce over halves and garnish each half with onions.
Makes 8 servings.

Nutritional information per serving:
425 calories; 26 percent fat (12.5 grams); 37 percent
carbohydrates; 37 percent protein; 1.25 grams fiber.

3. Plum-Glazed Chicken on Skewers

Ingredients:

1/4 cup green onions, finely chopped

2 tablespoons soy sauce

2 tablespoons sweet chili sauce

1 1/2 teaspoons gingerroot, grated

1 garlic clove, chopped

1/2 cup plum jam

2 pounds boneless chicken breast
cut into 2-inch chunks

1/2 pound zucchini, cut into 1-inch
slices

1 red onion, cut into thick slices

12 mushrooms

2 sweet red peppers, cut into 1-inch
strips

6 skewers

Directions:
Combine the first 6 ingredients in a medium-sized bowl and mix well. Add chicken and marinate for 15 minutes to several hours. Preheat grill (or broiler). In the meantime, prepare vegetables.

Alternate chicken and vegetables on skewers. Grill for 5 minutes on each side, or until chicken is no longer pink. Serve over rice pilaf.
Makes 6 servings.

Nutritional information per serving:
265 calories; 7 percent fat (2 grams); 37 percent
carbohydrates; 56 percent protein; 1.5 grams fiber.

4. *Roast Turkey with Herb Rub*

Ingredients:

3 tablespoons fresh rosemary,
  chopped, or 1 1/2 tablespoons
  dried rosemary

3 tablespoons fresh thyme, chopped,
  or 1 1/2 tablespoons dried thyme

3 tablespoons fresh tarragon,
  chopped, or 1 1/2 tablespoons
  dried tarragon

1 tablespoon ground pepper

1 1/2 teaspoons salt

One 18-to-20-pound turkey

Fresh herb sprigs (optional)

2 tablespoons vegetable oil

2 cups canned low-salt chicken broth

Directions:

Mix herbs, pepper, and salt in a small bowl. Pat turkey with paper towels until dry. Place on rack set in a large roasting pan. If not stuffing turkey, place herb sprigs in main cavity. If stuffing turkey, spoon stuffing loosely into main cavity. Brush turkey with oil. Rub herb mix all over turkey. (Can be prepared one day ahead if turkey is not stuffed. Cover and refrigerate. Let stand at room temperature for 1 hour before roasting.)

Position rack in lowest third of oven. Preheat oven to 425 degrees Fahrenheit. Pour 2 cups of broth into pan. Roast turkey 45 minutes, then remove turkey from oven and cover with foil. Reduce oven temperature to 350 degrees. Return turkey to oven. Baste with pan juices every hour until done. Continue roasting until meat thermometer inserted into thickest part of thigh registers 180 degrees, or, until juices run clear when thickest part of thigh is pierced with fork. Total cooking time: Approximately 4 hours, 20 minutes for stuffed turkey; approximately 3 hours, 50 minutes for non-stuffed turkey.

Transfer turkey to platter. Tent with foil and let stand for 30 minutes. Carve and serve.

Makes 16 servings.

Nutritional information
for a 3-ounce serving of breast meat:
161 calories; 35 percent fat (6.29 grams); 0 percent
carbohydrates; 65 percent protein; 0 grams fiber.

5. Mango Chicken

Ingredients:

1¹/₂ pounds boneless, skinless
    chicken thighs, fat trimmed and
    cut into 1-inch cubes

1¹/₂ teaspoons curry powder

¹/₂ cup Major Grey chutney

4 teaspoons fresh ginger, minced

¹/₂ cup green onions, greens only cut
    into 2-inch strips

1¹/₂ tablespoons lemon juice

³/₄ cup chicken broth

1 firm-ripe mango, peeled, pitted,
    and sliced into large chunks

3 cups cooked white rice (hot)

Salt

Directions:

Place chicken in 12-inch nonstick frying pan and cook over medium-high heat until lightly browned, stirring occasionally (about 12 minutes). Stir in curry and stir until chicken is coated. Add chutney, ginger, onions, lemon juice, and chicken broth. Top with mango, cover (stir occasionally), and simmer until chicken is tender, about 30 minutes.

Transfer cooked chicken and onions to a bowl and keep warm. Boil sauce uncovered over medium-high heat until reduced to about 1½ cups (about 5 minutes). Salt to taste. Pour sauce over chicken. Serve chicken mixture over rice.

Makes 4 servings.

Nutritional information per serving:
501 calories; 14 percent fat (7.6 grams); 54 percent
carbohydrates; 32 percent protein; 3.05 grams fiber.

6. Sautéed Shrimp and Vegetables

Ingredients:

2 tablespoons butter

²/₃ pound large, fresh shrimp

1 can chicken broth, canned

1¹/₂ cups onions, chopped

1¹/₂ cups cauliflower flowerets

1¹/₂ cups broccoli pieces

1 cup carrots, sliced

1 green pepper, seeded and sliced

¹/₄ cup sherry

1 tomato, chopped

1 tablespoon cornstarch

Salt and pepper to taste

Directions:

Melt butter in large saucepan and lightly sauté shrimp (approximately 5 minutes). Remove shrimp and place in a bowl. To the saucepan, add half of the chicken broth and the rest of the ingredients, except tomato and cornstarch. Simmer until vegetables are tender but crisp. Add tomato and shrimp. In a container, blend the second half of the chicken broth and cornstarch, then add to the vegetables, stirring over medium heat until broth thickens. Serve over rice or noodles.

Makes 4 servings.

Nutritional information per serving:
221 calories; 30 percent fat (7.5 grams); 33 percent
carbohydrates; 36 percent protein; 4.38 grams fiber.

7. Spicy Grilled Salmon with Ginger

Ingredients:

1/4 cup chopped fresh cilantro

1/3 cup hoisin sauce

2 tablespoons minced fresh ginger

1 teaspoon brown sugar

1 tablespoon chopped canned
    chipotle peppers

1/2 lemon

1 pound salmon fillet, 1-inch thick, or
    six 5-ounce salmon steaks

Fresh spinach, washed and stemmed

Directions:

Preheat grill or broiler. Stir together in a medium bowl the cilantro, hoisin, ginger, brown sugar, and peppers. Sprinkle lemon over salmon, then brush both sides of salmon with glaze mixture. Grill or broil until opaque in center, basting occasionally with remaining glaze (approximately 6 minutes per side). Transfer salmon to a plate of fresh spinach.

Makes 6 servings.

Nutritional information per serving:
284 calories; 50 percent fat (15.9 grams); 3 percent
carbohydrates; 47 percent protein; 0 grams fiber.

8. Paprika and Red Pepper Chicken

Ingredients:

1 tablespoon olive oil

10 large mushrooms, stemmed and
sliced

4 boneless, skinless chicken breasts,
cut into 1/2-inch strips

Salt and pepper

1 cup thinly sliced onion

4 garlic cloves, finely chopped

One 12-ounce jar roasted red
peppers, cut into strips

2 1/2 teaspoons paprika

1/4 teaspoon dried marjoram

1 teaspoon unbleached flour

1/2 cup chicken broth

2/3 cup plain, nonfat yogurt

3 tablespoons fresh parsley, chopped

Directions:

Heat 1 teaspoon olive oil in a large, nonstick skillet over medium-high heat. Add mushrooms and simmer 5 minutes. Season with salt and pepper to taste. Transfer mushrooms to platter. Increase heat to high and add chicken to skillet; stir until thoroughly cooked (about 10 minutes). Transfer to platter with mushrooms. Reduce heat to medium and add remaining oil, onion, and garlic. Sauté until transparent (about 5 minutes). Add peppers, paprika, and marjoram, and heat through (about 2 minutes). Sprinkle with flour and stir to coat. Add chicken broth, cover, and cook over low heat for 10 minutes. Uncover and let cool for 5 minutes.

Transfer half of pepper mixture to blender, add yogurt, and puree. Return to skillet. Stir in mushrooms and chicken. Stir, cover, and reheat over low heat for 10 minutes. Transfer to clean platter and garnish with parsley. Serve with couscous, pasta, or brown rice.

Makes 4 servings.

Nutritional information per serving:
246 calories; 21 percent fat (5.76 grams); 24 percent
carbohydrates; 55 percent protein; 2.74 grams fiber.

DESSERTS, CHOCOLATE, AND OTHER SWEETS

1. Pumpkin Mousse Pie

Ingredients:

1 (3.1-ounce) box Jell-O Vanilla
   Flavor (Fat-Free, Sugar-Free)
   Instant Pudding Mix

1²/₃ cups nonfat milk

4 ounces nonfat cream cheese

One 15-ounce can pumpkin

¹/₂ cup sugar

2 teaspoons pumpkin pie spice

2 teaspoons frozen fat-free whipped
   topping, thawed

One 6-ounce reduced-fat graham
   cracker Ready Crust Piecrust

Directions:

In a large bowl, combine instant pudding mix and milk. With a mixer, beat
on low speed for 2 minutes. Add the cream cheese, pumpkin, sugar, pumpkin pie spice, and whipped topping. Beat on low for 30 seconds. Pour into
piecrust. Refrigerate for at least 1 hour.
Makes 8 servings.

Nutritional information per serving:
296 calories; 10 percent fat (3.32 grams); 75 percent
carbohydrates; 15 percent protein; 2.49 grams fiber.

2. Apple-Cranberry Upside-down Pie

Ingredients:

PASTRY:

1 cup white flour

2 tablespoons wheat germ

2 tablespoons sugar

3 tablespoons butter

3 tablespoons ice water

FILLING:

6 cups Granny Smith or other tart,
   crisp apples (about
   2¹/₂ pounds), peeled, cored, and
   cut into ¹/₂-inch slices

1 cup fresh cranberries, halved

³/₄ cup sugar

¹/₄ teaspoon nutmeg

¹/₄ teaspoon orange zest

1 tablespoon white flour

1 tablespoon lemon juice

2 tablespoons butter

Directions:

Preheat oven to 425 degrees Fahrenheit. Combine flour, wheat germ, and sugar, in a medium-sized bowl. With a pastry blender, cut in butter until mixture resembles coarse crumbs. Sprinkle with water, 1 tablespoon at a time, mixing with a fork after each addition until pastry just holds together. Form into a ball, cover, and refrigerate for 15 minutes.

While pastry is in refrigerator, toss apples and cranberries with sugar, nutmeg, zest, and flour until mixture is thoroughly covered in flour; sprinkle with lemon juice. Set aside.

Roll pastry into an 11-inch circle on a lightly floured surface; cover with plastic wrap.

In a medium saucepan, melt butter over medium heat. Add apple mixture and heat until apples are just tender, stirring occasionally. Remove from heat. Arrange apple mixture in a deep-dish, 9-inch piepan so it is slightly mounded in the center. Place pastry on top of apples; tuck in edges. Cut slits in pastry to allow steam to escape.

Bake 25 minutes or until lightly browned. Remove from oven and allow to cool for 20 minutes. Invert onto a serving platter. Serve warm or at room temperature.

Makes 8 servings.

Nutritional information per serving:
240 calories; 18 percent fat (4.9 grams); 78 percent
carbohydrates; 4 percent protein; 2.72 grams fiber.

3. Civilized S'Mores

For those in search of the perfect comfort food, this dessert has all the memories of a childhood campfire, with almost no fat! And it takes less than 5 minutes to make.

Ingredients:

6 whole low-fat graham crackers

6 large marshmallows

6 teaspoons fat-free hot fudge sauce

Directions:

Break crackers in half. Place on a plate and top 6 halves with 1 marshmallow each. Spread the other 6 halves with 1 teaspoon of fudge sauce each. Microwave the marshmallow-topped crackers for 14 seconds or until they puff up to 1½ times or more of their original size. Quickly remove from microwave and place the fudge-topped halves on top of the hot marshmallow halves. Gently press down.

Makes 6 servings.

Nutritional information per serving:
70 calories; 9 percent fat (0.7 grams); 86 percent
carbohydrates; 4 percent protein; 0.2 grams fiber.

4. Frozen Vanilla Yogurt Pie with Berries

Ingredients:

½ of a ½ gallon of fat-free vanilla
    frozen yogurt
1 fat-free graham cracker piecrust
1 pint fresh or frozen berries
    (blueberries and raspberries are
    especially good)

⅓ cup sugar
Pinch of salt
1 tablespoon cornstarch
1 tablespoon water
1 tablespoon lemon juice
12 whole berries

Directions:

Soften yogurt and fill piecrust. Place in freezer in the morning. That night, rinse berries if fresh, and drain. Mix sugar, salt, and cornstarch in a saucepan. Add water and lemon juice and stir until dissolved. Add berries and bring to a boil, stirring gently. Boil for 2 minutes, until liquid is clear and slightly thickened. Try not to crush berries. Cool berries in refrigerator for 15 minutes. Remove pie from freezer and berries from refrigerator. Slice pie into 8 wedges, place on plates, and spoon sauce over top. Serve.

Makes 8 servings.

Nutritional information per serving:
310 calories; 10 percent fat (3.48 grams); 76 percent
carbohydrates; 14 percent protein; 2.5 grams fiber.

5. *Lemon Chiffon Pie*

The creamy, but delicate texture of this pie will satisfy your fat tooth, but it has almost no fat. You can make the lemon chiffon without the crust as a puddinglike mousse dessert, or you can top with various toppings. Instead of lemon zest, try chocolate shavings, fresh raspberries, or orange zest.

Ingredients:
1 cup hot water
1 1/2 tablespoons lemon juice
One 3-ounce box lemon Jell-O
   (sugar-free)
3/4 cup sugar

1 large container of fat-free cream
   cheese
1 can fat-free evaporated milk
2 teaspoons vanilla
2 fat-free graham cracker piecrusts
2 tablespoons lemon zest

Directions:
Mix water and lemon juice, then add Jell-O. Stir until thoroughly mixed. Set aside.

Using an electric mixer, blend sugar and cream cheese in a medium bowl until creamy. Add to lemon mixture and stir well.

In a large bowl and using an electric mixer, whip milk until it forms stiff peaks. Add vanilla and blend.

Add lemon mixture to milk, using low speed on an electric mixer or by hand until thoroughly blended.

Pour into piecrusts, top with lemon zest, and chill for 3 hours or more. Makes 16 servings.

Nutrition information per serving (pie):
190 calories; 14 percent fat (3 grams); 66 percent carbohydrates; 20 percent protein; 1 gram fiber.

Nutrition information per serving (pudding):
90 calories; less than 1 percent fat (0.04 grams); 65 percent carbohydrates; 34 percent protein; less than 1 gram fiber.

6. Chocolate Chip Cupcakes

Ingredients:

1 1/2 cups all-purpose,
    unbleached flour

1/2 cup granulated sugar

1/3 cup unsweetened cocoa powder

1 teaspoon baking powder

1/4 teaspoon salt

1/6 cup water

2/3 cup orange juice

2 tablespoons canola oil

2 teaspoons white vinegar

2 teaspoons vanilla extract

1/3 cup semisweet chocolate chips

2 teaspoons powdered sugar

Directions:

Preheat oven to 375 degrees Fahrenheit. Put paper liners in a muffin tin that holds 12 muffins.

Combine flour, sugar, cocoa, baking powder, and salt in a medium bowl. Make a well in the center of the flour mixture and set aside. Combine water, orange juice, canola oil, vinegar, and vanilla; pour into well in flour mixture. Stir until moistened. Fold in chocolate chips.

Spoon muffin batter evenly into paper-lined muffin pan so that each is approximately two-thirds filled. Bake for 15 minutes, or until wooden toothpick inserted into the center comes out clean. Remove from pans and place on a rack to cool. Sprinkle with powdered sugar.

Makes 12 servings.

Nutritional information per muffin:
144 calories; 25 percent fat (4 grams); 69 percent
carbohydrates; 6 percent protein; 1.5 grams fiber.

7. To-Die-For Low-Fat Brownies

While traditional brownies pack 280 calories and are 54 percent fat, this sinfully delicious treat has 37 percent fewer calories and is only 16 percent fat! Each brownie also supplies a hefty dose of iron and calcium. The problem is eating just one!

Ingredients:

Vegetable spray

2 cups granulated sugar

3/4 cup unsweetened cocoa powder

1 1/4 cups unbleached white flour

1/4 teaspoon salt

1 large egg plus one large egg white,
    lightly beaten

2 teaspoons vanilla extract

3 tablespoons butter, melted

7 ounces (one 6-ounce container
    plus 1 heaping tablespoon) low-
    fat vanilla yogurt

Directions:

Preheat oven to 350 degrees Fahrenheit. Using vegetable spray, lightly grease an 8" × 8" baking pan. Combine the sugar, cocoa, flour, and salt. Make a well in the middle of the dry ingredients and pour the eggs and vanilla into that center. Mix until all the dry ingredients have been combined. Add the butter and blend. Add the yogurt and blend until the mixture is a thick batter. Spread mixture evenly in pan. Bake for 55 minutes, or until sides pull away slightly from pan. Let cool before cutting.
Makes 16 brownies.

Nutritional information per brownie:
177 calories; 16 percent fat (3.2 grams); 77 percent
carbohydrates; 7 percent protein; 1.5 grams fiber.

Resources

AGING

The National Institute on Aging, P.O. Box 8057, Gaithersburg, MD 20898-8057. Call (800) 222-2225, from 8:30 A.M. to 5 P.M. EST, or (800) 222-4225 TDD. Free booklet: *In Search of the Secrets of Aging.*

CHRONIC FATIGUE SYNDROME

CFS Survival Association, P.O. Box 1889, Davis, CA 95617. (916) 756-9242.

Chronic Fatigue and Immune Dysfunction Syndrome (CFIDS) Association of America, P.O. Box 220398, Charlotte, NC 28222-0398. (800) 44-CFIDS. www.cfids.org

National Chronic Fatigue Syndrome Association (NCFS), P.O. Box 18426, Kansas City, MO 64133. Call (816) 931-4777 or the CFS Activation Network (CAN), (212) 627-5831.

DEPRESSION

Depression Awareness Recognition and Treatment (D/ART), a program of the National Institute of Mental Health. For free information, call (800) 421-4211. For brochures, call Isabella Davidoff at (301) 443-3720.

Depression and Related Affective Disorders Association (DRADA), Johns Hopkins University School of Medicine, Meyer 3-181, 600 N. Wolfe Street, Baltimore, MD 21287-7381. (410) 955-4647.

Depressives Anonymous, 329 E. 62nd Street, New York, NY 10021. Send a SASE for free information.

National Depressive and Manic Depressive Association (NDMDA), 730 N. Franklin, #301, Chicago, IL 60610. (800) 826-3632.

The National Foundation for Depressive Illness, 20 Charles Street, New York, NY 10014. Or, Box 32257, New York, NY 10116. Call (800) 248-4344 for recorded message on symptoms of depression and available pamphlets and referrals.

National Mental Health Association, 1021 Prince Street, Alexandria, VA 22314. Call (800) 969-6642 or (703) 684-7722.

EATING DISORDERS

American Anorexia/Bulimia Association, 418 E. 76th Street, New York, NY 10021. (212) 734-1114.

Anorexia Nervosa and Related Eating Disorders (ANRED), P.O. Box 5102, Eugene, OR 97405. (503) 344-1144.

Bulimia, Anorexia Self-Help, 6125 Clayton Avenue, Suite 215, St. Louis, MO 63139. Call (314) 567-4080 or (800) 726-3334 (crisis hot line).

National Anorexic Aid Society, 5796 Karl Road, Columbus, OH 43229. (614) 436-1112.

National Association of Anorexia Nervosa and Associated Disorders, Box 7, Highland Park, IL 60035. (708) 831-3438.

EXERCISE

American Alliance for Health, Physical Education, Recreation, and Dance, 1900 Association Drive, Reston, VA 22091. (703) 476-3400.

American College of Sports Medicine, P.O. Box 1440, Indianapolis, IN 46206. (317) 637-9200.

FOOD ALLERGIES

American Council on Science and Health, 1995 Broadway, 2nd floor, New York, NY 10023-5860. (212) 362-4919. Booklet: *Food Allergies;* $3.85.

General Foods: Consumer Response & Information Center, 250 North Street, White Plains, NY 10625. Free booklet: *Food Allergies & Intolerances.*

Superintendent of Documents, U.S. Government Printing Office, Washington, DC 20402. Booklet: *Cooking for People with Food Allergies,* G-246; $1.50.

HEADACHES

National Headache Foundation, 428 W. St. James Place, 2nd Floor, Chicago, IL 60614. (800) 843-2256.

HEALTHFUL EATING

The American Diabetes Association, 1660 Duke Street, Alexandria, VA 22314. (800) DIA-BETES.

The American Dietetic Association, 216 West Jackson Boulevard, Suite 800, Chicago, IL 60606-6995. Hot line (National Center of Nutrition and Dietetics, (800) 366-1655, 10 A.M. to 5 P.M., EST, Monday through Friday). Prerecorded messages from 9 A.M. to 9 P.M. seven days a week.

American Heart Association, 7272 Greenville Avenue, Dallas, TX 75231-4596. (800) 242-8721. Pamphlet: *The American Heart Association Diet: An Eating Plan for Healthy Americans;* free with SASE.) www.Americanheart.Org

Bulletin Office, 10B Agriculture Hall, Michigan State University, East Lansing, MI 48824-1039. (517) 355-0240. Booklet: *Shop Smart #5; 10¢.*

Consumer Information Center, Department 113-F, Pueblo, CO 81009. Free catalog of materials on health, exercise, and nutrition. www.pueblo.gsa.gov.

Food and Nutrition Information Center, National Agriculture Library, 10301 Baltimore Avenue, Room 304, Beltsville, MD 20705-2351. (301) 504-5719.

Food Marketing Institute, 800 Connecticut Avenue, NW, Washington, DC 20006. Pamphlet: *The Food Guide Pyramid: Beyond the Basic 4; 50¢* with SASE.

National Cancer Institute, 9000 Rockville Pike, Building 31, Room 10A24, Bethesda, MD 20892. Pamphlet: *Eat More Fruits & Vegetables: Five-a-Day for Better Health;* free with SASE.

LEARNING DISABILITIES

American Academy of Ophthalmology, P.O. Box 7424, San Francisco, CA 94120-7424. (415) 561-8500. Brochure: *Learning Disabilities: Dyslexia, Reading, and Perceptual Problems;* free with SASE.

American Academy of Pediatrics, Department of Publications, 141 Northwest Point Blvd., P.O. Box 747, Elk Grove Village, IL 60009-0747. (800) 433-9016. Pamphlet: *Learning Disabilities and Children: What Parents Need to Know;* free with SASE.

National Center for Learning Disabilities, 381 Park Avenue South, Suite 1401, New York, NY 10016-8806. Call (212) 545-7510; for toll-free information and referral: (888) 575-7373.

MENTAL HEALTH

Alzheimer's Association, 919 N. Michigan, Chicago, IL 60611. (800) 272-3900.

National Institute of Mental Health, U.S. Department of Health and Human Services,

5600 Fishers Lane, Rockville, MD 20857. (301) 443-4513. Call panic hot line (800) 647-2642 (Panic Attacks).

National Mental Health Association, Information Center, 1021 Prince Street, Alexandria, VA 22314. (703) 684-7722. 9 A.M. to 5 P.M., EST, Monday–Friday. Information available on clinical depression, the warning signs of mental illness, and local mental health services.

NEUROLOGICAL DISORDERS

National Institute of Neurological Disorders and Stroke, Building 31, Room 8A16, 31 Center Drive MSC 2540, Bethesda, MD 20892. (800) 352-9424.

National Organization for Rare Disorders, P.O. Box 8923, New Fairfield, CT 06812-8923. (800) 999-NORD.

PREMENSTRUAL SYNDROME (PMS)

National Women's Health Network, 514 10th Street NW, Washington, DC 20004. (202) 628-7814.

The National Women's Health Resource Center, 2440 M Street NW, No. 325, Washington, DC 20037. (202) 293-6045.

PMS Access, P.O. Box 259690, Madison, WI 53725-9690. PMS Access toll-free number (800) 222-4PMS. Provides coping tips, answers to questions, information packets, and charts to track symptoms. You can also get a newsletter for $18/yr. that contains articles on PMS.

SEASONAL AFFECTIVE DISORDER (SAD)

SAD Association, P.O. Box 989, Steyning BN44 3HG, England. (01903)-814942.

Society for Light Therapy and Biological Rhythms, 10200 West 44th Avenue, Wheatridge, CO 80033. (303) 422-7905 (e-mail: sltbr@resourcenter.com)

WHERE TO PURCHASE LIGHT FIXTURES:

The SunBox Company, 19217 Orbit Drive, Gaithersburg, MD 20879. (800) LITE-YOU or (548) 3868.

Apollo Light Systems, Inc., 352 West 1060, Orem, UT 84058. (800) 222-3296. http://www.bio-light.com.

Bio-Brite, Inc., 7315 Wisconsin Avenue, #1300 W., Bethesda, MD 20814-3202. (800) 621-LITE.

Enviro-Med, 1600 SE 141st Avenue, Vancouver, WA 98683. (800) 222-DAWN.

SLEEP DISORDERS

American Academy of Osteopathy, 3500 De Pauw Boulevard, Suite 1080, Indianapolis, IN 46268-1136. (317) 879-1881. Provides a list of local osteopathic physicians who specialize in manipulative therapy for people who can't sleep because of musculoskeletal pain, such as back or neck pain.

American Sleep Disorders Association, 6301 Bandel Road, Suite 101, Rochester, MN 55901. (507) 287-6006. Provides a list of accredited sleep disorders clinics in your area. www.asda.org

Better Sleep Council, P.O. Box 19534, Alexandria, VA 22320-0534. (703) 683-8371. www.bettersleep.org

National Sleep Foundation, 729 15th Street, 4th floor, Washington, DC 20005. (888) NSF-SLEEP. www.sleepfoundation.org.

STRESS

American Institute of Stress, 124 Park Avenue, Yonkers, NY 10703. (800) 24-RELAX.

Anxiety Disorders Association of America, Dept. B, P.O. Box 96505, Washington, DC 20077-7140. (301) 231-9350.

BOOKS:

Benson H: *The Relaxation Response.* New York, Avon, 1976.

Benson H: *Beyond the Relaxation Response.* New York, Putnam/Berkley, 1984.

Goleman D, Bennet-Goleman T: *The Relaxed Body Book.* New York, Doubleday, 1986.

Rifkin J: *Time Wars: The Primary Conflict in Human History.* New York, Henry Holt & Co., 1987.

Schor J: *The Overworked American: The Unexpected Decline in Leisure.* New York, Basic Books, 1991.

TAPES:

Ten Minutes to Relax. The Relaxation Company, 20 Lumber Road, Roslyn, NY 11576. (516) 621-2727.

ADDITIONAL RESOURCES

American Botanical Council, Box 201660, Austin, TX 78720. (512) 331-8868. www.HerbalGram.org.

American Holistic Medical Association, 4101 Lake Boone Trail, Suite 201, Raleigh, NC 27607. (919) 787-5181.

Center for Mind/Body Medicine, 5225 Connecticut Avenue, NW, Suite 414, Washington, DC 20015. (202) 966-7338.

Herb Research Foundation, 1007 Pearl Street, Suite 200, Boulder, CO 80302. (800) 748-2617. www.herbs.org/herbs.

National Institutes of Health, Office of Alternative Medicine (OAM) Clearinghouse, P.O. Box 8218, Silver Springs, MD 20907-8218. (800) 531-1794.

National Women's Health Network, 514 10th Street, NW, Suite 400, Washington, DC 20004. (202) 347-1140.

National Women's Health Resource Center, 2425 L Street, NW, 3rd floor, Washington, DC 20037. (202) 293-6045.

Omega Institute, 260 Lake Drive, Rhinebeck, NY 12572. (914) 266-4444.

U.S. Office of Alternative Medicine, National Institutes of Health, 9000 Rockville Pike, Building 31, Room 5B-38, Bethesda, MD 20892. (301) 402-2466.

Selected References

CHAPTER 1

Baldwin B, Sukhchai S: Intracerebroventricular injection of CCK reduces operant sugar intake in pigs. *Physl Behav* 1996;60:231–233.

Blundell J, Halford C: Serotonin and appetite regulation. *CNS Drugs* 1998;9:473–495.

Campfield L: Metabolic and hormone controls of food intake: Highlights of the last 25 years: 1972–1997. *Appetite* 1997;29:135–152.

Chow S, Sakai R, Fluharty S, et al: Brain oxytocin receptor antagonism disinhibits sodium appetite in preweanling rats. *Regul Pept* 1997;68:119–124.

Cohen B, Babb S, Yurgelun-Todd D, et al: Brain choline uptake and cognitive function in middle age. *Bio Psych* 1997;41:307.

Cummings S, Truong B, Gietzen D: Neuropeptide Y and somatostatin in the anterior piriform cortex alter intake of amino acid-deficient diets. *Peptides* 1998;19:527–535.

Ericsson M, Poston W, Foreyt J: Common biological pathways in eating disorders and obesity. *Addict Beha* 1996;21:733–743.

Foltin R, Haney M, Comer S, et al: Effect of fenfluramine on food intake, mood, and performance of humans living in a residential laboratory. *Physl Behav* 1996;59:295–305.

Heini A, Kirk K, Lara-Castro C, et al: Relationship between hunger-satiety feelings and various metabolic parameters in women with obesity during controlled weight loss. *Obes Res* 1998;6:225–230.

Hirschberg A: Hormonal regulation of appetite and food intake. *Ann Med* 1998;30:7–20.

Kaye W, Gendall K, Kye C: The role of the central nervous system in the psychoneuroendocrine disturbances of anorexia and bulimia nervosa. *Psych Cl N* 1998;21:381–397.

Kissileff H, Wentzlaff T, Guss J, et al: A direct measure of satiety disturbance in patients with bulimia nervosa. *Physl Behav* 1996;60:1077–1085.

Levine A, Billington C: Why do we eat? A neural systems approach. *Ann R Nutr* 1997;17:597–619.

Lieverse R, Masclee A, Jansen J, et al: Obese women are less sensitive for the satiety effects of bombesin than lean women. *Eur J Cl N* 1998;52:207–212.

Lin L, Umahara M, York D, et al: Beta caromorphins stimulate and enterostatin inhibits the intake of dietary fats in rats. *Peptides* 1998;19:325–331.

Mercer M, Holder M: Food cravings, endogenous opioid peptides and food intake: A review. *Appetite* 1997;29:325–352.

Olson G, Olson R, Kastin A: Endogenous opiates: 1995. *Peptides* 1996;17:1421–1466.

Rudski J, Billington C, Levine A: A sucrose-based maintenance diet increases sensitivity to appetite suppressant effects of naloxone. *Pharm Bio B* 1997;58:679–682.

Smith B, York D, Bray G: Effects of dietary preference and galanin administration in the paraventricular or amygdaloid nucleus on diet self-selection. *Brain Res B* 1996; 39:149–154.

Stricker E, Verbalis J: Central inhibition of salt appetite by oxytocin in rats. *Regul Pept* 1996;66:83–85.

Vandewater K, Vickers Z: Higher-protein foods produce greater sensory-specific satiety. *Physl Behav* 1996;59:579–583.

Wang J, Akabayashi A, Dourmashkin J, et al: Neuropeptide Y in relation to carbohydrate intake, corticosterone and dietary obesity. *Brain Res* 1998;802:75–88.

Wang J, Akabayashi A, Yu H, et al: Hypothalamic galanin: Control by signals of fat metabolism. *Brain Res* 1998;804:7–20.

Wolf G: Orexins: A newly discovered family of hypothalamic regulators of food intake. *Nutr Rev* 1998;56:172–173.

Woods S, Seeley R, Porte D, et al: Signals that regulate food intake and energy homeostasis. *Science* 1998;280:1378–1383.

CHAPTER 2

Blackburn G, Kanders B, Lavin P, et al: The effect of aspartame as part of a multidisciplinary weight-control program on short- and long-term control of body weight. *Am J Clin N* 1997;65:409–418.

Christensen L: The effect of carbohydrates on affect. *Nutrition* 1997;13:503–514.

Crovetti R, Santangelo A, Riso M, et al: Sweet taste reactivity and satiety. *Nutr Res* 1997;17:1417–1425.

Gendall K, Sullivan P, Joyce P, et al: Psychopathology and personality of young women who experience food cravings. *Addict Beh* 1997;22:545–555.

Glanz K, Basil M, Maibach E, et al: Why Americans eat what they do: Taste, nutrition, cost, convenience, and weight control concerns as influences on food consumption. *J Am Diet A* 1998;98:1118–1126.

Melanson K, Greenberg A, Ludwig D, et al: Blood glucose and hormonal responses to small and large meals in healthy young and older women. *J Geront A* 1998;53:8299–8305.

Pelchat M: Food cravings in young and elderly adults. *Appetite* 1997;28:103–113.

Pellegrain K, O'Neil P, Stellefson E, et al: Average daily nutrient intake and mood among obese women. *Nutr Res* 1998;18:1103–1112.

CHAPTER 3

Blass E: Milk-induced hypoalgesia in human newborns. *Pediatr* 1997;99:825–829.

Brooks S, Lampi B: Time course of enzyme changes after a switch from a high-fat to a low-fat diet. *Comp Bioc P* 1997;118:359–365.

Cooling J, Blundell J: Are high-fat and low-fat consumers distinct phenotypes? Differences in the subjective and behavioral response to energy and nutrient challenges. *Eur J Cl N* 1998;52:193–201.

Drewnowski A: Macronutrient substitutes and weight-reduction practices of obese, dieting, and eating disordered women. *Ann NY Acad* 1997;819:132–141.

Drewnowski A: Why do we like fat? *J Am Diet A* 1997;97(suppl):S58–S62.

Goldfarb A, Jamurtas A: Beta endorphin response to exercise: An update. *Sport Med* 1997;24:8–16.

Harber V, Sutton J, MacDougall J, et al: Plasma concentrations of beta endorphin in trained eumenorrheic and amenorrheic women. *Fert Steril* 1997;67:648–653.

Himaya A, Louis-Sylvestre J: The effect of soup on satiation. *Appetite* 1998;30:199–210.

Johnson R, Soultanakis R, Matthews D: Literacy and body fatness are associated with under-reporting of energy intake in US low-income women using the multiple-pass 24-hour recall: A doubly labeled water study. *J Am Diet A* 1998;98:1136–1140.

Karhunen L, Lappalaninen R, Haffner S, et al: Serum leptin, food intake and preferences for sugar and fat in obese women. *Int J Obes* 1998;22:819–821.

Katz D, Brunner R, St. Jeor S, et al: Dietary fat consumption in a cohort of American adults, 1985–1991: Covariates, secular trends, and compliance with guidelines. *Am J He Pro* 1998;12:382–390.

Kennedy K, Rains T, Shay N: Zinc deficiency changes preferred macronutrient intake in subpopulations of Sprague-Dawley outbred rats and reduces hepatic pyruvate kinase gene expression. *J Nutr* 1998;128:43–49.

Leibowitz S, Akabayashi A, Wang J: Obesity on a high-fat diet: Role of hypothalamic galanin in neurons of the anterior paraventricular nucleus projecting to the median eminence. *J Neurosc* 1998;18:2709–2719.

Leshem M: Salt preferences in adolescence is predicted by common prenatal and infantile mineralofluid loss. *Physl Behav* 1998;63:699–704.

Leshem M, Maroun M, Weintraub Z: Neonatal diuretic therapy may alter children preferences for salt taste. *Appetite* 1998;30:53–64.

Mantozoros C, Prasad A, Beck F, et al: Zinc may regulate serum leptin concentrations in humans. *J Am Col N* 1998;17:270–275.

Mattes R: The taste for salt in humans. *Am J Clin N* 1997;65(suppl):692S–697S.

Mercer M, Holser M: Food cravings, endogenous opioid peptides, and food intake: A review. *Appetite* 1997;29:325–352.

Miller D, Castellanos V, Shide D, et al: Effect of fat-free potato chips with and without nutrition labels on fat and energy intakes. *Am J Clin N* 1998;68:282–290.

Ookuma K, Barton C, York D, et al: Effect of enterostatin and kappa-opioids on macronutrient selection and consumption. *Peptides* 1997;18:785–791.

Pelchat M: Food cravings in young and elderly adults. *Appetite* 1997;28:103–113.

Radimer K, Harvey P: Comparison of self-report of reduced fat and salt foods with sales and supply data. *Eur J Cl N* 1998;52:380–383.

Rebro S, Patterson R, Kristal A, et al: The effect of keeping food records on eating patterns. *J Am Diet A* 1998;98:1163–1165.

Ricketts C: Fat preferences, dietary fat intake and body composition in children. *Eur J Cl N* 1997;51:778–781.

Rolls B: Fat and sugar substitutes and the control of food intake. *Ann NY Acad* 1997;819:180–193.

Sjostrom L, Rissanen A, Andersen T, et al: Randomized placebo-controlled trial of orlistat for weight loss and prevention of weight regain in obese patients. *Lancet* 1998; 352:167–172.

Sukala W: Pyruvate: Beyond the marketing hype. *Int J Sp Nu* 1998;8:241–249.

van Gaal L, Broom J, Enzi G, et al: Efficacy and tolerability of orlistat in the treatment of obesity: A 6-month dose-ranging study. *Eur J Cl Ph* 1998;54:125–132.

Wadden T, Considine R, Foster G, et al: Short- and long-term changes in serum leptin in dieting obese women: Effects of caloric restriction and weight loss. *J Clin End* 1998;83:214–218.

Wells A, Read N, Uvnas-Moberg K, et al: Influences of fat and carbohydrate on postprandial sleepiness, mood, and hormones. *Physl Behav* 1997;61:679–686.

CHAPTER 4

Barone J, Roberts H: Caffeine consumption. *Food Chem T* 1996;34:119–129.

Charlton K, Wolmarans P, Lombard C: Evidence of nutrient dilution with high sugar intakes in older South Africans. *J Hum Nu Di* 1998;11:331–343.

Christensen L; The effect of carbohydrates on affect. *Nutrition* 1997;13:503–514.

Cordain L: Does creatine supplementation enhance athletic performance? *J Am Col N* 1998;17:205–206.

Cunliffe A, Obeid O, Powell-Tuck J: Postprandial changes in measures of fatigue: Effect of a mixed or a pure carbohydrate or pure fat meal. *Eur J Cl N* 1997;51:831–838.

Engels H, Said J, Wirth J: Failure of chronic ginseng supplementation to affect work performance and energy metabolism in healthy adult females. *Nutr Res* 1996;16:1295–1305.

Engels H, Wirth J: No ergogenic effects of ginseng (panas ginseng C.A. Meyer) during graded maximal aerobic exercise. *J Am Diet A* 1997;97:1110–1115.

French J, Wainwright C, Booth D: Caffeine and mood: Individual differences in low-dose caffeine sensitivity. *Appetite* 1994;22:277–279.

Lloyd H, Rogers P, Hedderley D, et al: Acute effects on mood and cognitive performance of breakfast differing in fat and carbohydrate content. *Appetite* 1996;27:151–164.

Paz A, Berry E: Effect of meal composition on alertness and performance of hospital night-shift workers. *Ann Nutr M* 1997;41:291–298.

Scholz B, Gross R, Schultink W, et al: Anaemia is associated with reduced productivity of women workers even in less-physically-strenuous tasks. *Br J Nutr* 1997;77:47–57.

Wells A, Read N, MacDonald I: Effects of carbohydrate and lipid on resting energy expenditure, heart rate, sleepiness, and mood. *Physl Behav* 1998;63:621–628.

CHAPTER 5

Alberti-Fidanza A, Fruittini D, Servili M: Gustatory and food habit changes during the menstrual cycle. *Int J Vit N* 1998;68:149–153.

Boyd N, Lockwood G, Greenberg C, et al: Effects of a low-fat, high-carbohydrate diet on plasma sex hormones in premenopausal women: Results from a randomized controlled trial. *Br J Canc* 1997;76:127–135.

Buffenstein R, Poppitt S, McDevitt R, et al: Food intake and the menstrual cycle: A retrospective analysis, with implications for appetite research. *Physl Behav* 1995;58:1067–1077.

Chappell S, Hackney A: Associations between menstrual cycle phase, physical activity level, and dietary macronutrient intake. *Biol Sport* 1997;14:251–258.

Chuong C, Coulam C, Kao P, et al: Neuropeptide levels in premenstrual syndrome. *Fert Steril* 1985;44:760–765.

Chuong C, Dawson E, Smith E: Vitamin E levels in premenstrual syndrome. *Am J Obst G* 1990;163:1591–1595.

Dye L, Blundell J: Menstrual cycle and appetite control: Implications for weight regulation. *Hum Repr* 1997;12:1142–1151.

Dye L, Warner P, Bancroft J: Food craving during the menstrual cycle and its relationship to stress, happiness of relationship and depression: A preliminary enquiry. *J Affect D* 1995;34:157–164.

Kashuba A, Nafziger A: Physiological changes during the menstrual cycle and their effects on the pharmacokinetics and pharmacodynamics of drugs. *Clin Pharma* 1998; 34:203–218.

Landsdowne A, Provost S: Vitamin D_3 enhances mood in healthy subjects during winter. *Psychophar* 1998;135:319–323.

Lauretzen C, Reuter H, Repges R, et al: Treatment of premenstrual tension syndrome with vitex agnus castus: Controlled, double-blind study versus pyridoxine. *Phytomed* 1997;4:183–189.

Marean M, Cumming C, Fox E, et al: Fluid intake of women with premenstrual syndrome. *Women Heal* 1995;23:75–80.

Masuda A, Oishi T: Effects of restricted feeding on the light-induced body weight change and locomotor activity in the Djungarian hamster. *Physl Behav* 1995;58:153–159.

Perovic S, Muller W: Pharmacological profile of hypericum extract. *Drug Res* 1995; 45:1145–1148.

Rose D, Lubin M, Connolly J: Effects of diet supplementation with wheat bran on serum estrogen levels in the follicular and luteal phases of the menstrual cycle. *Nutrit* 1997;13:535–539.

Swedo S, Allen A, Glod C, et al: A controlled trial of light therapy for the treatment of pediatric seasonal affective disorder. *J Am A Chil* 1997;36:816–821.

Thys-Jacobs S, Starkey P, Bernstein D, et al: Calcium carbonate and the premenstrual syndrome: Effects on premenstrual and menstrual symptoms. *Am J Obst G* 1998; 179:444–452.

Wright K, Badia P, Myers B, et al: Caffeine and light effects on nighttime melatonin and temperature levels in sleep-deprived humans. *Brain Res* 1997;747:78–84.

CHAPTER 6

Adams P, Lawson S, Sanigorski A, et al: Arachidonic acid to eicosapentaenoic acid ratio in blood correlates positively with clinical symptoms of depression. *Lipids* 1996;31 (suppl):S157–S161.

Alpert J, Fava M: Nutrition and depression: The role of folate. *Nutr Rev* 1997;55:145–149.

Christensen L: The effect of carbohydrate on affect. *Nutrition* 1997;13:503–514.

Edwards R, Peet M, et al: Omega-3 polyunsaturated fatty acid levels in the diet and in red blood cell membranes of depressed patients. *J Affect D* 1998;48:149–155.

Edwards R, Peet M, Shay J, et al: Depletion of docosahexaenoic acid in red blood cell membranes of depressive patients. *Bioch Soc T* 1998;26:S142.

Fava M, Borus J, Alpert J, et al: Folate, vitamin B_{12}, and homocysteine in major depressive disorder. *Am J Psychi* 1997;154:426–428.

Haleem D, Yasmeen A, Haleem M, et al: 24h withdrawal following repeated administration of caffeine attenuates brain serotonin but not tryptophan in rat brain: Implications for caffeine-induced depression. *Life Sci* 1995;57:PL285–PL292.

Hawkes W, Hornbostel L: Effects of dietary selenium on mood in healthy men living in a metabolic research unit. *Biol Psychi* 1996;39:121–128.

Heuser I, Deuschle M, Lupa P, et al: Increased diurnal plasma concentrations of dehydroepiandrosterone in depressed patients. *J Clin End* 1998;83:30–33.

Hibbeln J: Fish consumption and major depression. *Lancet* 1998;351:1213.

Hillbrand M, Spitz R, VandenBos G: Investigating the role of lipids in mood, aggression, and schizophrenia. *Psychiat Serv* 1997;48:875–876,882.

Ledochowski M, Sperner B, Fuchs D: Lactose malabsorption is associated with early signs of mental depression in females. *Dig Dis Sci* 1998;43:2513–2517.

Maes M: Fatty acids, cytokines, and major depression. *Biol Psychi* 1998;43:313–314.

Nowak G: Alterations in zinc homeostasis in depression and antidepressant therapy. *Pol J Pharmacol* 1998;50:1–4.

Perovic S, Muller W: Pharmacological profile of hypericum extract. *Drug Res* 1995; 45:1145–1148.

Scully D, Kremer J, Meade M, et al: Physical exercise and psychological well being: A critical review. *Br J Sp Med* 1998;32:111–120.

Sutoo D, Akiyama K: The mechanism by which exercise modifies brain function. *Physl Behav* 1996;60:177–181.

Wells A, Read N, Laugharne J, et al: Alterations in mood and changing to a low-fat diet. *Br J Nutr* 1998;79:23–30.

Widmer J, Henrotte J, Raffin Y, et al: Relationship between erythrocyte magnesium, plasma electrolytes and cortisol, and intensity of symptoms in major depressed patients. *J Affect D* 1995;34:201–209.

Wurtman R, Wurtman J: Brain serotonin, carbohydrate-craving, obesity, and depression. *Obes Res* 1995;3 (suppl 4):477S–480S.

CHAPTER 7

Ascherio A, Willett W: Health effects of trans fatty acids. *Am J Clin N* 1997;66: 1006–1010.

Askew E: Environmental and physical stress and nutrient requirements. *Am J Clin N* 1995;61(suppl):631S–637S.

Banhegyi G, Braun L, Csala M, et al: Ascorbate and environmental stress: *Ann NY Acad* 1998;851:292–303.

Dantzer R: Stress and immunity: What have we learned from psychoneuroimmunology? *Acta Physiol Scand Suppl* 1997;640:43–46.

Durlach J, Bac P, Durlach V, et al: Magnesium status and ageing: An update. *Magnes Res* 1998;11:25–42.

Enig M: Trans fatty acids in diets and databases. *Cereal F W* 1996;41:58–63.

Hakim A, Ross G, Curb J, et al: Coffee consumption in hypertensive men in older middle-age and the risk of stroke: The Honolulu Heart Study. *J Clin Epid* 1998;51:487–494.

Henrotte J, Aymard N, Allix M, et al: Effect of pyridoxine and magnesium on stress-induced ulcers in mice selected for low or high blood magnesium levels. *Ann Nutr M* 1995;39:285–290.

Kamara K, Eskay R, Castonguay T: High-fat diets and stress responsivity. *Physl Behav* 1998;64:1–6.

Kelley D, Taylor P, Nelson G, et al: Dietary docohexaenoic acid and immunocompetence in young healthy men. *Lipids* 1998;33:559–566.

Lehmann E, Kinzler E, Friedemann J: Efficacy of a special kava extract (piper methysticum) in patients with states of anxiety, tension and excitedness on non-mental origin. *Phytomed* 1996;3:113–119.

McEwan B, Conrad C, Kuroda Y, et al: Prevention of stress-induced morphological and cognitive consequences. *Eur Neurops* 1997;7 (suppl 3):S323–S328.

Melchart D, Linde K, Worku F, et al: Immunomodulation with echinacea: A systematic review of controlled clinical trials. *Phytomedicine* 1994;1:245–254.

Mossad S, Machnin M, Medendorp S, et al: Zinc gluconate lozenges for treating the common cold. *Ann Int Med* 1996;125:81–88.

Rosch P: The stress-food-mood connection: Are there stress reducing foods and diets? *Stress Med* 1995;11:1–6.

Rousseau D, Moreau D, Raederstorff D, et al: Is a dietary n-3 fatty acid supplement able to influence the cardiac effect of the psychological stress? *Mol C Bioch* 1998;178:353–366.

Rudolph D, McAuley E: Cortisol and affective responses to exercise. *J Sport Sci* 1998;16:121–128.

Scully D, Kremer J, Meade M, et al: Physical exercise and psychological well being: A critical review. *Br J Sp Med* 1998;32:111–120.

Seelig M: Cardiovascular consequences of magnesium deficiency and loss: Pathogenesis, prevalence, and manifestations—Magnesium and chloride loss in refractory potassium repletion. *Am J Cardio* 1989;63:4G–21G.

Wells A, Read N, Laugharne J, et al: Alterations in mood after changing to a low-fat diet. *Br J Nutr* 1998;79:23–30.

CHAPTER 8

Allen R, Stabler S, Lindenbaum J: Relevance of vitamins, homocysteine and other metabolites in neuropsychiatric disorders. *Eur J Ped* 1998;157:S122–S126.

Baldewicz T, Goodkin K, Feaster D, et al: Plasma pyridoxine deficiency is related to increased psychological distress in recently bereaved homosexual men. *Psychos Med* 1998;60:297–308.

Benton D, Griffiths R, Haller J: Thiamine supplementation mood and cognitive functioning. *Psychophar* 1997;129:66–71.

Benton D, Parker P: Breakfast, blood glucose, and cognition. *Am J Clin N* 1998;67:S772–S778.

Berr C, Richard M, Rousel A, et al: Systemic oxidative stress and cognitive performance in the population-based EVA study. *Free Rad B* 1998;24:1202–1208.

Bro R, Shank L, McLaughlin T, et al: Effects of a breakfast program on on-task behaviors of vocational high school students. *J Educ Res* 1996;90:111–115.

Broadhurd C, Cunnane S, Crawford M: Dietary lipids and evolution of the human brain. *Br J Nutr* 1998;79:390–393.

Bruner A, Joffee A, Duggan A, et al: Randomized study of cognitive effects of iron supplementation in nonanemic iron deficient adolescent girls. *Lancet* 1996;348:992–996.

Chandler A, Walker S, Connolly K, et al: School breakfast improves verbal fluency in undernourished Jamaican children. *J Nutr* 1995;125:894–900.

Choma C, Sfoirzo G, Keller B: Impact of rapid weight loss on cognitive function in collegiate wrestlers. *Med Sci Spt* 1998;30:746–749.

Dichter D: Oxidative injury in the nervous system. *Act Neur Sc* 1998;98:145–153.

Furushiro M, Suzuki S, Shishido Y, et al: Effects of oral administration of soybean lecithin transphosphotidylated phosphatidylserine on impaired learning of passive avoidance in mice. *Jpn J Pharm* 1997;75:447–450.

Galduroz J, Carlini E: The effects of long-term administration of guarana on the cognition of normal, elderly volunteers. *Rev Paul Med* 1996;114:1073–1078.

Garcia M, Ward G, Ma Y, et al: Effect of docosahexaenoic acid on the synthesis of phosphatidylserine in rat brain in microsomes and C6 glioma cells. *J Neurochem* 1998; 70:24–30.

Godfrey K, Robinson S: Maternal nutrition, placental growth, and fetal programming. *P Nutr Soc* 1998;57:105–111.

Horwood L, Fergusson D: Breast-feeding and later cognitive and academic outcomes. *Pediatrics* 1998;101:E9–E99.

Joseph J, Denisova N, Fisher D, et al: Age-related neurodegeneration and oxidative stress. *Neurol Clin* 1998;16:747–755.

Kanofsky J: Thiamin status and cognitive impairment in the elderly. *J Am Col N* 1996; 15:197–198.

Kretsch M, Fong A, Green M, et al: Cognitive function, iron status, and hemoglobin concentrations in obese dieting women. *Eur J Cl N* 1998;52:512–518.

Kretsch M, Green M, Fong A, et al: Cognitive effects of a long-term weight reducing diet. *Int J Obes* 1997;21:14–21.

Lupien S, Gaudreau S, Techiteya B, et al: Stress-induced declarative memory impairment in healthy elderly subjects: Relationship to cortisol reactivity. *J Clin End* 1997; 82:2070–2075.

McCaddon A, Davies G, Hudson P, et al: Total serum homocysteine in senile dementia of Alzheimer type. *Int J Ger P* 1998;13:235–239.

Meck W, Williams C: Perinatal choline supplementation increases the threshold for thinking in spatial memory. *Neuroreport* 1997;8:3053–3059.

Murray C, Lynch M: Dietary supplementation with vitamin E reverses the age-related deficit in long term potentiation in dentate gyrus. *J Biol Chem* 1998;273: 2161–2168.

Packer L, Tritschler H, Wessel K: Neuroprotection by the metabolic antioxidant alpha-lipoic acid. *Free Rad B* 1997;22:359–378.

Paleologos M, Cumming R, Lazarus R: Cohort study of vitamin C intake and cognitive impairment. *Am J Epidem* 1998;148:45–50.

Paolisso G, Tagliamonte M, Rizzo M, et al: Oxidative stress and advancing age: Results from healthy centenarians. *J Am Ger So* 1998;46:833–838.

Parasrampuria J, Schwartz K, Petesch R: Quality control of dehydroepiandrosterone dietary supplement products. *J Am Med A* 1998;280:1565.

Perrig W, Perrig P, Stahelin H: The relation between antioxidants and memory performance in the old and very old. *J Am Ger So* 1997;45:718–724.

Pollitt E, Cuerto S, Jacoby E: Fasting and cognition in well- and undernourished schoolchildren: A review of three experimental studies. *Am J Clin N* 1998;67:S779–S784.

Sano M, Ernesto C, Thomas R, et al: A controlled trial of selegiline, alpha-tocopherol, or both as treatment for Alzheimer's disease. *N Eng J Med* 1997;336:1216–1222.

Snowden W: Evidence from an analysis of 2000 errors and omissions made in IQ tests by a small sample of school children, undergoing vitamin and mineral supplementation that speed of processing is an important factor in IQ performance. *Pers Indiv* 1997;22:131–134.

Tiwari B, Godbole M, Chattopadhyay N, et al: Learning disabilities and poor motivation to achieve due to prolonged iodine deficiency. *Am J Clin N* 1996;63:782–786.

Warburton D: Effects of caffeine on cognition and mood without caffeine abstinence. *Psychopharm* 1995;119:66–70.

Wyon D, Abrahamsson L, Jartelius M, et al: An experimental study of the effects of energy intake at breakfast on the test performance of 10-year-old children in school. *Int J F S M* 1997;48:5–12.

CHAPTER 9

Cangiano C, Laviano A, Del Ben M, et al: Effects of oral 5-hydroxy-tryptophan on energy intake and macronutrient selection in non-insulin dependent diabetic patients. *Int J Obes* 1998;22:648–654.

Chang H, Sei H, Morita Y: Effects of intravenously administered vitamin B_{12} on sleep in the rat. *Physl Behav* 1995;57:1019–1024.

Driver H, Taylor S: Sleep disturbances and exercise. *Sport Med* 1996;21:1–6.

Hansen M, Kapas L, Fang J, et al: Cafeteria diet-induced sleep is blocked by subdiaphragmatic vagotomy in rats. *Am J Physl* 1998;274:R168–R174.

Hibino G, Moritani T, Kawada T, et al: Caffeine enhances modulation of parasympathetic nerve activity in humans. *J Nutr* 1997;127:1422–1427.

Kiuchi T, Sei H, Seno H, et al: Effect of vitamin B_{12} on the sleep-wake rhythm following an 8-hour advance of the light-dark cycle in the rat. *Physl Behav* 1997;61:551–554.

Lin A, Uhde T, Slate S, et al: Effects of intravenous caffeine administrated to healthy males during sleep. *Depress Anxiety* 1997;5:21–28.

Mallick B, Gulyani S: Alterations in synaptosomal calcium concentrations after rapid eye movement sleep deprivation in rats. *Neuroscienc* 1996;75:729–736.

Mayer G, Kroger M, Meier-Ewert K: Effects of vitamin B_{12} on performance and circadian rhythm in normal subjects. *Neuropsych* 1996;15:456–464.

Reiter R: The pineal gland and melatonin in relation to aging: A summary of the theories and of the data. *Exp Geront* 1995;30:199–212.

Sicard B, Perault M, Enslen M, et al: The effects of 600mg of slow release caffeine on mood and alertness. *Aviat Sp En* 1996;67:859–862.

Sutoo D, Akiyama K: The mechanism by which exercise modifies brain function. *Physl Behav* 1996;60:177–181.

Tanabe K, Yamamoto A, Suzuki N, et al: Efficacy of oral magnesium administration on decreased exercise tolerance in a state of chronic sleep deprivation. *Jpn Circ J* 1998;62:341–346.

Vgontzas A, Bixler E, Tan T, et al: Obesity without sleep apnea is associated with daytime sleepiness. *Arch In Med* 1998;158:1333–1337.

Voderholzer U, Hornyak M, Thiel B, et al: Impact of experimentally induced serotonin deficiency by tryptophan depletion on sleep EEG in health subjects. *Neuropsych* 1998; 18:112–124.

Wells A, Read N, Idzikowski C, et al: Effects of meals on objective and subjective measures of daytime sleepiness. *J App Physl* 1998;84:507–515.

Wright K, Badia P, Myers B, et al: Caffeine and light effects on nighttime melatonin and temperature levels in sleep-deprived humans. *Brain Res* 1997;747:78–84.

CHAPTER 10

Barton C, Lin L, York D, et al: Differential effects of enterostatin, galanin, and opioids on high-fat diet consumption. *Brain Res* 1996;702:55–60.

Bell E, Castellanos V, Pelkman C, et al: Energy density of foods affects energy intake in normal-weight women. *Am J Clin N* 1998;67:412–420.

Blundell J, Lawton C, Cotton J, et al: Control of human appetite: Implications for the intake of dietary fat. *Ann R Nutr* 1996;16:285–319.

Campfield L: Metabolic and hormonal controls of food intake: Highlights of the last 25 years—1972–1997. *Appetite* 1997;29:135–152.

Drewnowski A: Taste preferences and food intake. *Ann R Nutr* 1997;17:237–253.

Galef B: Food selection: Problems in understanding how we choose foods to eat. *Neurosci B* 1996;20:67–73.

Geiselman P: Control of food intake: A physiologically complex, motivated behavioral system. *End Metab C* 1996;25:815–829.

Hahn N: The flavor of food? It's all in your head! *J Am Diet A* 1996;96:655–656.

Himaya A, Sylvestre J: The effect of soup on satiation. *Appetite* 1998;30:199–210.

Holt S, Miller J, Petocz P, et al: A satiety index of common foods. *Eur J Cl N* 1995; 49:675–690.

Krebs-Smith S, Cleveland L, Ballard-Barbash R, et al: Characterizing food intake patterns of American adults. *Am J Clin N* 1997;65:1264–1268.

Mattes R: Physiologic responses to sensory stimulation by food: Nutritional implications. *J Am Diet A* 1997;97:406–410,413.

Mela D: Consumer estimates of the percentage energy from fat in common foods. *Eur J Cl N* 1993;47:735–740.

Michener W, Rozin P: Pharmacological versus sensory factors in the satiation of chocolate craving. *Physl Behav* 1994;56:419–422.

Miller G, Groziak S: Impact of fat substitutes on fat intake. *Lipids* 1996;31:S293–S296.

Porrini M, Crovetti R, Riso P, et al: Effects of physical and chemical characteristics of food on specific and general satiety. *Physl Behav* 1995;57:461–468.

Reed D, Bachmanov A, Beauchamp G, et al: Heritable variation in food preferences and their contribution to obesity. *Behav Genet* 1997;27:373–387.

Reid M, Hetherington M: Relative effects of carbohydrates and protein on satiety: A review of methodology. *Neurosci B* 1997;21:295–308.

Rolls B: Sensory specific satiety. *Nutr Rev* 1986;44:93–101.

Schiffman S, Gatlin C: Clinical physiology of taste and smell. *Ann R Nutr* 1993; 13:405–436.

Shide D, Rolls B: Information about the fat content of preloads influences energy intake in healthy women. *J Am Diet A* 1995;95:993–998.

Teff K: Physiological effects of flavour perception. *Trends Food* 1996;7:448–452.

Tepper B: 6-n-propylthiouracil: A genetic marker for taste, with implications for food preference and dietary habits. *Am J Hu Gen* 1998;63:1271–1276.

Vandewater K, Vickers Z: Higher-protein foods produce greater sensory-specific satiety. *Physl Behav* 1996;59:579–583.

Warwick Z, Hall W, Pappas T, et al: Taste and smell sensations enhance the satiating effect of both a high-carbohydrate and a high-fat meal in humans. *Physl Behav* 1993; 53:553–563.

CHAPTER 11

Feunekes G, deGraaf C, vanStaveren W: Social facilitation of food intake is mediated by meal duration. *Physl Behav* 1995;58:551–558.

Grivetti L: Social determinants of food intake. *Ann NY Acad* 1997;819:121–131.

Hill J, Peters J: Environmental contributions to the obesity epidemic. *Science* 1998; 280:1371–1374.

Lahteenmaki L, Tuorila H: Three-factor eating questionnaire and the use and liking of sweet and fat among dieters. *Physl Behav* 1995;57:81–88.

Mela D: Eating behavior, food preferences, and dietary intake in relation to obesity and body weight status. *P Nutr Soc* 1996;55:803–816.

Nestle M, Wing R, Birch L, et al: Behavioral and social influences on food choice. *Nutr Rev* 1998;56:S50–S74.

Polivy J: Psychological consequences of food restriction. *J Am Diet A* 1996;96:589–592.

Pollard T, Steptoe A, Wardle J: Motives underlying healthy eating: Using the food choice questionnaire to explain variation in dietary intake. *J Biosoc Sc* 1998;30:165–179.

Shide D, Rolls B: Information about the fat content of preloads influences energy intake in healthy women. *J Am Diet A* 1995;95:993–998.

Uvnas-Morberg K: Endocrinologic control of food intake. *Nutr Rev* 1990;48:57–62.

Walcott-McQuigg J, Sullivan J, Dan A, et al: Psychosocial factors influencing weight control behavior of African-American women. *W J Nurs R* 1995;17:502–520.

CHAPTER 13

Ames B, Gold L: The causes and prevention of cancer: The role of environment. *Biotherapy* 1998;11:205–220.

Fernandez M, Pedraza V, Olea N: Estrogens in the environment: Is there a breast cancer connection. *Canc J* 1998;11:11–17.

Golden R, Noller K, Titus-Ernstoff L, et al: Environmental endocrine modulators and human health: An assessment of the biological evidence. *Cr R Toxic* 1998;28:109–227.

Schade G, Heinzow B: Organochlorine pesticides and polychlorinated biphenyls in human milk of mothers living in northern Germany. *Sci Total E* 1998;215:31–39.

Verma S, Goldin B: Effect of soy-derived isoflavonoids on the induced growth of MCF-7 cells by estrogenic environmental chemicals. *Nutr Cancer* 1998;30:232–239.

Warman P, Havard K: Yield, vitamin and minerals contents of organically and conventionally grown potatoes and sweet corn. *Agr Eco E* 1998;68:207–216.

Woese K, Lange D, Boess C, et al: A comparison of organically and conventionally grown foods: Results of a review of the relevant literature. *J Sci Food* 1997;74:281–293.

CHAPTER 14

Albertson A, Tobelmann R: Consumption of grain and whole-grain foods by an American population during the years 1990 to 1992. *J Am Diet A* 1995;95:703–704.

Benton D, Haller J, Fordy J: Vitamin supplementation for 1 year improves mood. *Neuropsychb* 1995;32:98–105.

Block G, Abrams B: Vitamin and mineral status of women of childbearing potential. *Ann NY Acad Sci* 1993;678:244–254.

Burton G, Traber M, Acuff R, et al: Human plasma and tissue alpha tocopherol concentrations in response to supplementation with deuterated natural and synthetic vitamin E. *Am J Clin N* 1998;67:669–684.

Dollahite J, Franklin D, McNew R: Problems encountered in meeting the Recommended Dietary Allowances for menus designed according to the Dietary Guidelines for Americans. *J Am Diet A* 1995;95:341–344.

Kennedy E, Ohls J, Carlson S, et al: The Healthy Eating Index: Design and Applications. *J Am Diet A* 1995;95:1103–1108.

Krebs-Smith S, Cleveland L, Ballard-Barbash R, et al: Characterizing food intake patterns of American adults. *Am J Clin N* 1997;65:1264–1268.

Kumar A, Aitas A, Hunter A, et al: Sweeteners, dyes, and other excipients in vitamin and mineral preparations. *Clin Pediat* 1996;35:443–450.

Mark S, Wang W, Fraumeni J, et al: Lowered risks of hypertension and cerebrovascular disease after vitamin and mineral supplementation: The Linxian Nutrition Intervention Trial. *Am J Epidem* 1996;143:658–664.

Mayne S: Antioxidant nutrients and cancer incidence and mortality: An epidemiologic perspective. *Adv Pharmacol* 1997;38:657–675.

Meydani S, Meydani M, Blumberg J, et al: Vitamin E supplementation and in vivo immune response in healthy elderly subjects. *J Am Med A* 1997;277:1380–1386.

Millen B, Quatromoni P, Franz M, et al: Population nutrient intake approaches dietary recommendations: 1991–1995 Framingham Nutrition Studies. *J Am Diet A* 1997;97:742–749.

Pennington J: Intakes of minerals from diets and foods. Is there a need for concern? *J Nutr* 1996;126:2304–2308.

Pennington J, Schoen S: Total diet study: Estimated dietary intakes of nutritional elements, 1982–1991. *Int J Vit N* 1996;66:350–362.

Zive M, Nicklas T, Busch E, et al: Marginal vitamin and mineral intakes of young adults: The Bogalusa Heart Study. *J Adoles H* 1996;19:39–47.

Index

PMS, 126; self-assessment quiz, 152; and sleep deficit, 217, 218; and sugar intake, 108, 109, 153, 154, 162–63, 197; and tryptophan, 155; and vitamin and mineral status, 159–62; and vitamin B$_6$, 158–59, 160–61. *See also* Seasonal Affective Disorder

desserts: gourmet coffee drinks as, 105–7; fat-free, 93; low-fat, low-calorie versions, 86; recipes, *380–85; in restaurants, 305; serving sizes, 346; shopping list, 299

dex-fenfluramine, 28

DHA *See* docosahexaenoic acid

DHEA (dehydroepiandro-sterone), 122–23, 138, 167, 214

diabetes, 109, 214

dibasic calcium phosphate, 323

diet: balanced, difficulty of achieving, 323–24, 325; and blood-glucose levels, 27, 112; changing gradually, 93, 274–77; long-range effects, xviii; neurotransmitters directly linked to, 13–20; self-assessment quiz, 33–43; and serotonin levels, 17. *See also* dieting; eating; Feeling Good Diet

dieting: and binge eating, 75, 259; and carbohydrate cravings, 56, 57, 63; and eating disorders, 29, 30, 259–60; and mental performance, 197–98; and overeating, 255–57; and serotonin levels, 46–47; starting over after, 258–59. *See also* quick-weight-loss diets

diet pills. *See* weight-loss medications

digestive tract, nerve chemicals released in, 25–26

dining out, 251, 303–5

dinner: for carbohydrate cravers, 64; and sleep, 224; for SAD, 145

Dip, Savory Cilantro, *351–52

docosahexaenoic acid (DHA), 156, 198–99, 211

dong quai, 138

dopa, 18

dopamine: and appetite control, 10; and galanin, 22; and mental performance, 207, 211, 212; as a mood and energy elevator, 16–18, 18, 112, 232, and PMS, 134, 138; and SAD, 144; and stress, 172, 176; and tyrosine, 16, 17–18, 18, 112, 215; and vitamin B$_6$, 158, 207

drowsiness, 108, 112–13

drugs. *See* medications; supplements

dysphoria, 51, 51

dysthymia, 151

eating: chemicals that influence, 9–11; healthy, tricks for, 265–66; mindfully, 246, 258; slowly, 93, 265; substituting other activities, 54, 55; unhealthy, 29–31; what makes us stop, 28–29. *See also* appetite regulation; diet; dieting; eating habits; emotional eating

eating disorders, 29–31: and CCK levels, 25, 29; due to dieting, 255, 259–60; early warning signs, 241; genetic causes, 30–31; and nerve chemicals, 239; and

sleep problems, 226; treatment, 31; and vitamin deficiencies, 159–60. *See also* anorexia; binge eating; bulimia; food addictions

eating habits: changing, 281–85; psychology of, 253–54. *See also* diet; eating

echinacea, 189

eggplant, snacks with, *111

Eggplant Caponata, *371

eggs, 209–10, 343

egg substitute, *100, *101, 103

Elimination Diet, 117

emotional eating, 61–62, 253–55, 257, 259; alternative activities, 55; curbing, 260–65; irrational beliefs underlying, 263

endorphins, 20, 22, 23–24; aspartame vs. sugar effect, 59–60; cravings caused by, 23–24, 25: for carbohydrate, 49–51; for chocolate, 84; for fat, 26, 73, 75, 179, 239; and depression, 154; and eating disorders, 29, 30, 31, 260; and exercise, 23, 121, 165; and food aromas, 71; and PMS, 125, 129–30; and SAD, 125; and skipping meals, 240; and stress, 253

energy, in foods. *See* calories

energy level, 95–123; and additives and preservatives, 118–19; and breakfast, 97–102, 100–101, 102, 103; chronic fatigue syndrome, 119–20, 121, 218; and coffee, 104–7; and food allergies, 115–18; herbs and supplements that boost, 122–23; and iron, 113–15, 116; and